CHART OF ACCOUNTS FOR HEALTH CARE ORGANIZATIONS

CRAHCA

CENTER FOR RESEARCH
IN AMBULATORY
HEALTH CARE ADMINISTRATION

Center for Research in Ambulatory Health Care Administration
104 Inverness Terrace East
Englewood, CO 80112-5306

ISBN: 1-56829-023-3

Library of Congress Catalog Card Number: 99-75205

Printed in the United States of America
10 9 8 7 6 5 4 3 2 1

Disclaimer

The **Center for Research in Ambulatory Health Care Administration** (CRAHCA), the research arm of the **Medical Group Management Association** (MGMA), prints publications that are intended to provide current and accurate information and are designed to assist readers in becoming more familiar with the subject matter covered. Such publications are distributed with the understanding that CRAHCA and MGMA do not render any legal, accounting or other professional advice. No representations nor warranties are made concerning the application of legal or other principles discussed by the author(s) to any specific fact situation, nor is any prediction made concerning how any particular judge, government official or other person will interpret or apply such principles. Specific factual situations should be discussed with professional advisors.

WARNING

The disk included with this book containing Excel files is protected by copyright law. Unauthorized reproduction or distribution of this program, or any portion of it, may result in severe civil and criminal penalties, and will be prosecuted to the maximum extent possible under law.

Dedications

To my mother, Anna Irene Peterson,
and my husband, Michael Glass,
you are the wind beneath my wings.

All my love, Kathryn

To Dr.s William Schonick and Milton Roemer,
wonderful mentors who never lost sight of the goal of improving the health and welfare of all people.

Neill F. Piland

Table of Contents

Preface ____ vii

About CRAHCA and MGMA ____ ix

Acknowledgments ____ xi

About the Authors ____ xv

Foreword ____ xix

1 Basic Guidelines: Accounting for Today's Health Care ____ 1

2 Coding Structure of the Chart of Accounts ____ 11

3 Balance Sheet Account Descriptions ____ 34

4 Income Statement Account Descriptions ____ 63

5 Adapting the Chart of Accounts to Activity-Based Costing ____ 107

6 Adapting the Chart of Accounts to Small Group Practices ____ 129

7 Adapting the Chart of Accounts to Not-for-Profit Health Care Organizations ____ 148

8 Adapting the Chart of Accounts to Community Health Centers ____ 159

9 Adapting the Chart of Accounts to Faculty Practice Plans ____ 171

10 Adapting the Chart of Accounts to Hospital-Based Physician Practices ____ 189

11 Adapting the Chart of Accounts to Integrated Delivery Systems ____ 202

12 Adapting the Chart of Accounts to the MGMA Surveys ____ 217

13 Adapting the Chart of Accounts to PSPA ____ 224

Glossary ____ **238**

Appendix—Table I ____ **251**

Table II ____ **275**

Table III ____ **299**

Table IV ____ **306**

Table V ____ **323**

Table VI ____ **330**

Index ____ **341**

Preface

Has health care accounting changed in the past 20 or so years? Have you noticed a greater need for detail in your chart of accounts structure and/or the need for additional accounts to track revenues and expenses that did not exist a decade ago? The answer to the above questions is an unequivocal YES for most health care organizations. We have heard our constituency loud and clear. This is the first major overhaul of the previous chart of accounts published by the Center for Research in Ambulatory Health Care Administration (CRAHCA). As an added bonus for those users who participate in the Medical Group Management Association (MGMA) surveys, this account structure closely mirrors that of the MGMA Cost Survey; thus, it will be much easier to follow the logic when completing the surveys.

As health care administrators increasingly focus on the costs of operating a practice with narrowing margins resulting from managed care, it would make sense that there would correspondingly be an increasing need for a cost-based chart of accounts. Leanne Travers and Rob Gold from Gold Consulting Group, Inc. in Needham, Massachusetts, designed a cost-based chart of accounts for their clients using CRAHCA's *Medical Group Practice Chart of Accounts* as the foundation.

According to Leanne Travers, Gold's challenge "was to design a cost-based chart of accounts that retained all of the traditional accounting capabilities as well as have the ability to produce accurate cost data at both a macro and micro level of detail." We believe that they have succeeded. This *Chart of Accounts for Health Care Organizations* (COA) is the result of their research and design along with the input from a wide variety of experts on the COA committee.

The scope of this COA is much broader than the one CRAHCA previously published. This edition addresses how to adapt this particular chart of accounts that was designed for a mid-size medical group practice to academic practices, community/migrant health centers, integrated delivery systems, hospital-based physician groups, not-for-profit health care organizations and small group practices. After reading the first few chapters that explain the basic concepts of the entire COA, you will zero in on the chapter that pertains to your specific type of organization to read how this COA can be adapted for use in your setting.

What is the target market of this publication? Up to now, CRAHCA has published chart of accounts references for small group practices. We expanded this COA so it can be used by health care organizations along the continuum of health care delivery entities. Contained in this publication are a shell, a summary and a detailed chart of accounts that can be easily adapted to a particular organization through expansion into sub-accounts or through roll-up into major account categories. The basic "shell" version of the COA can be used as a foundation by most any health care organization when building its own unique chart of accounts. At the other end of the spectrum is the full-blown, detailed COA as envisioned by Rob Gold who designed it for the mid-size and larger health care organizations. While the summary level COA may suffice for financial reporting, the detail level of this COA will allow the drill down necessary for managerial accounting analyses. The integrity of the account structure is maintained across the three levels of the COA, which makes it easy to expand or collapse account categories.

This publication is organized to first give a broad overview of the COA before directing the reader to the chapter that describes how to adapt the COA to a particular size and type of health care organization. The first half of the book describes the financial costing format design and gives a detailed description of each account. Armed with that knowledge, the reader skips to the chapter covering his or her type of organization. For those readers who currently use the *Medical Group Practice Chart of Accounts* and would like to make the switch to the *Chart of Accounts for Health Care Organizations,* we have included a crosswalk table in the back of the book. We also strongly encourage readers to load into their computers the electronic media included within this publication. The account descriptions have been added to the spreadsheets as line-item comments thus adding an element of interactivity to each level of the account structure.

The purpose of this COA is to give a wide range of health care organizations a model that will serve them across a variety of settings. As health care administration adjusts to the seemingly continual transitions of managed care, it would serve administrators and accountants well to have a standard chart of accounts that can be tweaked as their organization evolves. Many people view CRAHCA's previous version as the industry standard. We hope this new and very flexible version of the COA will set a new industry standard that will benefit an even wider array of organizations in health care administration through standardized reporting for benchmarking, surveys and research.

Neill F. Piland, Dr.P.H.
CRAHCA Research Director

Kathryn P. Glass, M.B.A., M.S.H.A.
CRAHCA Research Project Manager

About CRAHCA and MGMA

Founded in 1973 with funding from the W.K. Kellogg Foundation, the Center for Research in Ambulatory Health Care Administration (CRAHCA), also referred to as the Center for Research at the Medical Group Management Association (MGMA), is organized as a 501(c)(3) tax-exempt charitable organization as defined by the Internal Revenue Code. CRAHCA relies on foundation, corporate and government grants and revenue from education programs, publications and software, as well as interest from its endowment fund and services provided to MGMA. The CRAHCA endowment fund was established in 1978 and continues to grow through tax-deductible contributions from individuals and corporations.

As the research and development arm of the MGMA, CRAHCA conducts health services research, develops measurement tools and conducts educational seminars for the benefit of the entire health care industry. Its mission is to advance the art and science of medical group practice management to improve the health of our communities through health services research based largely in group practices and other health care delivery settings.

Since its founding in 1926, the MGMA has become the leading membership, education and research organization for professionals in medical practice management. MGMA is headquartered in Englewood, Colorado. MGMA's diverse membership includes administrators, CEOs and board members of health systems, physicians in management, office managers and many other management professionals from medical practices of all sizes and types, as well as from integrated health systems, hospital and medical school-affiliated practices and practice management organizations.

Acknowledgments

The Center for Research in Ambulatory Health Care Administration (CRAHCA) thanks the *many* contributors to this project. Without their individual research and expertise in the various topics covered in this book, these revisions and enhancements would not have been possible. A personal note of heartfelt thanks to both Rob Gold and Leanne Travers for their significant efforts in the expansion and revision of the previous *Medical Group Practice Chart of Accounts* upon which this publication is based. Rob, your incredible patience and unwavering positive attitude never ceased to amaze us. You have our eternal gratitude for your perseverance and for your willingness to make change after change after change...

Special thanks to Mickey O'Neal and the National CPA Healthcare Advisors Association who stepped in at the 11th hour to write a few chapters, edit a few chapters and provide additional insight into the account structure. Mickey, if it were not for you, this book would still be a project in process! Special thanks also to the Financial Management Society of the MGMA for its support and partial funding of this project's revisions and publishing.

Neill F. Piland, Dr.P.H.
CRAHCA Research Director

Kathryn P. Glass, M.B.A., M.S.H.A.
CRAHCA Research Project Manager

The following individuals, listed in alphabetical order, authored one or more sections of this publication:

Gil Bernhard, CPA, Senior Manager
Healthcare Services Group
American Express Tax and Business Services of New York, Inc.
New York, NY

Paul V. Calandrella, M.S., J.D.
Director of Finance and Human Resources
Brigham Surgical Group Foundation, Inc.
Brigham and Women's Hospital, Boston, MA

Beverly H. Donehoo, M.Ed., CMPE, Director
Banner HealthCare Solutions, Fairfax, VA

John R. Fernandez, Vice President of Surgical Services
Harvard Medical School
Department of Surgery
Brigham and Women's Hospital, Boston, MA

Robert J. Gold, M.S., CPA, President
Gold Consulting Group, Inc., PC, Needham, MA

Richard Gundling, FHFMA, CMA, Technical Director
Healthcare Financial Management Association, Washington, DC

Eric S. Holzberg, CPA, M.B.A., Managing Director
American Express Tax and Business Services of New York, Inc.
New York, NY

Lisa M. LaCourse, (Former) Technical Analyst
Healthcare Financial Management Association, Westchester, IL

Thomas M. (Mickey) O'Neal, CPA, President and Director
Auditing and Accounting
O'Neal, McGuinness & Company, PLLC, Houston, TX

Lisa E. Pieper, M.B.A., M.S.H.A., Project Manager
MGMA Survey Department, Englewood, CO

Hal Prink, FHFMA, Professional Development Director
Healthcare Financial Management Association, Westchester, IL

Leanne C. Travers, Consultant
Gold Consulting Group, Inc., PC, Needham, MA

In addition, the following individuals and organizations served on the Chart of Accounts for Health Care Organizations' advisory committee or otherwise reviewed and/or edited the account structure:

Jo Ellen Bertram, Controller
HealthSystems Minnesota, Minneapolis, MN

Leslie G. Eldenburg
Department of Accounting
College of Business and Public Administration
University of Arizona at Tucson, Tucson, AZ

Joe Havens, CPA
Horne CPA Group, Hattiesburg, MS

Frederick E. Hubbs, CMPE, Chief Operating Officer
Primary Medical Clinic, Odessa, TX

Marilyn Happold-Latham, CPA, FACMPE
Yergen & Meyer, LLP, Portland, OR

Jeffrey B. Milburn, CMPE, Senior Vice President, Chief Financial Officer
Colorado Springs Health Partners, PC, Colorado Springs, CO

National CPA Healthcare Advisors Association (HCAA)
Chicago, IL[1]

1 The National CPA Health Care Advisors Association (HCAA) is a nationwide network of CPA firms specifically selected for their experience in and commitment to serving the health care industry. HCAA members combine their expertise to provide the highest quality services to improve health care providers' practice management. For more information, please contact: HCAA, 111 East Wacker Drive, Suite 990, Chicago, Illinois 60601; phone 800.869.0491; or visit their web site at www.hcaa.com.

Ernest J. Pavlock, Ph.D., CPA, President
JPM Associates, Ltd., Reston, VA

Naomi S. Soderstrom, Ph.D.
College of Business
University of Colorado at Denver, Denver, CO

The following CRAHCA and MGMA personnel reviewed and significantly supported the administrative efforts of this publication:

Meg Bayerl
CRAHCA Research Assistant

David Gans, M.S.H.A., CMPE
MGMA Survey Operations Director

Kerstin B. Lynam
CRAHCA Operations Manager

About the Authors

In Alphabetical Order:

Gil Bernhard, CPA

With over 10 years of experience in the health care field, Gil Bernhard has acquired expertise in health care reporting and reimbursement issues. Mr. Bernhard consults on financial management, installation of general ledger accounting software systems and internal controls for health centers and other not-for-profit corporations. Along with his financial management services for health care organizations, Mr. Bernhard supervises and reviews the preparation of specialized cost reports specific to ambulatory care facilities reimbursement and financial reports required for filing with the U.S. Department of Health and Human Services (i.e., UDS and FSR). Mr. Bernhard is a frequent lecturer for the National Association of Community Health Centers (NACHC) and for various state primary care associations on the issue of health care finance and reporting requirements for community health centers.

Paul V. Calandrella, M.S., J.D.

Mr. Calandrella's current position is director of Finance and Human Resources for Brigham Surgical Group Foundation, Inc. (BSG), a multi-specialty physician organization affiliated with Brigham and Women's Hospital. He also serves as compliance officer for BSG. Mr. Calandrella has 13 years experience in finance and administration in both industry and non-profit sectors. He has a bachelor of science degree in accounting, a master of science degree in computer information systems and a juris doctorate degree. He was also admitted to the Massachusetts Bar.

Beverly H. Donehoo, M.Ed., CMPE

Beverly Donehoo, a former practice administrator, is director of Banner Health-Care Solutions in Fairfax, Virginia. She is also the developer of Profit Point, an RVU-based software management tool that performs the type of financial benchmarking and cost accounting functions described in this book. Ms. Donehoo is a certified medical practice executive and holds a master's degree from the University of North Carolina and a postgraduate certificate from Georgetown University in health care management.

John R. Fernandez

Mr. Fernandez has worked at Brigham and Women's Hospital (BWH) since 1992. His positions have ranged from administrator of the Trauma, Burn and Critical Care Division to director of the BWH Cardiovascular Service Line to interim executive director of the Department of Surgery to his current position as vice president of Surgical Services. As interim executive director of the Department of Surgery, Mr. Fernandez was responsible for the operations of the department, which encompasses more than 70 surgeons, 10 managers and more than 200 research and administrative staff. His responsibilities included acting as the department's liaison with BWH senior management, while also serving as the director of the Cardiovascular Service Line and administrative director for the Cardiac Vascular Surgery Divisions. He was promoted to vice president of Surgical Services in October 1998.

Kathryn P. Glass, M.B.A., M.S.H.A.

Since January 1995, Kathryn Glass has worked for the Medical Group Management Association (MGMA) and its research arm, the Center for Research in Ambulatory Health Care Administration (CRAHCA). As a research project manager for CRAHCA, Ms. Glass is involved with numerous projects, such as the Chart of Accounts for Health Care Organizations, a nationwide program on cost effectiveness for community health centers and the Physician Services Practice Analysis (PSPA) software program and comparison database. Ms. Glass holds two master's degrees from the University of Colorado at Denver: an M.B.A. and an M.S.H.A. (Master of Science in Health Care Administration).

Robert J. Gold, M.S., CPA

Rob Gold, CPA holds both a B.S. and M.S. degree in accounting from the Wharton School, University of Pennsylvania. With over 15 years of experience in the health care field, Mr. Gold specializes in servicing the health care industry. His primary focus is consulting physicians and physician practice groups. As a shareholder and managing principal of R.J. Gold & Company, P.C. he provides multi-faceted services for businesses as well as individuals. The firm is a full service professional corporation of Certified Public Accountants. Prior to his current position, he was a manager with Ernst & Young in New York and New Jersey and also has been a manager of Corporate Accounting at Wheelabrator-Frye, Inc. in New Hampshire.

As president of Gold Consulting Group, Inc. since 1994, he provides health care management consulting services focused on physician organization financial systems, financial and operations management and information systems.

Richard L. Gundling, FHFMA, CMA

Richard Gundling is the technical director and content specialist for the Healthcare Financial Management Association (HFMA). He also serves as staff liaison to the Principles and Practices Board of the HFMA. Before joining HFMA in January 1995, Mr. Gundling served in many fiscal departments in hospitals as budget and reimbursement analyst, director of Budget and Reimbursement and as chief financial officer. In addition to these positions, he was a controller for a large home health agency.

Eric S. Holzberg, CPA, M.B.A.

Eric Holzberg has over 12 years of experience and is a nationally recognized expert in health care finance and managed care. He is a frequent lecturer at seminars across the country on health care finance, managed care, health care mergers and acquisitions, the implementation of patient information systems and community-based health care. Mr. Holzberg specializes in strategic planning, cost evaluation and reduction, organizational development, feasibility analysis, reimbursement and information systems. Mr. Holzberg participated in workgroups for two bureaus—Primary Health Care (BPHC) and the U.S. Department of Health and Human Services (DHHS). One workgroup focused on redesigning the BPHC Primary Care Effectiveness Review and the other on overcoming the barriers to cost competitiveness for health centers.

Lisa M. LaCourse

At the time that Ms. LaCourse wrote her chapter, she was a technical analyst for the Healthcare Financial Management Association (HFMA), working out of its Washington, D.C. office. She specializes in medical group practices, patient financial services and long-term care issues. Prior to joining HFMA, Ms. LaCourse managed physician billing for over 65 hospital-based physicians at a D.C. hospital. While there, she contributed to the complete redesign of the chart of accounts for those practices. Ms. LaCourse has a bachelor's degree in mechanical and aerospace engineering from Princeton University.

Thomas M. (Mickey) O'Neal, CPA

Mr. O'Neal is the founder, principal and current president of O'Neal, McGuinness and Company, P.L.L.C. (OMC), Accountants and Management Consultants, located in Houston, Texas. He was a founder and executive committee member of the National CPA Healthcare Advisors Association, a national trade association providing education, marketing and networking services to CPAs serving the health care industry. Mr. O'Neal received his bachelor of business administration degree from the University of Houston in 1975 and became a certified public accountant in 1978. Prior to establishing his own accounting practice, he was a manager in the Emerging Business Services Group of Coopers and Lybrand. Memberships include the Medical Group Management Association, the National IPA Coalition, the American Institute of Certified Public Accountants and the Texas Society of Certified Public Accountants, Houston Chapter.

Lisa E. Pieper, M.B.A., M.S.H.A.

Lisa Pieper is a senior project manager in the Survey Operations Department at Medical Group Management Association (MGMA). She has been with MGMA for nine years and has managed MGMA's physician and faculty compensation and productivity and cost surveys. During her 15 years in the health care field she also worked in provider contracting, marketing and client relations. Her educational background includes a bachelor of arts in political science from Augustana College and a master's in business administration and master's of science in health administration from the University of Colorado at Denver.

Harold L. Prink, FHFMA

Hal Prink has served as the director of Professional Development at Healthcare Financial Management Association (HFMA) since 1995. Previously, he was education director at the Medical Management Association (MGMA) for 15 years and served as a research project director for the Center for Reasearch in

Ambulatory Health Care Administration (CRAHCA) on a grant from the Robert Wood Johnson Foundation. Mr. Prink was also the CFO for Mariposa County Department of Health Services, which included fiscal responsibility for a 500-bed county hospital, numerous primary-care centers and the veternary center. He holds a B.S.B.A. (Bachelor of Science in Business Administration) degree in accounting from the University of Denver.

Leanne C. Travers

Ms. Travers is a consultant with the Gold Consulting Group, Inc., a national firm established in 1994 that focuses on the implementation and/or upgrading of physician organization financial systems, operations and management. Prior to joining the Gold Consulting Group, Inc., Ms. Travers was a surgical group administrator in the Harvard University teaching hospital systems. Her previous professional experience included financial, administration and operations management in the private and public sectors. She has a particular expertise in financial, operations and computer systems management and development.

The Gold Consulting Group, Inc. services provider organizations throughout the country by designing and implementing cost and allocation systems that specifically conform to the unique information and analysis requirements of each group.

Foreword

The health care industry continues to be a volatile environment. Competitive pressures in the marketplace have forced medical groups to enter into an age of networking, consolidating and risk sharing. Medical groups are joining provider networks under various contractual relationships, acquiring other providers, and entering into risk-sharing contracts with insurers and other providers.

As a result of these relationships, medical group administrators and financial managers must have prompt access to relevant and reliable financial information if they want to make good business decisions and meet the demands of outside parties, including owners, creditors and the Internal Revenue Service. Information about a practice's cost of providing care, for example, is essential to the successful negotiation and management of capitated (prepaid) contracts because capitated rates may be significantly lower than equivalent fee-for-service rates.

The chart of accounts in this text will provide administrators and financial managers with the necessary framework for organizing financial information clearly and at a level of detail that is meaningful and useful. It will provide the foundation from which financial statements and management reports can be developed. The model chart of accounts is an important tool for building a medical group financial accounting system that will give administrators and financial managers the knowledge they need for sound decision making, thus improving and maintaining the quality of care provided and achieving better economic results.

Richard L. Clarke, FHFMA
President and CEO
Healthcare Financial Management Association

1

Basic Guidelines: Accounting for Today's Health Care

Thomas M. (Mickey) O'Neal, CPA

Background

Over a period of many years, the accounting profession has developed standards of financial reporting for external users of financial statements. These principal users include:

- Financing institutions
- Internal Revenue Service (IRS)
- State and federal regulatory authorities
- Third-party payers
- HMOs

Increasingly, third-party users of medical practice financial statements also include investors and holders of publicly traded securities of companies with ownership interests in medical practice operations. An adequate financial reporting system would not be complete without also providing financial reports to the administrator and physician-owners of the organization and the managers of responsibility centers.

Financial reporting for internal users is not bound by the accounting principles that guide external financial reporting. This is due, in part, to the fact that internal financial reports are designed to meet the specific needs of management and are not intended for external review.

Development of Accounting Standards

The accounting profession has developed standards for measuring transactions as a result of two very different occurrences:

- The evolution of accepted practice
- Authoritative pronouncements by rule-making bodies

Over generations of economic activity, financial statements have evolved that provide useful financial information. However, because of variations among industries, differences in accounting standards for measurement of assets, liabilities, revenues and expenses have occurred. Because of the diversity in accounting practices, the accounting profession has issued accounting standards through its committees and its governing body, which is now called the Financial Accounting Standards Board (FASB). Created in 1973, the FASB is an independent board comprising CPAs, business executives, financial analysts and educators. The FASB researches problems in financial reporting as they arise, identifying the principal issues involved and possible solutions. Through the rule-making process a body of accounting standards has been developed and those standards are referred to as Generally Accepted Accounting Principles (GAAP). The major strength of the GAAP guidelines is that, as the complexity of business operations increases, these principles are continually re-examined and revised to keep pace with the changing environment.

Conceptual Framework for Financial Reporting

In an attempt to develop a conceptual framework (or a constitutional document) for financial reporting, the FASB developed a statement of objectives of financial reporting. Financial reporting means the general purpose financial statements, and other information that relates directly to the financial statements, that are prepared for external users who do not have the authority to identify the specific financial information they want. These users must instead rely upon the information management communicates to them.

The FASB's main objectives of financial reporting stress that information provided to external users should be useful in making investment, credit and similar decisions. Further, financial reports should assist the user in assessing future cash flows and analyzing past performance, as well as presenting financial position and changes therein.

A second objective or statement issued by the FASB outlines the qualitative characteristics of accounting information. Decision usefulness is identified as the most important qualitative characteristic. To be useful, accounting information must be both **relevant** and **reliable**. Relevant information has the capacity to influence a user to make a decision. It may have predictive value when used to evaluate future events or feedback value that confirms or corrects expectations. In any case, the information must be timely enough to have the potential of influencing the decision. According to the FASB, reliable accounting information must be neutral, possess representational faithfulness; it also must be verifiable. In brief, this means that if accounting information is to be reliable, it must be free from error and bias, represent what it purports to represent and be verifiable by different accountants using the same objective data and measurement techniques.

Qualities identified by the FASB as supporting both relevance and reliability are **comparability** and **consistency**. Financial statements of the organization should be comparable over time and, to a lesser extent, be comparable to similar organizations.

The FASB has issued other statements or components of the conceptual framework, and it promises to issue still others in the near future. Among them are statements dealing with the definition of accounting elements (assets, liabilities, revenues, expenses, etc.), their measurement, and the criteria for their recognition in accounting records. When the conceptual framework is complete, it should serve as a general constitution that the FASB can use to evaluate financial accounting standards already issued and to evaluate alternative proposed standards in the future. In any event, it has emphasized that accounting information should have decision usefulness based on the criteria of relevance and reliability.

Accounting Methods

Generally Accepted Accounting Principles

Generally Accepted Accounting Principles (GAAP) are based upon the accrual accounting method.

Accrual: An accounting system where revenues are recorded as earned when services are performed rather than when cash is received. Expenses are recorded in the period during which they are incurred, that is, when the asset or service is used, regardless of when the goods or services are paid for. Costs for goods and services that will be used to produce revenues in the future (inventory) are reported as assets and recorded as expenses in future periods. The accrual balance sheet includes not only the assets and liabilities resulting from cash transactions but also includes accounts receivable from patients, prepayments and deferrals of expenses, accruals of purchased medical services and accounts payable to suppliers.

Accrual accounting follows the principle of matching revenues with their related expenses and is based on GAAP. Some of the more important GAAP guidelines are as follows:

1. Historical Cost Basis — Assets and liabilities are recorded at their original cost or the value of the consideration given. Cost is a more reliable measurement of value and can be objectively determined much easier than other valuation methods.

2. Revenue from the sale of goods and/or services is recognized when the organization has delivered goods or performed services and is entitled

to collect fees. The general rule for professional service firms under accrual accounting is to recognize revenue when services are performed. If collection of those revenues becomes doubtful, an estimate of the uncollectable amount can be made in the form of an allowance for doubtful accounts. This recognizes an expense for the bad debt and adjusts the value of the receivable balance at the end of the period.

3. Recognition of expenses depends on the nature of the expense:

   - Costs directly related to specific revenue, such as eyeglasses or contacts in an optical department, are carried as an asset (inventory) until revenue is recognized for the sale of those items. At that point, the cost of the eyeglasses and contacts are treated as an expense (cost of goods sold);
   - Long-lived assets generally have no direct relationship between the cost of the asset and revenue generated. Therefore, expense recognition involves the use of a systematic and rational plan of allocating a portion of the cost of the asset to specific time periods. This process is called depreciation (for tangible assets) and amortization (for non-tangible assets such as goodwill); and
   - Other examples of costs that have no direct relationship to particular revenue or long-lived assets are interest expense and advertising and marketing expenses. These types of expenses should be recognized in the period in which they were incurred.

The accrual accounting method provides for a more accurate measurement of the sources and uses of an organization's resources than the cash method of accounting. This is because the revenues are matched with the corresponding expenses when they occur. Thus, measurement accuracy is enhanced for expense and revenue recognition. Expenses are recorded as they are incurred or consumed in the generation of patient revenue, regardless of when payments are received. Under the accrual method, cash receipts and payments do not always correspond with the time period when revenues and expenses are recorded in the organization's accounts. The delivery of patient services and resource consumption are the determining points for revenue and expense recognition on the accrual basis of accounting.

Other Accounting Methods

Accounting methods that are not GAAP, but may be used for specific reporting purposes, are termed an "Other Comprehensive Basis of Accounting" (OCBOA). The list of OCBOA accounting methods is quite extensive. Those that are applicable to medical practices and will be addressed here include the following:

- The Cash Basis of Accounting

- The Modified Cash Basis of Accounting
- The Income Tax Basis of Accounting

The Cash Basis of Accounting

Cash: An accounting method where revenues are recognized when cash is received and expenses are recognized when cash is paid. Receivables, payables, accruals and deferrals arising from operations are not recognized, although still tracked in supporting records. On a pure cash basis, long-lived (fixed) assets are expensed when acquired, leaving cash and investments as the only assets and borrowings and payroll withholdings as the only liabilities. This pure cash method of accounting is rarely used as fixed assets are capitalized and depreciated by most entities. The exceptions are certain governmental and quasi-governmental organizations.

Cash basis of accounting can not be used for audited financial statements because GAAP requires the use of accrual-based accounting. A CPA (in the U.S.) must prepare audited financial statements. The role of the CPA as an auditor is to attest that the financial statements of an entity designed for external use present fairly the financial position and results of operations of that entity in conformity with this body of GAAP. Many organizations do not normally need audited financial statements and *The Chart of Accounts for Health Care Organizations* can be used for cash, modified cash or accrual-based methods.

A reason for strictly using the cash-basis method would be to facilitate income tax return filing and to avoid having two methods of bookkeeping.

Since tax laws permit the delay of reporting revenue until cash is collected, the cash method is the most commonly used in medical organizations. If the cash basis is used, it may be necessary to produce supplemental management reports related to production, adjustments and accounts receivable to generate a meaningful measure of performance. An important advantage that can be overlooked when only a cash method is used is the ability to generate meaningful performance measurements strictly from the financial statements. An organization can have two sets of books — a cash set and an accrual set — however, this is rarely ever operationally efficient. The more common solution is to keep the books on the cash method of accounting and to produce supplemental management reports related to production, adjustments and accounts receivable management.

Cash-basis accounting is most appropriate when the following conditions are present:

- The level of operations is stable with minimal seasonal variations.
- The amount of patient receivables does not change dramatically from month to month, and the age of these receivables does not change materially during the year.

- Long-lived assets are leased rather than purchased, and rental expense is paid monthly.
- Supply inventories are replenished as used.
- Large expenses (such as insurance premiums) are paid monthly rather than yearly.
- No substantial inventories are maintained by the practice.

Even though the accrual method presents the clearest and most complete picture of the organization's financial performance, there are four concerns about using the accrual method that administrators frequently raise:

- Measuring income for tax purposes
- Measuring income for distribution to physicians
- Measuring the financial position of the organization for buy-in or buy-out by physicians
- Measuring the financial position of the group for credit evaluation

The concern over financial statement presentation and differences in cash and accrual methods arises because the same statements are required to serve many objectives. The evaluation of performance and financial position, determination of income subject to taxes, determination of cash available for distribution to physicians and determination of financial position for physician buy-in and buy-out require different information. Therefore, the use of cash, modified cash or accrual accounting methods are dependent on the goals and objectives of the organization. If there are multiple goals and objectives, then different methods may have to be used concurrently.

As the cash basis facilitates income tax reporting for professional service companies, the accrual method provides for proper matching of revenues and expenses, especially for comparison purposes. In order to have a better reporting method upon which to evaluate management, the accrual method can be adopted for internal reporting purposes, while the cash basis can continue to be used for income tax reporting.

Additional Accounting Method for Internal Management Purposes

Modified cash is an accounting system that is primarily a cash-basis system, but allows the cost of long-lived (fixed) assets to be expensed through depreciation. This system is essentially what is used for income tax reporting for most medical practices and is commonly referred to as the Income Tax Method of Accounting. The modified cash system recognizes inventories of goods intended for resale as assets. Under a modified cash system, buildings and equipment purchases, leasehold improvements and insurance premium payments applicable to more than one accounting period are normally recorded as assets. Costs for these assets are allocated to accounting periods in a systematic manner over the length of time the practice benefits from the assets.

The modified cash method alters "pure" cash-basis accounting using additional accounts in the recording of long-lived assets, payables and receivables related to borrowing and investing of cash. This method recognizes the following as assets:

- Inventories of goods intended for resale as assets
- Purchases of buildings and equipment
- Leasehold improvements
- Accumulation of cash value of life insurance policies

Costs of these assets are charged against revenues in a rational and systematic manner over the length of time the medical organization benefits from their use by using depreciation and amortization accounts.

Assumptions and Characteristics of Financial Statements

The business environment in which a medical organization operates influences the form and content of financial statements. The following assumptions are an integral part of this influence: **entity, going concern, accounting period, objectivity and monetary unit.** Likewise, the following characteristics influence financial presentations: **relevance, reliability, full disclosure, conservatism, consistency, comparability and timeliness.**

Assumptions

Entity—The entity assumption refers to reporting the activity of a business enterprise as a separate and distinct organization. Accounting information should pertain only to the economic activities of the individual business and should be separate from the personal financial affairs of the owners or any other businesses in which the owners may be involved. Accordingly, entities, as specific areas of interest defined by the owners or managers, establish boundaries for elements to be included in the financial statements. A number of entities can be identified for a particular organization. One entity may be the legal organization owning and operating the business (corporation, partnership, not-for-profit, etc.). Another may be a part of the organization for which responsibility has been defined (each specialty or department). Yet another possibility is a combination of legal entities representing the larger economic entity (consolidation of the individual medical practice, the management services organization and the realty corporation). Financial statements may be prepared for each type of entity.

An organization operating more than one entity may use the same chart of accounts by using the entity field of the coding structure to identify each entity. Using uniform accounts for all entities allows financial statements to be combined into a set of financial statements for the organization as a whole.

Going-concern (Continuity of Business Life) — It is assumed that the business will continue operations in the future unless otherwise stated in the financial statement disclosures. Were it not for this assumption asset and liabilities values would need to be adjusted to approximate a liquidation value. Assets benefiting future periods under GAAP are expensed over those future periods. If the organization was not expected to continue as a viable business operation, the assets may have to be written down to a nominal realizable value in the current period. Most medical practices do not retain substantial amounts of assets or retained earnings. On their face, presented on the cash or income tax basis of accounting, many medical practices look insolvent.

Accounting Period — Since it is assumed that entities have an indefinite life, it is necessary to establish an arbitrary time frame on businesses to make a periodic accounting and reporting for determining financial performance. Therefore, a division of a business' existence into time periods such as months, quarters or years is used to report results of operations for these periods. Estimates and judgments about revenues and expenses to reflect their status for a given time period must be pro-rated based on this concept of an annual accounting. Expenses such as depreciation and amortization must be pro-rated in interim financial statements.

Objectivity — Business activity involves an exchange of goods or services at a specified price agreed upon by the parties in the exchange. The normal accounting procedure is to record these transactions at their cost, which is measured by the value of the resource given in exchange. The resource is usually cash. It is an objective and verifiable measure of the consideration used to record a transaction. Financial transactions are assumed to be measured by objective criteria such as the U.S. dollar. Likewise, subjective evaluation is not to be used to measure financial transactions.

Monetary Units — In the United States accounting systems measure and report the results of transactions and events in dollars that represent the value of the resources exchanged at the time of their acquisition. The monetary unit enables assets, liabilities, revenues and expenses to be measured and presented in the financial statements. Further, the assumption is made that the monetary unit of measure is unchanging in terms of its purchasing power — an assumption that is unrealistic in the real world. The accounting profession has not yet decided upon a feasible way to adjust accounting data for price level changes.

Characteristics

Relevance — To be relevant, accounting information must be capable of invoking the user to make a decision. But, the various users of financial statements have different needs. For example, lenders are interested in the firm's ability to repay its loan. Owners and managers are interested in the organization's ability to provide quality care and generate an adequate income stream to its owners while remaining financially strong. Although general-purpose financial statements may meet creditors' needs, these statements may have to be supplemented with internal reports and nonfinancial data to meet the needs of owners and managers.

Reliability — Reliability is the quality of information that gives assurance it is reasonably free of error and bias and users can depend on it to truly represent the economic conditions or events in question. To be reliable, accounting information must be capable of eliciting a high degree of consensus among independent measurers who use the same measurement methods.

Full Disclosure — The financial statements must present a complete picture of the organization's financial position, results of operations, changes in equity and cash flows. Since the financial statements are considered general-purpose presentations, they are intended to fulfill the needs of all external users who do not have access to the organization's internal records. Thus, financial statements should include all information that would influence the users' decisions. This is normally accomplished in financial statements intended for external reporting purposes by the addition of explanatory statement headings as well as detailed footnotes. These footnotes will normally detail the organization's accounting policies as well as provide detailed analysis of certain assets and liabilities, such as property and equipment or notes payable.

Conservatism — Conservatism is an accounting guideline to follow in difficult situations. In developing accounting measurements and techniques, the accounting profession has attempted to prevent overstatements of periodic earnings and financial position. Thus, a conservative practice in accrual accounting is to estimate and record an allowance for uncollectable accounts. This helps to reduce their value as carried on the books based on the historical experience of bad debts or contractual adjustments. But the recognition rule for losses is less rigid; losses are recorded when there is the first sign of their likelihood to occur. There is nothing in the conservative convention urging accountants to deliberately understate assets or earnings. Rather, the rule means that, when in doubt, choose the solution that will be least likely to overstate assets and earnings. In a medical practice, widespread use of cash-basis accounting is predicated on conservatism.

Consistency — Consistency occurs when an accounting entity applies the same accounting treatment from period to period to similar accounting events. This practice ensures comparability of accounting data among the various periods. Consistency does not mean that the business cannot switch from one acceptable method of accounting to another. When it can be demonstrated that another method is preferable to the current one, it is permissible to adopt the new one, for both tax and financial reporting purposes. However, it is generally not acceptable to switch back and forth among acceptable methods — once a switch is made, that method should remain permanent. The impact of any change in accounting methods must be disclosed in the financial statements.

Comparability — Because many accounting measurements are influenced by the assumption that organizations will have long lives, it is necessary to be sure that information prepared for short periods of time is comparable. Accounting conventions have evolved to provide comparable results of operations and financial position in interim financial statements. Likewise financial statement formats are anticipated to remain relatively unchanged from period to period to assure comparability among periods. Accounts are expected to be classified under comparable headings for different periods to avoid distorting an organization's results of operations for external reporting purposes.

Timeliness — The financial statements must be timely to be of any value to the user. The older the data, the less useful it becomes in measuring and predicting the organization's future. Medical practices are very time sensitive in that significant changes in the operations of an entity may go unnoticed, and extensive problems can occur if financial data is not presented in a timely manner.

2

Coding Structure of the Chart of Accounts

Rob Gold, M.S., CPA

Introduction

The *Chart of Accounts for Health Care Organizations* is the core component to a financial reporting framework that applies to physician organizations of all sizes — from a single practitioner practice to a large multi-specialty, multi-sited physician practice and beyond to structured physician organizations. The goal was to build upon the chart of accounts as set forth in the previous edition of the *Medical Group Practice Chart of Accounts*, published in 1996, and provide a financial tool that any practice/organization could utilize immediately and easily adopt to the particular practice setting. Flexibility of structure for the Chart of Accounts continues to be a basic key component, but at the same time a re-thinking of the current use of financial information, with the continued expansion of the prepaid/capitation component of health care practice, requires both a vertical and horizontal evolution of the chart of accounts.

The *Chart of Accounts for Health Care Organizations* is designed to assist in reporting financial transactions incurred and the distribution of this information into a relevant grouping of accounts that will serve as the first tier of financial analysis for health care organizations. A chart of accounts facilitates the assignment process of transactions to asset, liability, equity, income and expense accounts. In the past, the primary reason for financial reported data through a chart of accounts was to determine a practice's level of profitability. Today there is a greater need to accumulate financial data to allow for the reporting and analysis of detailed costing information — by practice, entity, physician, cost centers (billing, occupancy, administrative, as example), specialties and service centers (locations). All of this information can be obtained by designing and implementing a comprehensive chart of accounts built out horizontally from a complete basic core chart of accounts. The information available from the chart of accounts is now a required component for financial analysis and practice management purposes along with detailed patient and billing data from practice management systems. The marriage of this information allows for current, as well as historical analysis, managed care contract review and negotiation support to practice organization budgeting and projections. The revised chart of account framework should work to serve as the backbone to satisfying financial reporting needs.

The *Chart of Accounts for Health Care Organizations* has been revised to allow for continued participation in various comparative data studies, such as the annual Medical Group Management Association Cost Survey, which enables an organization to financially benchmark itself with and against other organizations for multiple levels of comparison. The annual cost survey will be referenced for the new chart of accounts format to the numerical ranges of accounting and financial data requested for the survey.

Coding Structure

The basic account field presented in this section has been designed as a four-digit field and serves as the core field, or basic field, in the expanded chart of account framework. In the next section the expanded account framework will be introduced and used to build the financial data gathering structure into a reporting tool for analysis purposes. The purpose of the core account or basic field is to serve as the common denominator for all organizations to the extent possible. The chart has been revised to provide a vertical numerical coding system as extensive as possible to accommodate the following: organizations with straightforward reporting needs and organizations that are able to utilize the same core coding system and then expand horizontally with additional coding fields to allow for sophisticated and complex financial data gathering and reporting. To anticipate the financial needs of smaller physician practices/organizations a summary version of the chart of accounts has also been designed. The approach used for the summary version allows for subsequent expansion to the general detailed version with little modification required because of the alignment of account descriptions and numbers between the two versions.

Basic Field

The four-digit field is the central element to the financial data gathering process. It serves to describe the fundamental nature of the accounts (assets, liability, equity, revenues or expenses) and allows further recording of activity within. The design is an ordering process to allow for a defined account to receive and record each financial activity that takes place within an organization. This basic design also retains the informational objectives of financial managerial needs, as well as financial reporting through financial statements and tax compliance reporting.

Summary Categories

The first digit of the basic field identifies the major financial statement category. This component, although modified slightly, has been maintained from the previous chart of account guidelines.

Basic field — Financial categories

Account Number	Description
1000	Assets
2000	Liabilities
3000	Owners' Equity
4000	Revenues
4500	Adjustments and Allowances
5000	Operating Expenses — Salary & Fringe Benefits
6000-7000	Services and General Expenses
8000	Provider-Related Expenses
9000	Nonoperating Revenues and Expenses; Income Taxes & Other Expenses

The second digit of the basic field identifies the primary classification of accounts within the major financial statement categories (of the first digit). Again, this component has been maintained from the previous chart of account guidelines but has been modified as shown.

Statement of financial position accounts

Account Number	Description
1000	Assets
1100-1500	Current Assets
1600	Investments and Long-Term Receivables
1700-1800	Non-Current Tangible Assets
1900	Intangible and Other Assets
2000	Liabilities
2100-2300	Current Liabilities
2400	Long-Term Liabilities
3000	Owners' Equity

The third and fourth digits of the basic field have been retooled in the following vertical account approach to allow for a breakdown of reporting needs. Typically these digits identify sub-accounts for organizations that need more detail for financial recording. The approach followed was to use similar third and fourth digits when possible to denote correlations between certain accounts (for example: Account #1751 — furniture and equipment and the related accumulated depreciation Account #1851 — furniture and equipment), and related accounts in different second digit primary classification of account areas (for example: Account #5640 — books and subscriptions [ancillary providers] and Account #8240 — books and subscriptions [physician]).

Income Statement Accounts

Account Number	Description
4000	Revenues
4100-4400	Gross Charges/Professional Fees/Prepaid & Capitation
4500	Adjustments
4500-4800	Gross Charges — Discount/Adjustments
5000	Operating Expenses — Salary and Fringe Benefits
5100	Physician — Salaries *
5200	Physician — Employee-Related Expenses* ***(See Accounts 8100-8400)**
5300	Midlevel Providers — Salaries *
5400	Midlevel Providers — Employee-Related Expenses*
5500	Ancillary Staff — Salaries
5600	Ancillary Staff — Employee-Related Expenses
5700	Employee — Salaries
5800	Employees — Employee-Related — Expenses
5900	Temporary Employee Salaries and Benefits
6000-7000	Services and General Expenses
6100-6400	Office and Administration Expense
6500-6600	Billing Expense
6700	Bad Debt Expense
7000	Clinical Expense
7500	Occupancy Expense
7600	Cost of Goods Sold
7700	Purchased Services/Management Fees
7800	Purchased Services for HMO/PPO Patients – Professional and Medical
8000	Provider-Related Expenses
8100	Physicians — Salaries
8200	Physicians — Employee-Related Expenses
8300	Midlevel Providers — Salaries
8400	Midlevel Providers — Employee — Other Expenses
9000	Nonoperating Revenues & Expenses, Income Taxes & Extraordinary Items
9100	Nonoperating Revenues
9200	Nonoperating Expenses
9300	Other Income Expenses

Chart Format

This Chart of Accounts has been created to allow for the rollup of detailed accounts into the first and/or second digits of the basic field. The design approach was to provide a ready-to-use format with enough detail to minimize the need to build a chart from the ground up. The account detail presented might appear to provide some level of duplication, but this has been deliberate in that the basic one column or vertical presentation of the chart of accounts provides the framework for recording all organizational financial activity along major revenue and expense categories often without needing the requirement of an expanded chart of account number. What is important to remember is that no two organizations' financial data gathering and reporting needs are exactly the same, so the model chart of accounts as presented should be tailored to that organization's particular requirements. After financial information is gathered, an organization should not hesitate to expand the chart of accounts to fit any particular detailed reporting required. The chart of accounts presented is still only a guideline or tool, never an absolute and rigid required model.

The presentation of provider-related salaries and expense (physician/ midlevel) accounts in the chart is a departure from the traditional financial statement approach. This has been done in order to address the importance of capturing expense financial data for a cost-based or managerial-financial prospective. For those organizations wanting to analyze their financial data to better understand the cost of providing health care services this format helps to present on a current basis this data for review. Further, for those organizations that are of a not-for-profit nature or those that prefer a different presentation, provision has been made to report these accounts in their more traditional location under the 5000 account category (5100-5400).

Consideration should be given to those situations where a fifth (5th) digit in the chart of accounts basic field would provide more detail for sub-account reporting. This added digit would appear at the end of the currently proposed core field and allow for up to 10 accounts below any currently listed account (for example #### 0 to 9). Although not presented in the chart of accounts as listed, this added vertical flexibility should not be overlooked when needed.

To facilitate future ability to participate in cost survey studies the presented basic account numbering should be retained even with any accounts considered not needed or just eliminated without renumbering the remaining accounts. As this presented chart of account format has continued to evolve over the years, this process of evolution will continue as health care financial needs continue to change and more data is needed to base financial management and reimbursement contract decisions. The goal is to provide the tools so that an organization can independently and internally record and analyze its financial transactions in a clear, logical and precise manner.

The two chart of account formats presented here are the General Detailed Format and General Summary Format designed to accommodate both the larger physician organization and the smaller physician practice, respectively.

Chart of Accounts — General — Detailed Format

Account Number	Description
	BALANCE SHEET
1000	**ASSETS**
1100	Cash
1110	Cash — Banks
1111	General Checking Accounts
1112	Payroll Checking Accounts
1113	Other Checking Accounts
1120	Cash — On hand
1121	Change Fund
1122	Petty Cash
1130	Cash — Restricted
1200	Marketable Securities & Short-Term Investments
1210	Valuation Allowance — Short-Term Investments
1300	Accounts Receivable
1301	Accounts Receivable — Fee-for-Service Amounts
1302	Accounts Receivable — Prepaid Contracts
1320	Allowance for Estimated uncollectable Receivables
1321	Allowance for Bad Debts — Patient Accounts
1322	Allowance for Contractual Adjustments
1323	Allowance for Bad Debts —Third-Party Payers
1324	Allowance for Charity Care
1340	Notes Receivable — Short-Term
1345	Managed Care Contract— Bonus/Withhold
1350	Other Short-Term Receivables
1351	Interest Receivables
1352	Intercompany Receivables
1353	Due from Employees
1354	Due from Related Parties
1400	Supply Inventories
1401	Drugs and Medication
1402	Medical Supplies
1403	Administrative Supplies
1404	Forms
1405	Housekeeping and Maintenance Supplies
1406	Linen Supplies
1407	Other Supplies
1420	Ancillary Department Supplies
1500	Prepaid Expenses
1501	Prepaid Interest
1502	Prepaid Insurance
1503	Prepaid Rent
1504	Prepaid Taxes
1505	Prepaid Dues
1506	Other Prepaid Expenses
1550	Other Current Assets
1600	**INVESTMENTS — LONG-TERM RECEIVABLES**
1610	Long-Term Receivables
1630	Long-Term Investments
1635	Valuation Allowance — Long-Term Investments
1640	Investments in Affiliates
1650	Property Held for Future Use
1700	**PROPERTY, FURNITURE, FIXTURES & EQUIPMENT**
1710	REAL PROPERTY
1711	Land
1712	Land Improvements
1713	Buildings

Detailed Format (Continued)

Account Number	Description
1714	Capital Leases — Buildings
1715	Leasehold Improvements
1716	Construction in Progress
1717	Other Real Property
1750	**FURNITURE, FIXTURES & EQUIPMENT**
1751	Furniture and Fixtures
1752	Capital Leases — Furniture and Fixtures
1753	Equipment
1754	Capital Leases — Equipment
1755	Medical Equipment
1756	Capital Leases — Medical Equipment
1760	Computer
1761	Computer — Hardware
1762	Computer — Software
1763	Computer — Other
1770	Capital Leases — Computer
1771	Capital Leases — Computer — Hardware
1772	Capital Leases — Computer — Software
1773	Capital Leases — Computer — Other
1780	Vehicles
1781	Vehicles
1782	Capital Leases — Vehicles
1790	Ancillary Service Equipment
1791	Laboratory Equipment
1792	Radiology Equipment
1793	Physical Therapy Equipment
1794	Diagnostic Equipment
1795	Capital Leases — Ancillary Service Equipment
1796	Capital Leases — Laboratory Equipment
1797	Capital Leases — Radiology Equipment
1798	Capital Leases — Physical Therapy Equipment
1799	Capital Leases — Diagnostic Equipment
1800	**ACCUMULATED DEPRECIATION — PROPERTY, FURNITURE, ETC.**
1810	ACCUMULATED DEPRECIATION — REAL PROPERTY
1812	Accum Depreciation — Land Improvements
1813	Accum Depreciation — Buildings
1814	Accum Depreciation — Capital Leases — Buildings
1815	Accum Depreciation — Leasehold Improvements
1817	Accum Depreciation — Other Real Property
1850	ACCUMULATED DEPRECIATION — FURNITURE, FIXTURES & EQUIPMENT
1851	Accum Depreciation — Furniture & Fixtures
1852	Accum Depreciation — Capital Leases — Furniture & Fixtures
1853	Accum Depreciation — Equipment
1854	Accum Depreciation — Capital Leases — Equipment
1855	Accum Depreciation — Medical Equipment
1856	Accum Depreciation — Capital Leases — Medical Equipment
1860	Accumulated Depreciation — Computer
1861	Accum Depreciation — Computer — Hardware
1862	Accum Depreciation — Computer — Software
1863	Accum Depreciation — Computer — Other
1870	Accum Depreciation — Capital Leases — Computer
1871	Accum Depreciation — Capital Leases — Computer Hardware
1872	Accum Depreciation — Capital Leases — Computer Software
1873	Accum Depreciation — Capital Leases — Computer Other
1880	Accumulated Depreciation — Vehicles
1881	Accum Depreciation — Vehicles
1882	Accum Depreciation — Capital Leases — Vehicles

Detailed Format (Continued)

Account Number	Description
1890	Other Accumulated Depreciation — Ancillary Service Equipment
1891	Accum Depreciation — Laboratory Equipment
1892	Accum Depreciation — Radiology Equipment
1893	Accum Depreciation — Physical Therapy Equipment
1894	Accum Depreciation — Diagnostic Equipment
1895	Accumulated Depreciation — Capital Leases — Ancillary Service Equipment
1896	Accum Depreciation — Capital Leases — Laboratory Equipment
1897	Accum Depreciation — Capital Leases — Radiology Equipment
1898	Accum Depreciation — Capital Leases — Physical Therapy Equipment
1899	Accum Depreciation — Capital Leases — Diagnostic Equipment
1900	**INTANGIBLE AND OTHER ASSETS**
1910	Organization Costs
1915	Accumulated Amortization — Organization Costs
1920	Goodwill
1925	Accumulated Amortization — Goodwill
1930	Other Intangible Assets
1940	Deposits
1950	Noncurrent Expenses Paid in Advance
1951	Noncurrent Interest Paid in Advance
1952	Noncurrent Insurances Paid in Advance
1953	Noncurrent Rent Paid in Advance
1954	Noncurrent Taxes Paid in Advance
1955	Noncurrent Dues Paid in Advance
1956	Other Noncurrent Expenses Paid in Advance
1960	Other Assets
1961	Cash Surrender Value of Life Insurance Policies
2000	**LIABILITIES**
2100	**CURRENT LIABILITIES — PAYABLE**
2110	Accounts Payable
2120	Bank Overdrafts Payable
2130	Other Current Liabilities Payable
2131	Intercompany Accounts Payable
2132	Accounts Payable — Employee
2133	Accounts Payable — Related Parties
2134	Accounts Payable — Other
2160	Contract Claims Payable
2200	**CURRENT LIABILITIES — PAYROLL**
2210	Payroll Tax Withholdings Payable
2211	Federal Income Tax Withholdings Payable
2212	State Income Tax Withholdings Payable
2213	FICA/Medicare Withholdings Payable
2214	Local Tax Withholdings Payable
2215	Other Tax Withholdings Payable
2220	Insurance Withholdings Payable
2221	Health Insurance Withholdings Payable
2222	Life Insurance Withholdings Payable
2223	State Disability Insurance Withholdings Payable
2224	Other Insurance Withholdings Payable
2230	Other Payroll Withholdings Payable
2231	401(k) Withholdings Payable
2232	Cafeteria Plan Withholdings Payable
2233	Court Mandated Child Support Withholdings Payable
2234	Other Payroll Withholdings Payable
2250	Accrued Payroll Liabilities
2251	Accrued Payroll

Detailed Format (Continued)

Account Number	Description
2252	Accrued Vacation, Holiday & Sick Pay (Compensated Absences)
2253	Accrued FICA/Medicare Taxes Payable
2255	Accrued Federal Unemployment Taxes Payable
2256	Accrued Retirement Plan Contribution
2257	Other Accrued Payroll Liabilities
2260	Other Payroll Liabilities
2300	**CURRENT LIABILITIES — OTHER**
2310	Accrued Liabilities — Nonpayroll
2311	Accrued Rent
2312	Accrued Interest
2313	Accrued Insurance
2314	Accrued Income Taxes (Federal/State)
2315	Accrued Property Taxes
2316	Accrued Franchise Taxes
2317	Other Accrued Liabilities
2320	Notes and Loans Payable
2321	Current Notes and Loans Payable — Vendors
2322	Current Notes and Loans Payable — Employees
2323	Current Notes and Loans Payable — Stockholders/Partners
2324	Current Other Notes and Loans Payable
2325	Bank Working Capital Line Outstanding
2330	Long-Term Debt — Current Portion
2331	Capital Lease Obligation — Current Portion
2332	Construction Contracts Payable
2333	Other Loans Payable — Current Portion
2340	Advances from Settlements Due to Third-Party Agencies
2350	Patient Deposits
2360	Claims Payable Incurred But Not Reported
2361	Incurred But Not Reported Claims — Commercial
2362	Incurred But Not Reported Claims — Medicare
2363	Incurred But Not Reported Claims — Medicaid
2365	Other Claims Incurred But Not Reported
2370	Deferred Revenue
2371	Deferred Revenue — Fee for Service
2372	Deferred Revenue — Capitated or Prepaid Plan
2375	Other Deferred Revenue
2380	Deferred Income Taxes — Current Portion
2390	Other Current Liabilities
2400	**LONG-TERM LIABILITIES**
2410	Long-Term Notes Payable
2420	Construction Loans
2430	Capital Lease Obligation — Long-Term Portion
2450	Deferred Third-Party Revenue
2451	Deferred Third-Party Revenue — Medicare
2452	Deferred Third-Party Revenue — Medicaid
2453	Deferred Third-Party Revenue — Other
2460	Deferred Compensation
2465	Severance Plan
2470	Deferred Income Taxes — Long-Term Portion
2480	Other Long-Term Liabilities
	OWNERS' EQUITY ACCOUNTS
3000	**PARTNERS' EQUITY (PARTNERSHIP)**
3010	Contributed Capital (Each Partner)
3020	Undistributed Earnings
3030	Partners' Drawing Accounts (Each Partner)
3040	Current Income/Loss

Detailed Format (Continued)

Account Number	Description
3000	**STOCKHOLDERS' EQUITY (CORPORATION)**
3010	Preferred Stock
3020	Common Stock
3030	Capital Contributed in Excess of Par
3040	Donated Capital
3050	Allowance for Change in Net Unrealized Gains/Losses on Investments
3060	Dividends and Distributions
3070	Retained Earnings — Unappropriated
3075	Retained Earnings — Appropriated
3080	Current Income/Loss
3090	Treasury Stock
3000	**NET ASSETS (NOT-FOR-PROFIT EQUITY)**
3010	Unrestricted Net Assets
3030	Temporarily Restricted Net Assets
3040	Permanently Restricted Net Assets
3050	Current Surplus/Deficit
3000	**LIMITED LIABILITY COMPANY/PARTNERSHIP**
3010	Members' Capital/Limited Partners' Interest
3020	Members' Distributions/Limited Partners' Distributions
3030	Current Income/Loss
	INCOME STATEMENT ACCOUNTS
4000	**REVENUES**
4100	**GROSS CHARGES**
4110	Gross Charges — Fee-for-Services (FFS)
4120	Gross Charges — Discounted FFS Contracts
4130	Gross Charges — FFS Equivalents for Capitation Plan Benefits
4140	Other Gross Charges
4150	Other Revenue
4200	Fees Collected
4210	Fees Collected — FFS
4220	Fees Collected — FFS for Managed Care
4230	Capitated Premium Revenues — Commercial
4240	Capitated Premium Revenues — Medicare
4250	Capitated Premium Revenues — Medicaid
4260	Capitated Premium Revenues — Other
4270	Risk Sharing Revenue
4271	Hospital Risk Sharing — Commercial
4272	Hospital Risk Sharing — Medicare
4273	Hospital Risk Sharing — Medicaid
4274	Hospital Risk Sharing — Pharmacy
4275	Hospital Risk Sharing — Other
4280	Other Managed Care Collected Revenues
4281	Copayments
4282	Coordination of Benefits
4283	Other Prepaid Professional Fees Collected
4290	Recoveries
4291	Reinsurances Recoveries
4292	Bad Debt Recovery
4300	Patient Refunds
4400	Fees Collected — Other Revenue
4410	Sales — Medical Related
4420	Patient Records Copying Reimbursement
4430	Fees Collected — Other
4450	Donations Received (Operating Revenue)
4460	Research/Clinical Studies Income

Detailed Format (Continued)

Account Number	Description
4470	Grant Revenue
4480	Miscellaneous Income
4490	Operating Subsidy Income
4500	**ADJUSTMENTS**
4510	Gross Charges — FFS Discount/Adjustment
4520	Gross Charges — Discounted FFS Contracts Adjustments
4530	Gross Charges — FFS Equivalents for Cap Plan Patients/Adjustment
4540	Other Gross Charges/Adjustments
4550	Other Revenue Discount/Adjustment
4600	Financial Hardship Care Discount/Adjustment
4610	Courtesy Discount/Adjustment
4620	Employee Discount/Adjustment
4630	Charity Care Discount/Adjustment
4700	Third-Party Settlements
4800	Provision for Cash-Basis Conversion
5000	**OPERATING EXPENSES — SALARY AND FRINGE BENEFITS**
5100	**PHYSICIAN — SALARIES ***
5100	**PHYSICIAN-EMPLOYEE-RELATED EXPENSES *** ***(See Accounts 8100 - 8400)**
5300	**MIDLEVEL PROVIDERS — SALARIES ***
5400	**MIDLEVEL PROVIDERS — EMPLOYEE-RELATED EXPENSES ***
5500	**ANCILLARY STAFF — SALARIES**
5510	Salaries — Radiology
5520	Salaries — Laboratory
5530	Salaries — Optical
5540	Salaries — Physical Therapy
5550	Salaries — Other Ancillary Services BONE DENSITY
5600	**ANCILLARY STAFF — EMPLOYEE-RELATED EXPENSES**
5610	Payroll Taxes (Ancillary)
5611	Payroll Taxes — FICA/Medicare (Ancillary)
5612	Payroll Taxes — Federal Unemployment Insurance (Ancillary)
5613	Payroll Taxes — State Unemployment Insurance (Ancillary)
5614	Payroll Taxes — Other (Ancillary)
5620	Insurance (Ancillary)
5621	Insurance — Health (Ancillary)
5622	Insurance — Dental (Ancillary)
5623	Insurance — Life (Ancillary)
5624	Insurance — Disability (Ancillary)
5625	Insurance — Workers' Compensation (Ancillary)
5626	Insurance — Other (Ancillary)
5630	Pension and Retirement Benefits (Ancillary)
5631	Pension (Ancillary)
5632	Deferred Compensation (Ancillary)
5633	Severance Plan (Ancillary)
5635	Professional Development (Ancillary)
5640	Books and Subscriptions (Ancillary)
5645	Dues and Memberships (Ancillary)
5650	Licenses (Ancillary)
5655	Meetings (Ancillary)
5660	Travel (Ancillary)
5665	Medical Reimbursement Plan (Ancillary)
5670	Vehicles (Ancillary)
5675	Parking (Ancillary)

Detailed Format (Continued)

Account Number	Description
5680	Telephones (Ancillary)
5685	Beepers (Ancillary)
5690	Meals and Entertainment (Ancillary)
5695	Other Benefits (Ancillary)
5700	**EMPLOYEES — SALARIES**
5710	Salaries — General Administrative
5715	Salaries — Business Office -GEN
5720	Salaries — Managed Care Administrative
5725	Salaries — Information Services
5730	Salaries — Housekeeping/Maintenance/Security
5735	Salaries — Medical Receptionist
5740	Salaries — Medical Secretaries/Transcribers
5745	Salaries — Medical Records
5750	Salaries — Other Administrative Support
5755	Salaries — Registered Nurses
5760	Salaries — Licensed Practical Nurses
5765	Salaries — Medical Assistants/Nurses' Aids
5800	**EMPLOYEES — EMPLOYEE-RELATED EXPENSES**
5810	Payroll Taxes (Other)
5811	Payroll Taxes — FICA/Medicare (Other)
5812	Payroll Taxes — Federal Unemployment Insurance (Other)
5813	Payroll Taxes — State Unemployment Insurance (Other)
5814	Payroll Taxes — Other (Other)
5820	Insurance (Other)
5821	Insurance — Health (Other)
5822	Insurance — Dental (Other)
5823	Insurance — Life (Other)
5824	Insurance — Disability (Other)
5825	Insurance — Workers' Compensation (Other)
5826	Insurance — Other (Other)
5830	Pension and Retirement Benefits (Other)
5831	Pension (Other)
5832	Deferred Compensation (Other)
5833	Severance Plan (Other)
5835	Professional Development (Other)
5840	Books and Subscriptions (Other)
5845	Dues and Memberships (Other)
5850	Licenses (Other)
5855	Meetings (Other)
5860	Travel (Other)
5865	Medical Reimbursement Plan (Other)
5870	Vehicles (Other)
5875	Parking (Other)
5880	Telephones (Other)
5885	Beepers (Other)
5890	Meals and Entertainment (Other)
5895	Other Benefits (Other)
5900	Temporary Employee Salaries
5901	Physician Salaries
5902	Midlevel Provider Salaries

Detailed Format (Continued)

Account Number	Description
5903	Ancillary Staff Salaries
5904	Administrative and Other Staff
5910	Temporary Employee Benefits
5911	Physician Benefits
5912	Midlevel Provider Benefits
5913	Ancillary Staff Benefits
5914	Administrative and Other Staff
6000	**SERVICES AND GENERAL EXPENSE**
6100	Office and Administrative Expense
6110	Equipment Rentals (Admin)
6115	Equipment Maintenance (Admin)
6120	Telephones (Admin)
6130	Postage (Admin)
6140	Courier and Overnight Delivery (Admin)
6150	Security
6160	Library/Books and Subscriptions
6170	Advertising and Marketing
6180	General Business and Other Insurance
6181	Officers' and Directors' Liability
6182	Other Liability
6183	Reinsurance for Capitation Contracts
6184	Keyman and Overhead Insurance
6185	Malpractice Insurance
6186	Physicians
6187	Midlevel Providers
6188	Ancillary and Clinical Staff
6189	Global Coverage
6190	Printing (Admin)
6200	Copying (Admin)
6210	Medical Forms
6220	Answering Service
6230	Meals and Entertainment
6240	Cafeteria
6250	Employee Relations
6260	Physician Recruitment
6270	Nonphysician Recruitment
6300	Depreciation/Amortization
6301	Furniture and Fixtures
6302	Capital Leases
6303	Equipment
6304	Computers
6305	Vehicles
6306	Amortization
6307	Other Depreciation
6310	Accounting Services
6320	Legal Services
6330	Actuarial Services
6340	Pension Administration Expense
6350	Consulting Services
6360	Other Professional Services
6370	Medical Transcription
6380	Payroll Services
6390	Business Transportation
6400	General Supplies
6410	Taxes — Excise and Other Business Taxes
6420	Computer Supplies
6430	Computer Software

Detailed Format (Continued)

Account Number	Description
6440	Other Office and Administrative Expense
6500	Billing Expense
6510	Equipment Rentals (Billing)
6515	Equipment Maintenance (Billing)
6520	Electronic Data Processing (Billing)
6530	Telephones (Billing)
6540	Postage (Billing)
6550	Courier and Overnight Delivery (Billing)
6560	Printing (Billing)
6570	Copying (Billing)
6580	Depreciation
6600	General Services
6650	Other Billing Expense
6700	Bad Debt Expense
6710	Accounts Receivable Write-Offs
6720	Collection Agency Write-Offs
6730	Collection Expenses
7000	**CLINICAL EXPENSE**
7010	Drugs and Medications
7020	Medical Supplies
7021	Radiology
7022	Laboratory
7023	Other Ancillary Supplies
7030	Linen Supplies
7040	Uniforms and Laundry
7050	Patient Education
7060	Photography
7070	Biohazardous Waste Removal
7100	Equipment Rentals (Clinical)
7110	Equipment Maintenance (Clinical)
7120	Telephones (Clinical)
7130	Postage (Clinical)
7140	Medical Record Supplies
7150	Other Clinical Expense
7160	Depreciation (Clinical)
7161	General Clinical
7162	Radiology
7163	Laboratory
7500	Occupancy Expense
7510	Rent/Lease
7520	Condominium Assessments/Monthly Maintenance Fees
7530	General Maintenance
7540	Utilities
7541	Utilities — Water
7542	Utilities — Electricity
7543	Utilities — Waste Disposal
7544	Other Utilties
7550	Property Taxes
7560	Housekeeping/Maintenance Services
7570	Other Occupancy Expense
7580	Insurance (Occupancy)
7590	Depreciation (Occupancy)
7595	Amortization — Leasehold Improvements (Occupancy)
7600	Cost of Goods Sold — Medical Related

Detailed Format (Continued)

Account Number	Description
7700	**PURCHASED SERVICES/MANAGEMENT FEES**
7710	Medical Directorships
7720	General and Administrative Expense — Purchased Services
7730	Management Fees — MSO/PPMC
7731	Management Fees — Commercial
7732	Management Fees — Medicare
7733	Management Fees — Medicaid
7734	Management Fees — Other
7740	Management Company Incentive
7800	Purchased Services for HMO/PPO Patients — Professional and Medical
7810	FFS Purchased Services for HMO/PPO Patients
7811	FFS Purchased Services — Commercial
7812	FFS Purchased Services — Medicare
7813	FFS Purchased Services — Medicaid
7814	FFS Purchased Services — Other
7815	FFS Purchased Services for HMO/PPO Patients — Hospital Inpatient
7816	FFS Purchased Services for HMO/PPO Patients — Hospital Emergency Room
7817	FFS Purchased Services for HMO/PPO Patients — Ambulance
7818	FFS Purchased Services for HMO/PPO Patients — Out-of-Area Emergency Care
7819	FFS Purchased Services for HMO/PPO Patients — Other Professional and Medical
7850	Sub-capitation Payments — Primary Care
7851	Sub-capitation Payments — Primary Care — Commercial
7852	Sub-capitation Payments — Primary Care — Medicare
7853	Sub-capitation Payments — Primary Care — Medicaid
7854	Sub-capitation Payments — Primary Care — Other
7860	Sub-capitation Payments — Specialty Care
7861	Sub-capitation Payments — Specialty Care — Commercial
7862	Sub-capitation Payments — Specialty Care — Medicare
7863	Sub-capitation Payments — Specialty Care — Medicaid
7864	Sub-capitation Payments — Specialty Care — Other
7870	Sub-capitation Payments — Hospitals
7880	Sub-capitation Payments — Other
8000	**PROVIDER-RELATED EXPENSES**
8100	**PHYSICIAN — SALARIES**
8110	Salaries, Distributions and Incentives (Physician)
8120	Salaries — Owner/Stockholder (Physician)
8130	Distributions and Incentives (Physician)
8140	Global/Capitation Distributions (Physician)
8150	Employee Salaries (Physician)
8160	Employee Incentives (Physician)
8170	Administrative Salaries (Physician)
8180	Other Compensation (Physician)
8200	**PHYSICIAN — EMPLOYEE-RELATED EXPENSES**
8210	Payroll Taxes (Physician)
8211	Payroll Taxes — FICA/Medicare (Physician)
8212	Payroll Taxes — Federal Unemployment Insurance (Physician)
8213	Payroll Taxes — State Unemployment Insurance (Physician)
8214	Payroll Taxes — Other (Physician)
8220	Insurance (Physician)
8221	Insurance — Health (Physician)
8222	Insurance — Dental (Physician)
8223	Insurance — Life (Physician)
8224	Insurance — Disability (Physician)
8225	Insurance — Workers' Compensation (Physician)
8226	Insurance — Other (Physician)

Detailed Format (Continued)

Account Number	Description
8227	Insurance — Officers' Life (Physician)
8230	Pension and Retirement Benefits (Physician)
8231	Pension (Physician)
8232	Deferred Compensation (Physician)
8233	Severance Plan (Physician)
8235	Professional Development (Physician)
8240	Books and Subscriptions (Physician)
8245	Dues and Memberships (Physician)
8250	Licenses (Physician)
8255	Meetings (Physician)
8260	Travel (Physician)
8265	Medical Reimbursement Plan (Physician)
8270	Vehicles (Physician)
8271	Leased Motor Vehicles (Physician)
8275	Parking (Physician)
8280	Telephones (Physician)
8285	Beepers (Physician)
8290	Meals and Entertainment (Physician)
8295	Other Benefits (Physician)
*	
8300	**MIDLEVEL PROVIDERS — SALARIES**
8310	Salaries, Distributions and Incentives (Midlevel)
8320	Salaries — Owner/Stockholder (Midlevel)
8330	Distributions and Incentives (Midlevel)
8340	Global/Capitation Distribution (Midlevel)
8350	Employee Salaries (Midlevel)
8360	Employee Incentives (Midlevel)
8370	Administrative Salaries (Midlevel)
8380	Other Compensation (Midlevel)
8400	**MIDLEVEL PROVIDERS — EMPLOYEE-RELATED EXPENSES**
8410	Payroll Taxes (Midlevel)
8411	Payroll Taxes — FICA/Medicare (Midlevel)
8412	Payroll Taxes — Federal Unemployment Insurance (Midlevel)
8413	Payroll Taxes — State Unemployment Insurance (Midlevel)
8414	Payroll Taxes — Other (Midlevel)
8420	Insurance (Midlevel)
8421	Insurance — Health (Midlevel)
8422	Insurance — Dental (Midlevel)
8423	Insurance — Life (Midlevel)
8424	Insurance — Disability (Midlevel
8425	Insurance — Worker's Compensation (Midlevel)
8426	Insurance — Other (Midlevel)
8430	Pension and Retirement Benefits (Midlevel)
8431	Pension (Midlevel)
8432	Deferred Compensation (Midlevel)
8433	Severance Plan (Midlevel)
8435	Professional Development (Midlevel)
8440	Books and Subscriptions (Midlevel)
8445	Dues and Memberships (Midlevel)
8450	Licenses (Midlevel)
8455	Meetings (Midlevel)
8460	Travel (Midlevel)
8465	Medical Reimbursement Plan (Midlevel)
8470	Vehicles (Midlevel)
8475	Parking (Midlevel)
8480	Telephones (Midlevel)
8485	Beepers (Midlevel)

* 8296 Personal Computers
8297 Contributions

Detailed Format (Continued)

Account Number	Description
8490	Meals and Entertainment (Midlevel)
8495	Other Benefits (Midlevel)
9000	**NONOPERATING REVENUE & EXP; INCOME TAXES & OTHER EXP**
9100	Nonoperating Revenues
9110	Interest Income
9120	Income from Long-Term Investments
9130	Property Rentals
9140	Unrealized Gains and Losses — Investments
9150	Realized Gains and Losses — Investments
9160	Donations Received (Nonoperating Revenue)
9170	Nonoperating Subsidy Income
9200	Nonoperating Expense
9210	Interest Expense
9220	Contributions/Donations Expense
9230	Current Income Tax Expense (Recovery)
9231	Current Income Taxes — Federal
9232	Current Income Taxes — State
9233	Current Income Taxes — Other
9240	Deferred Income Tax Expense (Recovery)
9241	Deferred Income Taxes — Federal
9242	Deferred Income Taxes — State
9243	Deferred Income Taxes — Other
9300	Other Income/Expense

Chart of Accounts — General — Summary Format

Account Number	Description
	BALANCE SHEET
1000	**ASSETS**
1100	Cash
1200	Marketable Securities & Short-Term Investments
1300	Accounts Receivable
1320	Allowance for Estimated Uncollectable Receivables
1350	Other Short-Term Receivables
1353	Due from Employees
1354	Due from Related Parties
1400	Supply Inventories
1500	Prepaid Expenses
1550	Other Current Assets
1600	**INVESTMENTS — LONG-TERM RECEIVABLES**
1700	**PROPERTY, FURNITURE, FIXTURES & EQUIPMENT**
1710	REAL PROPERTY
1711	Land
1713	Buildings
1715	Leasehold Improvements
1750	FURNITURE, FIXTURES & EQUIPMENT
1751	Furniture & Fixtures
1753	Equipment
1754	Capital Leases — Equipment
1760	Computer
1770	Capital Leases — Computer
1780	Vehicles
1790	Ancillary Service Equipment
1795	Capital Leases — Ancillary Service Equipment
1800	**ACCUMULATED DEPRECIATION — PROPERTY, FURNITURE, ETC.**
1810	ACCUMULATED DEPRECIATION — REAL PROPERTY
1813	Accum Depreciation — Buildings
1815	Accum Depreciation — Leasehold Improvements
1850	ACCUM DEPRECIATION — FURNITURE, FIXTURES & EQUIPMENT
1851	Accum Depreciation — Furniture and Fixtures
1853	Accum Depreciation — Equipment
1854	Accum Depreciation — Capital Leases — Equipment
1860	Accum Depreciation — Computer
1870	Accum Depreciation — Capital Leases — Computer
1880	Accum Depreciation — Vehicles
1890	Other Accum Depreciation — Ancillary Service Equipment
1895	Accum Depreciation — Capital Leases — Ancillary Service Equipment
1900	**INTANGIBLE AND OTHER ASSETS**
1910	Organization Costs
1915	Accumulated Amortization — Organization Costs
1940	Deposits
1960	Other Assets
2000	**LIABILITIES**
2100	CURRENT LIABILITIES — PAYABLES
2110	Accounts Payable
2130	Other Current Liabilities Payable

Summary Format (Continued)

Account Number	Description
2200	**CURRENT LIABILITIES — PAYROLL**
2210	Payroll Tax Withholdings Payable
2250	Accrued Payroll Liabilities
2300	**CURRENT LIABILITIES — OTHER**
2310	Accrued Liabilities — Nonpayroll
2320	Notes and Loans Payable
2325	Bank Working Capital Line Outstanding
2330	Long-Term Debt — Current Portion
2331	Capital Lease Obligation — Current Portion
2333	Other loans Payable — Current portion
2400	**LONG-TERM LIABILITIES**
2410	Long-Term Notes Payable
2430	Capital Lease Obilgation — Long-Term Portion
2440	Other Loans Payable — Long-Term Portion
	Owners' Equity Accounts
3000	**PARTNERS' EQUITY (PARTNERSHIP)**
3010	Contributed Capital (Each Partner)
3030	Partners' Drawing Accounts (Each Partner)
3040	Current Income/Loss
3000	**STOCKHOLDERS' EQUITY (CORPORATION)**
3010	Preferred Stock
3020	Common Stock
3060	Dividends and Distributions
3070	Retained Earnings — Unappropriated
3080	Current Income/Loss
3090	Treasury Stock
3000	**NET ASSETS (NOT-FOR-PROFIT EQUITY)**
3010	Unrestricted Net Assets
3030	Temporarily Restricted Net Assets
3040	Permanently Restricted Net assets
3050	Current Surplus/Deficit
3000	**LIMITED LIABILITY COMPANY/PARTNERSHIP**
3010	Members' Capital/Limited Partners' Interest
3020	Members' Distributions/Limited Partners' Distributions
3030	Current Income/Loss
	INCOME STATEMENT ACCOUNTS
4000	**REVENUES**
4100	Gross Charges
4110	Gross Charges — Fee-for-Service (FFS)
4120	Gross Charges — Discounted FFS Contracts
4130	Gross Charges — FFS Equivalent for Capitation Plan Patients
4140	Other Gross Charges
4150	Other Revenue
4200	Fees Collected
4210	Fees Collected — FFS

Summary Format (Continued)

Account Number	Description
4220	Fees Collected — FFS for Managed Care
4230	Capitated Premium Revenues — Commercial
4240	Capitated Premium Revenues — Medicare
4250	Capitated Premium Revenues — Medicaid
4260	Capitated Premium Revenues — Other
4270	Risk Sharing Revenue
4280	Other Managed Care Collected Revenues
4290	Recoveries
4300	Patient Refunds
4400	Fees Collected — Other Revenue
4410	Sales — Medical Related
4420	Patient Records Copying Reimbursement
4430	Fees Collected — Other
4450	Donations Received (Operating Reveunue)
4460	Research/Clinical Sudies Income
4470	Grant Revenue
4480	Miscellaneous Income
4490	Operating Subsidy Income
4500	**ADJUSTMENTS**
4510	Gross Charges — FFS Discount/Adjustment
4520	Gross Charges — Discounted FFS Contracts Discount/Adjustment
4530	Gross Charges — FFS Equivalent for Cap Plan Patients/Adjustment
4540	Other Gross Charges/Adjustments
4550	Other Revenue Discount/Adjustment
4600	Financial Hardship Care Discount/Adjustment
4610	Courtesy Discount/Adjustment
4620	Employee Discount/Adjustment
4700	Third-Party Settlements
4800	Provision for Cash-Basis Conversion
5000	**OPERATING EXPENSES — SALARY AND FRINGE BENEFITS**
5100	PHYSICIAN — SALARIES *
5200	PHYSICIAN — EMPLOYEE-RELATED EXPENSES * ***(See Accounts 8100-8400)**
5300	MIDLEVEL PROVIDERS — SALARIES *
5400	MIDLEVEL PROVIDERS — EMPLOYEE-RELATED EXPENSES *
5500	**ANCILLARY STAFF — SALARIES**
5600	**ANCILLARY STAFF — EMPLOYEE-RELATED EXPENSES**
5610	Payroll Taxes (Ancillary)
5620	Insurance (Ancillary)
5630	Pension and Retirement Benefits (Ancillary)
5635	Professional Development (Ancillary)
5640	Books and Subscriptions (Ancillary)
5645	Dues and Memberships (Ancillary)
5650	Licenses (Ancillary)
5655	Meetings (Ancillary)
5660	Travel (Ancillary)
5665	Medical Reimbursement Plan (Ancillary)
5670	Vehicles (Ancillary)

Summary Format (Continued)

Account Number	Description
5680	Telephones (Ancillary)
5685	Beepers (Ancillary)
5690	Meals and Entertainment (Ancillary)
5700	**EMPLOYEES — SALARIES**
5800	**EMPLOYEES — EMPLOYEE-RELATED EXPENSE**
5810	Payroll Taxes (Other)
5820	Insurance (Other)
5830	Pension and Retirement Benefits (Other)
5835	Professional Development (Other)
5840	Books and Subscriptions (Other)
5845	Dues and Memberships (Other)
5850	Licenses (Other)
5855	Meetings (Other)
5860	Travel (Other)
5865	Medical Reimbursement Plan (Other)
5870	Vehicles (Other)
5875	Parking (Other)
5880	Telephones (Other)
5885	Beepers (Other)
5890	Meals and Entertainment (Other)
5900	Temporary Employee Salaries
5910	Temporary Employee Benefits
6000	**SERVICES AND GENERAL EXPENSE**
6100	Office and Administrative Expense
6110	Equipment Rentals (Admin)
6115	Equipment Maintenance (Admin)
6120	Telephones (Admin)
6130	Postage (Admin)
6180	General Business and Other Insurance
6185	Malpractice Insurance
6240	Cafeteria
6250	Employee Relations
6300	Depreciation/Amortization
6310	Accounting Services
6320	Legal Services
6340	Pension Administration Expense
6370	Medical Transcription
6380	Payroll Services
6410	Taxes — Excise and Other Business Taxes
6500	Billing Expense
6700	Bad Debt Expense
7000	Clinical Expense
7500	Occupancy Expense
7510	Rent/Lease
7530	General Maintenance
7540	Utilities
7550	Property Taxes
7560	Housekeeping/Maintenance Services
7580	Insurance (Occupancy)
7590	Depreciation (Occupancy)

Summary Format (Continued)

Account Number	Description
7595	Amortization — Leasehold Improvements (Occupancy)
7600	Cost of Goods Sold — Medical Related
7700	**PURCHASED SERVICES/MANAGEMENT FEES**
7800	Purchased Services for HMO/PPO Patients — Professional and Medical
8000	**PROVIDER-RELATED EXPENSE**
8100	**PHYSICIAN — SALARIES**
8110	Salaries, Distributions and Incentives (Physician)
8200	**PHYSICIAN — EMPLOYEE-RELATED EXPENSES**
8210	Payroll Taxes (Physician)
8220	Insurance (Physician)
8230	Pension and Retirement Benefits (Physician)
8235	Professional Development (Physician)
8240	Books and Subscriptions (Physician)
8245	Dues and Memberships (Physician)
8250	Licenses (Physician)
8255	Meetings (Physician)
8260	Travel (Physician)
8265	Medical Reimbursement Plan (Physician)
8270	Vehicles (Physician)
8275	Parking (Physician)
8280	Telephones (Physician)
8285	Beepers (Physician)
8290	Meals and Entertainment (Physician)
8295	Other Benefits (Physician)
8300	**MIDLEVEL PROVIDERS — SALARIES**
8310	Salaries, Distributions and Incentives (Midlevel)
8400	**MIDLEVEL PROVIDERS — EMPLOYEE-RELATED EXPENSES**
8410	Payroll Taxes (Midlevel)
8420	Insurance (Midlevel)
8430	Pension and Retirement Benefits (Midlevel)
8435	Professional Development (Midlevel)
8440	Books and Subscriptions (Midlevel)
8445	Dues and Memberships (Midlevel)
8450	Licenses (Midlevel)
8455	Meetings (Midlevel)
8460	Travel (Midlevel)
8465	Medical Reimbursement Plan (Midlevel)
8470	Vehicles (Midlevel)
8475	Parking (Midlevel)
8480	Telephones (Midlevel)
8485	Beepers (Midlevel)
8490	Meals and Entertainment (Midlevel)
8495	Other Benefits (Midlevel)
9000	**NONOPERATING REVENUE AND EXPENSES; INCOME TAXES & OTHER EXPENSES**
9110	Interest Income
9210	Interest Expense
9220	Contributions/Donations Expense

Summary Format (continued)

Account Number	Description
9230	Current Income Tax Expense (Recovery)
9240	Deferred Income Tax Expense (Recovery)
9300	Other Income/Expense

For the physician practice or organization that does not fall into the general format, guidelines have been provided in later chapters to show any tailored reporting needs. Refer to the chapter that best fits your organizational operation and function.

See Table I in the Appendix for a complete reference listing of the chart of accounts and the corresponding accounting basis available to be used by medical practices/organizations. As discussed in the section "Basic Guidelines: Accounting for Today's Health Care," it is not always clear whether an entity is using what is referred to as the cash basis of accounting. In reality, the pure cash basis of accounting is rarely used and in operation the modified cash basis of accounting is being followed with its more comprehensive inclusion of accounts. Unfortunately, over the years there has been a blurring of terms employed to describe these actual two accounting methods used by management. To even further complicate matters there are those in practice who feel that capitalized leases (assets), their related liabilities and some accounts receivable accounts should be included in the modified cash method. This all translates into a word of caution and a required moment of pause as each organization reviews and implements Table I.

See Table II (Tables I - IV are in the Appendix) for a complete reference-table listing of the chart of accounts and the corresponding type of entity that can utilize the accounts.

See Table III for a complete cross-reference-table listing of the chart of account numbers as set forth in the *Medical Group Practice Chart of Accounts*, 1st Edition, 1996, to the current revised chart of accounts.

See Table IV for an annual *MGMA Cost Survey* questionnaire mapping tool to bridge your financial results and Chart of Accounts to the current Chart of Accounts and Cost Survey format.

See Tables V and VI (respectively) for a listing of the balance sheet accounts and income statement accounts in alphabetical order. The balance sheet accounts are alphabetized within the categories of assets, liabilities and owners' equity. The income statement accounts are alphabetized within the categories of revenue and expense.

3

Balance Sheet Account Descriptions

Kathryn P. Glass, M.B.A., M.S.H.A.

Balance Sheet

The balance sheet is also known as the Statement of Financial Position because it lists the organization's assets, liabilities and owners' equity (capital) at a particular point in time. It is a snapshot of the financial situation on a given date.

1000 ASSETS

Assets are resources owned by the business. Assets may be tangible (physical in nature) such as land, buildings and equipment, a direct right to tangible property such as amounts due from patients and third-party agencies. Or, they may be intangible such as goodwill, patents, licenses and leaseholds.

Current assets are cash and other assets that are expected to be converted to cash, sold or consumed in the normal course of operations within one year.

Long-term assets are assets that are not expected to be converted to cash, sold or otherwise consumed in the normal course of operations within one year.

Accounts are numbered to reflect degree of asset liquidity. The lower numbers are the most liquid; the higher numbers are the least liquid.

1100 Cash

1110 Cash — Banks

Cash on deposit in banks that is immediately available for current operations. Cash restricted for other than general operating purposes should be included in Account 1130 — Cash — Restricted.

1111 General Checking Accounts

Cash on deposit in banks that is immediately available for general purposes.

1112 Payroll Checking Accounts

Cash on deposit in banks that is immediately available for payroll transactions.

1113 Other Checking Accounts

Cash on deposit in banks that is immediately available for other disbursements.

1120 Cash — On Hand

Unrestricted cash on hand covers both a change fund (sub-account 1121) and/or a petty cash fund (sub-account 1122). These funds may reside in either this general account or in the sub-accounts 1121 or 1122.

1121 Change Fund

Cash on hand that is used to support daily operational patient/sale operations.

1122 Petty Cash

Cash on hand that is available and used to periodically reimburse for miscellaneous amounts expended.

1130 Cash — Restricted

Cash restricted for other than general operating purposes. Previous versions of the chart of accounts categorized this account as a Long-Term Investment. However, cash is most commonly considered a current asset and not a long-term asset, therefore it has been reclassified in this particular chart of accounts. Even though the cash may be restricted for use with noncurrent budget items, it may still be expended within one year.

If particular restrictions place the use of cash beyond one year, consideration should be made to list the account within the Account 1600 — Investments — Long-Term Receivables section. If so, this account should include cash and claims to cash that are:

- Restricted as to withdrawal or use for other than current operations
- Designated for expenditure in the acquisition or construction of noncurrent assets
- Required to be segregated for the liquidation of long-term debts
- Required by a donor-imposed restriction that limits their use to long-term purposes.

1200 Marketable Securities & Short-Term Investments

Short-term investments are intended to be used to finance current operations, including savings accounts, marketable securities, U.S. Government securities, certificates of deposit and other securities that are traded regularly. Securities not intended to be used to finance current operations should be included in a sub-account of 1630 — Long-Term Investments.

1210 Valuation Allowance — Short-Term Investments

Adjustments to short-term investments to reflect the unrealized appreciation or depreciation in the fair market value of the investment at the end of the period. At the end of the period, changes in the fair market value of equity and debt securities of a not-for-profit medical organization should be recorded here.

Changes in the fair market value of equity securities and debt securities (that are not intended to be held until maturity) of a for-profit medical organization should be recorded here. For-profit medical organizations that intend to hold debt securities until maturity should record them at amortized cost and not use the valuation accounts.

1300 Accounts Receivable

In general, the accounts receivable represent the open account amounts (debts) owed to the organization by other entities (including customers, patients and third-party payers) as a result of the services provided to its customers and patients.

1301 Accounts Receivable — Fee-for-Service Amounts

Amounts owed to the organization by patients, third parties, employer groups, unions, individuals, subscribers and others. This account is usually a control account for individual accounts receivable balances that may be contained in a subsidiary ledger.

1302 Accounts Receivable — Prepaid Contracts

Amounts owed to the organization by HMOs (Health Maintenance Organizations) and other prepaid plans. This account is usually a control account for individual accounts receivable balances that may be contained in a subsidiary ledger.

1320 Allowance For Estimated uncollectable Receivables

Estimated amount of uncollectable receivables. A historical analysis of bad debt write-offs as well as contractual adjustments is usually required to determine periodic credits to this account.

1321 Allowance for Bad Debts — Patient Accounts

Estimated amount of uncollectable receivables from patient accounts. A historical analysis of bad debt write-offs is usually required to determine periodic credits to this account.

1322 Allowance for Contractual Adjustments

Estimated adjustments for third-party agencies. A historical analysis of contractual adjustments is usually required to determine periodic credits to this account.

1323 Allowance for Bad Debts — Third-Party Payers

Estimated amount of uncollectable receivables from third-party payers. Credits to this account are usually generated based on specific knowledge of troubled payers and related negotiations for payment.

1324 Allowance for Charity Care

An account that tracks the patient services in which payment was neither sought nor collected by request of an authority (such as a physician or executive manager) within the organization or hospital.

1340 Notes Receivable — Short Term

Amounts owed to the organization by other entities where the obligation is represented by a note with a maturity of one year or less.

1345 Managed-Care Contract — Bonus/Withhold

Typically used in capitation contracts or other risk-sharing arrangements, a withhold is a percentage of the primary care capitation rate that is withheld every month and used to cover the cost overruns (excess medical expenses) in referral or organizational services. The account is reconciled at year-end. If the entire amount of the withhold was not required to cover cost overruns, the remainder may be distributed or kept in the account to fund the risk pool as determined by contract terms. This account reflects the bonus/withhold amount earned, not received.

Managed care contracts may also have provisions for a bonus that would be paid after the accounts were reconciled at year-end. Bonuses are commonly linked to the achievement of predetermined goals typically based on either total plan performance or on the reduction of medical expenses.

1350 Other Short-Term Receivables

Short-term receivables not recorded elsewhere. For example, interest that has been earned but not yet received may be recorded here or in sub-account 1351.

1351 Interest Receivables

Interest that has been earned but not yet received.

1352 Intercompany Receivables

Amounts owed to the organization by other entities consolidated for financial reporting purposes.

1353 Due from Employees

Amounts owed to the organization by its employees, including physician-owners.

1354 Due from Related Parties

Amounts owed to the organization by related entities including entities under common ownership or control.

1400 Supply Inventories

Costs of unused supplies are recorded here. The organization should establish an inventory policy defining which items are charged to an inventory account at the date of purchase and which items are expensed as acquired. At the organization's discretion, sub-accounts 1401 - 1407 may be used to delineate the supply categories. Supplies specific to ancillary departments may be recorded in Account 1420 — Ancillary Department Supplies.

1401 ***Drugs and Medications***

1402 ***Medical Supplies***

1403 ***Administrative Supplies***

1404 ***Forms***

1405 ***Housekeeping and Maintenance Supplies***

1406 ***Linen Supplies***

1407 ***Other Supplies***

1420 Ancillary Department Supplies

Costs of unused supplies and inventory of goods held for resale that are distinct to an ancillary department that include all items to be sold in a retail setting of the organization. (See Account 7600 — Cost of Goods Sold — Medical Related, for applying expenses of inventory after sales are made.) The type of department may be identified either by using Account 1420 with specific department designated by the responsibility center field or by designating sub-accounts under 1420.

Suggested sub-accounts may be set up for each department as follows if the organization requires more detailed accounts:

1430 - 1439 ***Radiology***

1440 - 1449 ***Laboratory***

1450 - 1459 ***Optical***

1460 - 1469 ***Physical Therapy***

1470 - 1479 ***Other Ancillary***

1500 Prepaid Expenses

Payments for goods or services that will benefit future operations. At the organization's discretion, sub-accounts 1501 - 1509 may be used for additional detail if needed.

1501 ***Prepaid Interest***

1502 ***Prepaid Insurance***

1503 ***Prepaid Rent***

1504 ***Prepaid Taxes***

1505 ***Prepaid Dues3***

1506 ***Other Prepaid Expenses***

1550 Other Current Assets

Current assets not recorded elsewhere.

1600 INVESTMENTS — LONG-TERM RECEIVABLES

Long-term investments in securities, property (not used for operations), and receivables due beyond one year. Assets recorded in these accounts will not be used to finance operations.

1610 Long-Term Receivables

Receivables that will mature beyond one year.

1630 Long-Term Investments

Long-term investments not included in Account 1200 — Marketable Securities and Short-Term Investments.

1635 Valuation Allowance — Long-Term Investments

Adjustments to long-term investments to reflect the unrealized appreciation or depreciation in the fair market value of the investment at the end of the period. At the end of the period, changes in the fair market value of equity and debt securities of a not-for-profit medical organization should be recorded here.

Changes in the fair market value of equity securities and debt securities (that are not intended to be held until maturity) of a for-profit medical organization should be recorded here. The corresponding credit should be recorded in Account 3050 — Allowance for Change in Net Unrealized Gains and Losses on Investments or Account 9140 — Unrealized Gains and Losses — Investments, depending on the classification of the investment and whether the medical organizations that intend to hold debt securities until maturity should record them at amortized cost and not use the valuation allowance accounts.

1640 Investments In Affiliates

Investments in affiliated companies.

1650 Property Held For Future Use

Investments in land, buildings, vehicles and/or equipment not currently used in organizational operations but held for future use.

1700 PROPERTY, FURNITURE, FIXTURES & EQUIPMENT

This account is for noncurrent, tangible assets that generally have a useful life in excess of one year. Assets may be classified as real property under Account 1710 or as furniture, fixtures and equipment under Account 1750. Amortization/ depreciation for these assets are shown in the Account 1800 category.

1710 REAL PROPERTY

1711 Land

Acquisition value or cost of land owned by an organization. If land is purchased, this account includes the purchase price and other costs, such as legal fees and excavation costs, which may be necessary to put the land in condition for its intended use. This account also should include the costs of off-site improvements or assessments, such as charges for sewer and water lines, assessments for paving and sidewalks, and any other land-related expenditures of a nondepreciable nature. Land does not deteriorate with use or with the passage of time; therefore, no depreciation is charged. If land is acquired by gift, this account reflects its appraised value at the time of acquisition.

1712 Land Improvements

All land-related expenditures for organizational operations that are amortized or depreciated to Account 7590 — Depreciation — Occupancy over their useful lives. For example, the cost of on-site sewer and water lines, parking lots, shrubbery, fences and sidewalks may be charged to this account.

1713 Buildings

Acquisition value or cost of buildings plus the cost of any subsequent additions. Architectural, consulting and legal fees applicable to acquisition or construction should be charged to this account.

1714 Capital Leases — Buildings

Initial cost measured by the present value of future lease payments, not in excess of fair market value and excluding all interest, financing charges, maintenance and taxes for building acquired under a capital lease.

A capital lease meets any of the following criteria:

- Lease transfers ownership to lessee during or at the end of the lease term.
- Lease contains a bargain purchase option.
- Lease term (including any bargain renewal options) is 75 percent or more of estimated economic life of property.
- Present value of the minimum lease payments (excluding tax credits and executory costs, for example, maintenance, taxes and insurance) equals 90 percent or more of fair market value of leased property, minus investment tax credit.

The initial cost of a depreciable asset capitalized under a capital lease should be amortized to its residual value over the term of the lease or over the life of the asset if the lease transfers title.

1715 Leasehold Improvements

Costs of any depreciable improvements to leased land or buildings. For financial reporting purposes, depreciation should be charged for the estimated life of the improvement or the remaining term of the lease, whichever is shorter. For tax purposes the estimated life is considered to be 39 years.

1716 Construction in Progress

Costs pertaining to new structures that have not yet been placed in service. At the time the structure is placed in service, its total cost is transferred to the appropriate asset account.

1717 Other Real Property

Real property that does not fit the above categories and that is used in the operations of the organization.

1750 FURNITURE, FIXTURES & EQUIPMENT

Costs of furniture, fixtures and equipment. A common criterion for capitalization is a unit cost of $500 or more, with smaller items expensed in the supplies accounts (under Account 6000 series — Services and General Expense). Each organization should determine rules for the capitalizing or expensing of the costs of furniture, fixtures and equipment. Sub-accounts 1751 - 1790 may be used to further delineate the cost categories.

Other criteria for capitalization are:

- A unit cost sufficiently large to justify the cost of control incident to an equipment or property ledger.
- Depreciable life of two years or more but less than the life of buildings to which the equipment or fixtures may be affixed.
- Used in organizational operations.
- Sufficient individuality and size to make control feasible by means of identification tags or numbers.

In this chart of accounts, equipment acquired under a lease and capitalized as an asset is included with the sub-accounts labeled as capital leases.

1751 Furniture and Fixtures

1752 Capital Leases — Furniture and Fixtures

1753 Equipment

1754 Capital Leases — Equipment

1755 Medical Equipment

1756 Capital Leases — Medical Equipment

1760 Computer

1761 Computer — Hardware

1762 Computer — Software

Software should only be capitalized if it has a useful life in excess of one year. The original acquisition costs or license agreements would be capitalized here. Fees to renew or upgrade software, which represent an annual fee for upgrades or maintenance should be expensed as incurred.

1763 Computer — Other

1770 Capital Leases — Computer

1771 Capital Leases — Computer Hardware

1772 Capital Leases — Computer Software

1773 Capital Leases — Computer — Other

1780 Vehicles

1781 Vehicles

1782 Capital Leases — Vehicles

1790 Ancillary Service Equipment

1791 Laboratory Equipment

1792 Radiology Equipment

1793 Physical Therapy Equipment

1794 Diagnostic Equipment

1795 Capital Leases — Ancillary Service Equipment

1796 Capital Leases — Laboratory Equipment

1797 Capital Leases — Radiology Equipment

1798 Capital Leases — Physical Therapy Equipment

1799 Capital Leases — Diagnostic Equipment

1800 ACCUMULATED DEPRECIATION — PROPERTY, FURNITURE, ETC.

As a general rule, depreciation is used to record the consumption or utilization over time of *tangible* property. Accumulated depreciation is a contra-account to the related fixed asset. Depreciation expense is recorded periodically as a charge against earnings in the statement of operations and the offsetting entry is recorded as accumulated depreciation. This contra-asset account tracks the sum of the accumulated depreciation of Account 1700 - 1799.

1810 ACCUMULATED DEPRECIATION — REAL PROPERTY

Contra-asset accounts used to accumulate the sum of depreciation recorded for real property. (Note that the last two digits of each accumulated depreciation account match the last two digits of the related asset account.)

1812 Accumulated Depreciation — Land Improvements

Accumulation of total depreciation/amortization for Account 1712 — Land Improvements.

1813 Accumulated Depreciation — Buildings

Accumulation of total depreciation for Account 1713 — Buildings.

1814 Accumulated Depreciation — Capital Leases — Buildings

Accumulation of total depreciation for Account 1714 — Capital Leases — Buildings.

1815 Accumulated Depreciation — Leasehold Improvements

Accumulation of total depreciation for Account 1715 — Leasehold Improvements.

1817 Accumulated Depreciation — Other Real Property

Accumulation of total depreciation for Account 1717 — Other Real Property.

1850 ACCUMULATED DEPRECIATION — FURNITURE, FIXTURES & EQUIPMENT

Contra-asset accounts used to accumulate the sum of depreciation recorded for furniture, fixtures and equipment.

1851 Accumulated Depreciation — Furniture and Fixtures

Accumulation of total depreciation for Account 1751 — Furniture and Fixtures.

1852 Accumulated Depreciation — Capital Leases — Furniture and Fixtures

Accumulation of total depreciation for Account 1752 — Capital Leases — Furniture and Fixtures.

1853 Accumulated Depreciation — Equipment

Accumulation of total depreciation for Account 1753 — Equipment.

1854 Accumulated Depreciation — Capital Leases — Equipment

Accumulation of total depreciation for Account 1754 — Capital Leases — Equipment.

1855 Accumulated Depreciation — Medical Equipment

Accumulation of total depreciation for Account 1755 — Medical Equipment.

1856 Accumulated Depreciation — Capital Leases — Medical Equipment

Accumulation of total depreciation for Account 1756 — Capital Leases — Medical Equipment.

1860 Accumulated Depreciation — Computer

Accumulation of total depreciation for Account 1760 — Computer.

1861 Accumulated Depreciation — Computer Hardware

Accumulation of total depreciation for Account 1761 — Computer Hardware.

1862 Accumulated Depreciation — Computer Software

Accumulation of total depreciation for Account 1762 — Computer Software.

1863 Accumulated Depreciation — Other Computer

Accumulation of total depreciation for Account 1763 —- Other Computer.

1870 Accumulated Depreciation — Capital Leases — Computer

Accumulation of total depreciation for Account 1770 — Capital Leases — Computer.

1871 Accumulated Depreciation — Capital Leases — Computer Hardware

Accumulation of total depreciation for Account 1771 — Capital Leases — Computer Hardware.

1872 Accumulated Depreciation — Capital Leases — Computer Software

Accumulation of total depreciation for Account 1772 — Capital Leases — Computer Software.

1873 Accumulated Depreciation — Capital Leases — Other Computer

Accumulation of total depreciation for Account 1773 — Capital Leases — Other Computer.

1880 Accumulated Depreciation — Vehicles

Accumulation of total depreciation for Account 1780 — Vehicles.

1881 Accumulated Depreciation — Vehicles

Accumulation of total depreciation for Account 1781 — Vehicles.

1882 Accumulated Depreciation — Capital Leases Vehicles

Accumulation of total depreciation for Account 1782 — Capital Leases — Vehicles.

1890 Other Accumulated Depreciation — Ancillary Service Equipment

Accumulation of total depreciation for Account 1790 — Ancillary Service Equipment.

1891 Accumulated Depreciation — Laboratory Equipment

Accumulation of total depreciation for Account 1791 — Laboratory Equipment.

1892 Accumulated Depreciation — Radiology Equipment

Accumulation of total depreciation for Account 1792 — Radiology Equipment.

1893 Accumulated Depreciation — Physical Therapy Equipment

Accumulation of total depreciation for Account 1793 — Physical Therapy Equipment.

1894 Accumulated Depreciation — Diagnostic Equipment

Accumulation of total depreciation for Account 1794 — Diagnostic Equipment.

1895 Accumulated Depreciation — Capital Leases — Ancillary Service Equipment

Accumulation of total depreciation for Account 1795 — Capital Leases — Ancillary Service Equipment.

1896 Accumulated Depreciation — Capital Leases — Laboratory Equipment

Accumulation of total depreciation for Account 1796 — Capital Leases — Laboratory Equipment.

1897 Accumulated Depreciation — Capital Leases — Radiology Equipment

Accumulation of total depreciation for Account 1797 — Capital Leases — Radiology Equipment.

1898 Accumulated Depreciation — Capital Leases — Physical Therapy Equipment

Accumulation of total depreciation for Account 1798 — Capital Leases — Physical Therapy Equipment.

1899 Accumulated Depreciation — Capital Leases — Diagnostic Equipment

Accumulation of total depreciation for Account 1799 — Capital Leases — Diagnostic Equipment.

1900 INTANGIBLE AND OTHER ASSETS

Costs of property rights without physical substance that will benefit future operations of the organization. Intangible assets are purchased from external sources, provide future benefit and are relatively long-lived. Other assets include long-term prepayments, deferred charges and assets not included in other categories.

1910 Organization Costs

Costs incurred in the original incorporation and start up of a business operation. These costs are generally amortized over a period of five years.

1915 Accumulated Amortization — Organization Costs

As a general rule, amortization is used to record the consumption or utilization over time of ***intangible*** property. Accumulated amortization is a contra-account to the related intangible asset. Amortization expense is recorded periodically as a charge against earnings in the statement of operations and the offsetting entry is recorded as accumulated amortization. This contra-asset account tracks the sum of the accumulated amortization of Account 1910.

1920 Goodwill

Excess of costs over the fair market value of identifiable assets in the purchase of an entire organization.

1925 Accumulated Amortization — Goodwill

This contra-asset account tracks the sum of the accumulated amortization of Account 1920. These costs are generally amortized over a period not to exceed 40 years. For tax purposes the period of amortization might be considered to be no less than 15 years.

1930 Other Intangible Assets

Intangible assets not recorded elsewhere.

1940 Deposits

Costs incurred for amounts paid as a down payment on a purchase or contract such as on real estate/office leases, deposits for utility services and advances for the purchase of furniture and equipment. This account is not intended to be used for bank or cash deposits.

1950 Noncurrent Expenses Paid In Advance

Costs incurred (payments) for goods or services that will benefit future operations (beyond a year). Sub-accounts could be set up to reflect, for instance, the following categories:

1951 Noncurrent Interest Paid in Advance

1952 Noncurrent Insurance Paid in Advance

1953 Noncurrent Rent Paid in Advance

1954 Noncurrent Taxes Paid in Advance

1955 Noncurrent Dues Paid in Advance

1956 Other Noncurrent Expenses Paid in Advance

1960 Other Assets

Costs incurred and not classified above that would have an anticipated life in excess of one year.

1961 Cash Surrender Value of Life Insurance Policies

Amounts that recognize the accumulated build-up in value inside a life insurance policy that could be used for loan purposes and/or that would be available upon the termination of a policy.

EXHIBIT 3.1

Account Number	Description
1000	**ASSETS**
1100	Cash
1110	Cash — Banks
1111	General Checking Accounts
1112	Payroll Checking Accounts
1113	Other Checking Accounts
1120	Cash — On hand
1121	Change Fund
1122	Petty Cash
1130	Cash — Restricted
1200	Marketable Securities & Short-Term Investments
1210	Valuation Allowance — Short-Term Investments
1300	Accounts Receivable
1301	Accounts Receivable — Fee-for-Service Amounts
1302	Accounts Receivable — Prepaid Contracts
1320	Allowance for Estimated uncollectable Receivables
1321	Allowance for Bad Debts — Patient Accounts
1322	Allowance for Contractual Adjustments
1323	Allowance for Bad Debts — Third-Party Payers
1324	Allowance for Charity Care
1340	Notes Receivable — Short Term
1345	Managed Care Contract — Bonus/Withhold
1350	Other Short-Term Receivables
1351	Interest Receivables
1352	Intercompany Receivables
1353	Due from Employees
1354	Due from Related Parties
1400	Supply Inventories
1401	Drugs and Medications
1402	Medical Supplies
1403	Administrative Supplies
1404	Forms
1405	Housekeeping and Maintenance Supplies
1406	Linen Supplies
1407	Other Supplies
1420	Ancillary Department Supplies
1500	Prepaid Expenses
1501	Prepaid Interest
1502	Prepaid Insurance
1503	Prepaid Rent
1504	Prepaid Taxes
1505	Prepaid Dues
1506	Other Prepaid Expenses
1550	Other Current Assets
1600	**INVESTMENTS — LONG-TERM RECEIVABLES**
1610	Long-Term Receivables
1630	Long-Term Investments
1635	Valuation Allowance — Long-Term Investments
1640	Investments in Affiliates
1650	Property Held for Future Use
1700	**PROPERTY, FURNITURE, FIXTURES & EQUIPMENT**
1710	REAL PROPERTY
1711	Land
1712	Land Improvements
1713	Buildings
1714	Capital Leases — Buildings

Exhibit 3.1 continued

Account Number	Description
1715	Leasehold Improvements
1716	Construction in Progress
1717	Other Real Property
1750	FURNITURE, FIXTURES & EQUIPMENT
1751	Furniture and Fixtures
1752	Capital Leases — Furniture and Fixtures
1753	Equipment
1754	Capital Leases — Equipment
1755	Medical Equipment
1756	Capital Leases — Medical Equipment
1760	Computer
1761	Computer — Hardware
1762	Computer — Software
1763	Computer — Other
1770	Capital Leases — Computer
1771	Capital Leases — Computer — Hardware
1772	Capital Leases — Computer — Software
1773	Capital Leases — Computer — Other
1780	Vehicles
1781	Vehicles
1782	Capital Leases — Vehicles
1790	Ancillary Service Equipment
1791	Laboratory Equipment
1792	Radiology Equipment
1793	Physical Therapy Equipment
1794	Diagnostic Equipment
1795	Capital Leases — Ancillary Service Equipment
1796	Capital Leases — Laboratory Equipment
1797	Capital Leases — Radiology Equipment
1798	Capital Leases — Physical Therapy Equipment
1799	Capital Leases — Diagnostic Equipment
1800	**ACCUMULATED DEPRECIATION — PROPERTY, FURNITURE, ETC.**
1810	ACCUMULATED DEPRECIATION — REAL PROPERTY
1812	Accum Depreciation —Land Improvements
1813	Accum Depreciation — Buildings
1814	Accum Depreciation — Capital Leases — Buildings
1815	Accum Depreciation — Leasehold Improvements
1817	Accum Depreciation — Other Real Property
1850	ACCUM DEPRECIATION — FURNITURE, FIXTURES & EQUIPMENT
1851	Accum Depreciation — Furniture and Fixtures
1852	Accum Depreciation — Capital Leases — Furniture and Fixtures
1853	Accum Depreciation — Equipment
1854	Accum Depreciation — Capital Leases — Equipment
1855	Accum Depreciation — Medical Equipment
1856	Accum Depreciation — Capital Leases — Medical Equipment
1860	Accum Depreciation — Computer
1861	Accum Depreciation — Computer — Hardware
1862	Accum Depreciation — Computer — Software
1863	Accum Depreciation — Computer — Other
1870	Accum Depreciation — Capital Leases — Computer
1871	Accum Depreciation — Capital Leases — Computer Hardware
1872	Accum Depreciation — Capital Leases — Computer — Other
1880	Accum Depreciation — Vehicles
1881	Accum Depreciation — Vehicles
1882	Accum Depreciation — Capital Leases — Vehicles
1890	Other Accum Depreciation — Ancillary Service Equipment
1891	Accum Depreciation — Laboratory Equipment
1892	Accum Depreciation — Radiology Equipment

Exhibit 3.1 continued

Account Number	Description
1893	Accum Depreciation — Physical Therapy Equipment
1894	Accum Depreciation — Diagnostic Equipment
1895	Accum Depreciation — Capital Leases — Ancillary Service Equipment
1896	Accum Depreciation — Capital Leases — Laboratory Equipment
1897	Accum Depreciation — Capital Leases — Radiology Equipment
1898	Accum Depreciation — Capital Leases — Physical Therapy Equip.
1899	Accum Depreciation — Capital Leases — Diagnostic Equipment
1900	INTANGIBLE AND OTHER ASSETS
1910	Organization Costs
1915	Accumulated Amortization — Organization Costs
1920	Goodwill
1925	Accumulated Amortization — Goodwill
1930	Other Intangible Assets
1940	Deposits
1950	Noncurrent Expenses Paid in Advance
1951	Noncurrent Interest Paid in Advance
1952	Noncurrent Insurance Paid in Advance
1953	Noncurrent Rent Paid in Advance
1954	Noncurrent Taxes Paid in Advance
1955	Noncurrent Dues Paid in Advance
1956	Other Noncurrent Expenses Paid in Advance
1960	Other Assets
1961	Cash Surrender Value of Life Insurance Policies

2000 LIABILITIES

Liabilities are debts or obligations owed by the organization to creditors. These debts arise as a result of the purchase of goods and services from others on credit and through cash borrowings to finance business operations. Liabilities are also obligations of responsibility to transfer other assets or provide services to another entity.

2100 CURRENT LIABILITIES — PAYABLES

Liabilities that mature and require payment from current assets or through the creation of other liabilities within one year.

2110 Accounts Payable

Amounts on an open account owed by the organization to outside persons or entities for goods and services received by the organization. These accounts are usually control accounts for individual accounts payable balances that may be contained in a subsidiary ledger.

2120 Bank Overdrafts Payable

Overdrafts on bank accounts having no other free balances in amounts sufficient to offset.

2130 Other Current Liabilities Payable

2131 Intercompany Accounts Payable

Amounts owed by the organization to other entities consolidated for financial reporting purposes.

2132 Accounts Payable — Employees

Amounts owed to the organization by its employees.

2133 Accounts Payable — Related Parties

Amounts owed to the organization by related parties including entities under common ownership or control.

2134 Accounts Payable — Other

Other current liabilities payable not recorded elsewhere.

2160 Contract Claims Payable

This account is related to Account 2360 — Claims Payable Incurred But Not Reported. Once determined or invoiced, the contract claims from Account 2360 should be transferred to this account. Contract Claims Payable records amounts owed by the organization to providers outside the organization for medical services to patients assigned to the organization. At the organization's discretion, sub-accounts 2161 - 2169 may be used to record contract claims by an individual entity as contra-accounts to 2361 - 2369.

2200 CURRENT LIABILITIES — PAYROLL

Liabilities related to payroll and/or for amounts withheld from employees or otherwise accrued.

2210 Payroll Tax Withholdings Payable

Actual liabilities for Payroll Tax Withholdings. These accounts are credited for amounts withheld from employees and are debited when payment is made to the appropriate agency, authority or plan. At the organization's discretion, sub-accounts 2211 - 2216 may be used to record individual categories of withholdings payable.

2211 Federal Income Tax Withholdings Payable

2212 State Income Tax Withholdings Payable

2213 FICA/Medicare Tax Withholdings Payable

2214 Local Tax Withholdings Payable

2215 Other Tax Withholdings Payable

Other Tax Withholdings Payable not recorded elsewhere, such as income tax garnishments on employees or taxes imposed by other taxing authorities.

2220 Insurance Withholdings Payable

2221 Health Insurance Withholdings Payable

2222 Life Insurance Withholdings Payable

2223 State Disability Insurance Withholdings Payable

2224 Other Insurance Withholdings Payable

2230 Other Payroll Withholdings Payable

2231 401(k)Withholdings Payable

2232 Cafeteria Plan Withholdings Payable

2233 Court Mandated Child Support Withholdings Payable

2234 Other Payroll Withholdings Payable

Other Payroll Withholdings Payable not recorded elsewhere, such as charitable organizations, savings program, union dues, parking fees, employee social clubs and other payroll withholdings.

2250 Accrued Payroll Liabilities

Actual or estimated liabilities for payroll obligations. These accounts are credited when the payroll expense is incurred and are debited when payment is made to the appropriate employee, agency or authority. At the organization's discretion, sub-accounts 2251 - 2257 may be used to record individual categories of accrued payroll liabilities.

2251 ***Accrued Payroll***

2252 ***Accrued Vacation, Holiday, & Sick Pay (Compensated Absences)***

2253 ***Accrued FICA/Medicare Taxes Payable***

2254 ***Accrued State Unemployment Taxes Payable***

2255 ***Accrued Federal Unemployment Taxes Payable***

2256 ***Accrued Retirement Plan Contribution***

2257 ***Other Accrued Payroll Liabilities***

2260 Other Payroll Liabilities

2300 CURRENT LIABILITIES — OTHER

Current liabilities not included in Accounts 2100 - 2200.

2310 Accrued Liabilities — Nonpayroll

Current liabilities accrued at the end of an accounting period to reflect the proper amount of expenses for the organization under the accrual basis of accounting. Generally, no invoices or other billings are received within the accounting period, and the liability for these items is estimated or obtained from other sources.

2311 ***Accrued Rent***

2312 ***Accrued Interest***

2313 ***Accrued Insurance***

2314 ***Accrued Income Taxes (Federal/State)***

2315 ***Accrued Property Taxes***

2316 ***Accrued Franchise Taxes***

2317 ***Other Accrued Liabilities***

2320 Notes and Loans Payable

2321 ***Current Notes and Loans Payable — Vendors***

2322 ***Current Notes and Loans Payable — Employees***

2323 ***Current Notes and Loans Payable — Stockholders/Partners***

2324 ***Current Other Notes and Loans Payable***

2325 ***Bank Working Capital Line Outstanding***

2330 Long-Term Debt — Current Portion

2331 Capital Lease Obligation — Current Portion

2332 Construction Contracts Payable

2333 Other Loans Payable — Current Portion

2340 Advances From Settlements Due To Third-Party Agencies

Amounts owed to third-party agencies for current financing and other advances that are due and payable within one year. At the organization's discretion, sub-accounts 2341 - 2344 may be used to record amounts owed to individual third-party agencies. Sub-accounts 2345 - 2349 may be used to record amounts owed to third-party agencies arising from reimbursement settlements.

An example of a settlement due to a third-party agency would include amounts owed Medicare or Medicaid resulting from overpayments because of inaccurate claims.

2350 Patient Deposits

Amounts paid by patients in advance of specific services such as OB/GYN pre-delivery payments or plastic surgery deposits. This account is not to be used for payments received under a capitation plan.

2360 Claims Payable Incurred But Not Reported

Incurred But Not Reported (IBNR) is also referred to as IBNP (which tracks claims "received but not paid"). This is used as a liability account to record an estimation of the amounts owed to providers outside the organization for medical services to prepaid patients of the organization for which invoices have not been received. These are normally estimated using historical lag factors. When invoiced, the claims should be transferred to Account 2160 — Contract Claims Payable. Some consideration should also be given to setting up a revenue reserve account to accumulate funds to pay IBNR.

2361 Incurred But Not Reported Claims — Commercial

Account used to record the organization's liability for unpaid referral care provided to prepaid patients for whom the organization receives capitation payments under commercial contracts. Alternatively, accounts 2361 - 2369 can be used to categorized IBNR claims by type of claim (professional, inpatient, ancillary service) or by contract depending upon the entity's tracking and reporting needs.

2362 Incurred But Not Reported Claims — Medicare

Account used to record the organization's liability for unpaid referral care provided to prepaid patients for whom the organization receives capitation payments under Medicare contracts.

2363 Incurred But Not Reported Claims — Medicaid

Account used to record the organization's liability for unpaid referral care provided to prepaid patients for whom the organization receives capitation payments under Medicaid contracts.

2365 Other Claims Incurred But Not Reported

Other accrued claims not reported elsewhere.

2370 Deferred Revenue

Revenue received in one period applicable to services to be rendered at some future time.

2371 Deferred Revenue — Fee-for-Service

An account used only with cash basis accounting to convert accounts receivable (Accounts 1300 - 1302) from accrual basis to cash basis. This account may be used in lieu of Account 4800 — Provision for Cash Basis Conversion.

2372 Deferred Revenue — Capitated or Prepaid Plan

Revenue received in one period from capitated or prepaid plans applicable to services to be rendered in some future period.

2375 Other Deferred Revenue

Revenue received in one period that is applicable to services to be rendered in some future period. Any deferred revenue that is not earned within one year is treated as a long-term liability.

2380 Deferred Income Taxes — Current Portion

Timing difference between tax on income reported in financial statements and tax on income reported in the tax return, when the timing difference is related to a current asset.

2390 Other Current Liabilities

Current liabilities not recorded elsewhere. This account may include possible contingent liabilities (such as from a lawsuit).

2400 LONG-TERM LIABILITIES

Liabilities that will mature and require payment at some future date beyond one year.

2410 Long-Term Notes Payable

Notes payable that mature more than one year from financial statement date. The current portion of any long-term liability should be included in Account 2330 — Long-Term Debt — Current Portion, except those obligations to be refinanced or paid from a sinking fund. A sinking fund is an actual depository account established to liquidate a specific liability.

2420 Construction Loans

Loans during construction stages that mature more than one year from financial statement date.

2430 Capital Lease Obligation — Long-Term Portion

Present value of future lease payments, excluding interest and finance charges, that will be made beyond one year on leases that have been capitalized. Refer to Account 1714 — Capital Leases — Buildings for capitalization criteria.

2440 Other Loans Payable — Long-Term Portion

Other long-term loans payable, including the mortgage payable. The current portion of mortgage payable should be entered under Account 2333 — Other Loans Payable — Current Portion.

2450 Deferred Third-Party Revenue

Timing differences or difference in accounting methods between financial statements and third-party reimbursement accounting methods.

At the organization's discretion, sub-accounts that may be set up include:

2451 ***Deferred Third-Party Revenue — Medicare***

2452 ***Deferred Third-Party Revenue — Medicaid***

2453 ***Deferred Third-Party Revenue — Other***

2460 Deferred Compensation

Liability for compensation to physicians and employees whose payment is being deferred until some future date.

2465 Severance Plan

Liability for severance plans to physicians and employees whose payment is being deferred until some future date.

2470 Deferred Income Taxes — Long-Term Portion

Timing difference between tax on income reported in financial statements and tax on income reported in the tax return, when the timing difference is related to a noncurrent asset.

2480 Other Long-Term Liabilities

Liabilities that will mature beyond one year and are not included above.

EXHIBIT 3.2

Account Number	Description
2000	**LIABILITIES**
2100	CURRENT LIABILITIES — PAYABLE
2110	Accounts Payable
2120	Bank Overdrafts Payable
2130	Other Current Liabilities Payable
2131	Intercompany Accounts Payable
2132	Accounts Payable — Employees
2133	Accounts Payable — Related Parties
2134	Accounts Payable — Other
2160	Contract Claims Payable
2200	CURRENT LIABILITIES — PAYROLL
2210	Payroll Tax Withholdings Payable
2211	Federal Income Tax Withholdings Payable
2212	State Income Tax Withholdings Payable
2213	FICA/Medicare Tax Withholdings Payable
2214	Local Tax Withholdings Payable
2215	Other Tax Withholdings Payable
2220	Insurance Withholdings Payable
2221	Health Insurance Withholdings Payable
2222	Life Insurance Withholdings Payable
2223	State Disability Insurance Withholdings Payable
2224	Other Insurance Withholdings Payable
2230	Other Payroll Withholdings Payable
2231	401(k) Withholdings Payable
2232	Cafeteria Plan Withholdings Payable
2233	Court Mandated Child Support Withholdings Payable
2234	Other Payroll Withholdings Payable
2250	Accrued Payroll Liabilities
2251	Accrued Payroll
2252	Accrued Vacation, Holiday, & Sick Pay (Compensated Absences)
2253	Accrued FICA/Medicare Taxes Payable
2254	Accrued State Unemployment Taxes Payable
2255	Accrued Federal Unemployment Taxes Payable
2256	Accrued Retirement Plan Contribution
2257	Other Accrued Payroll Liabilities
2260	Other Payroll Liabilities
2300	CURRENT LIABILTIES — OTHER
2310	Accrued Liabilities — Nonpayroll
2311	Accrued Rent
2312	Accrued Interest
2313	Accrued Insurance
2314	Accrued Income Taxes (Federal/State)
2315	Accrued Property Taxes
2316	Accrued Franchise Taxes
2317	Other Accrued Liabilities
2320	Notes and Loans Payable
2321	Current Notes and Loans Payable — Vendors
2322	Current Notes and Loans Payable — Employees
2323	Current Notes and Loans Payable — Stockholders/Partners
2324	Current Other Notes and Loans Payable
2325	Bank Working Capital Line Outstanding
2330	Long-Term Debt — Current Portion
2331	Capital Lease Obligation — Current Portion
2332	Construction Contracts Payable
2333	Other Loans Payable — Current Portion
2340	Advances from Settlements Due to Third-Party Agencies

Exhibit 3.2 continued	
Account Number	Description
2350	Patient Deposits
2360	Claims Payable Incurred But Not Reported
2361	Incurred But Not Reported Claims — Commercial
2362	Incurred But Not Reported Claims — Medicare
2363	Incurred But Not Reported Claims — Medicaid
2365	Other Claims Incurred But Not Reported
2370	Deferred Revenue
2371	Deferred Revenue — Fee-for-Service
2372	Deferred Revenue — Capitated or Prepaid Plan
2375	Other Deferred Revenue
2380	Deferred Income Taxes — Current Portion
2390	Other Current Liabilities
2400	LONG-TERM LIABILITIES
2410	Long-Term Notes Payable
2420	Construction Loans
2430	Capital Lease Obligation — Long-Term Portion
2440	Other Loans Payable — Long-Term Portion
2450	Deferred Third-Party Revenue
2451	Deferred Third-Party Revenue — Medicare
2452	Deferred Third-Party Revenue — Medicaid
2453	Deferred Third-Party Revenue — Other
2460	Deferred Compensation
2465	Severance Plan
2470	Deferred Income Taxes — Long-Term Portion
2480	Other Long-Term Liabilities

3000 — OWNERS' EQUITY ACCOUNTS

Owners' equity is a residual interest or claim of the owners to the assets after creditor claims are settled. (Legally, creditors are first in line to receive reimbursement.) Owners' equity derives from two sources:

- Contributed Capital, which is the investment of cash or other assets by the owner or owners
- Retained earnings, the accumulative results of income, less losses and withdrawals over the years

The 3000 series of accounts are to be used regardless of the type of entity for which this chart of accounts is being used. Different accounts are designated below based on the following entity types:

- General Partnership
- Corporation
- Not-For-Profit Organization
- Limited Liability Entity (Corporation or Partnership)

3000 PARTNERS' EQUITY (PARTNERSHIP)

Net assets of the partnership; that is, the excess of the partnership entity's assets over its liabilities. The balances in these accounts are the cumulative results of the partners' investments, earnings and losses, and withdrawals.

A partnership is a legal entity where two or more individuals have agreed that they will share profits and losses and assets and liabilities, although not necessarily on an equal basis. The partnership agreement is typically formalized in writing.

3010 Contributed Capital (Each Partner)

Amounts invested by the partners. Sub-accounts should be established for each partner.

3020 Undistributed Earnings

Difference between revenues and expenses allocated to the partners as earned capital. This account tracks the prior year's net earnings/losses. Sub-accounts should be established for each partner. This account may be combined for financial reporting purposes into Account 3010 — Contributed Capital at the end of the period.

3030 Partners' Drawing Accounts (Each Partner)

Withdrawals made by a partner during an operating period, typically one year. This account is closed at year-end into Account 3020 — Undistributed Earnings.

3031 Cash Distributions

3032 Estimated Tax Payments

Partnership payment of partner's estimated tax payments treated as distributions.

3033 Health Insurance Premiums

Partnership payment of partner's health insurance premiums treated as distributions.

3034 Other Payments Treated as Partner Distributions

3035 Property Distributions

3040 Current Income/Loss

This account tracks the current year's net earnings/losses. The account is closed out at year-end into Account 3020 — Undistributed Earnings.

EXHIBIT 3.3

Account Number	Description
3000	**PARTNERS' EQUITY (PARTNERSHIP)**
3010	Contributed Capital (Each Partner)
3020	Undistributed Earnings
3030	Partners' Drawing Accounts (Each Partner)
3031	Cash Distributions
3032	Estimated Tax Payments
3033	Health Insurance Premiums
3034	Other Payments Treated as Partner Distributions
3035	Property Distributions
3040	Current Income/Loss

3000 STOCKHOLDERS' EQUITY (CORPORATION)

Net assets of the corporation; that is, the excess of the corporate entity's assets over its liabilities. The balances in these accounts are the cumulative result of the owners' investments and the equity originating from net earnings retained by the corporation.

A for-profit organization recognized by law as a business entity separate and distinct from its shareholders. A *business* corporation is a legal entity whose shareholders need ***not*** be licensed to practice the profession practiced by the corporation.

A *professional* corporation is a legal entity whose shareholders must typically all be licensed to practice in the same profession as that practiced by the organization.

A medical practice organized as a corporation can either be an 'C' corporation or an 'S' corporation as designated by the Internal Revenue Code. The primary difference between these two types of entities as it impacts the owners' equity section of accounts is the way in which distributions and certain expenses are categorized.

3010 Preferred Stock

Preferred stock is a type of stock whose holders are given certain priority over common stockholders in the payment of dividends and liquidation/termination of the entity. Usually the dividend rate is fixed at the time of stock issue.

3020 Common Stock

Common stock is a type of stock whereby equity claims are held by the "residual owners" of the organization who are the last to receive any distribution of earning or assets. It represents the stated or par value of stock issued to owners.

3030 Capital Contributed In Excess Of Par

This is capital contributed by owners in excess of the par or stated value of the capital stock.

3040 Donated Capital

This refers to assets contributed to the corporation that increase owners' equity.

3050 Allowance For Change In Net Unrealized Gains/Losses On Investments

For-profit medical organizations should record changes in fair market value of investments that are classified as "available for sale" in this account. The corresponding credit is Account 1210 — Valuation Allowance — Short-Term Investments or Account 1635 — Valuation Allowance — Long-Term Investments.

3060 Dividends And Distributions

'C' Corporations

Distribution to owners of retained earnings paid in cash, shares of stock or property. This account is closed into Account 3070 — Retained Earnings — Unappropriated at the end of the fiscal year.

'S' Corporations

Distributions to owners of accumulated retained earnings paid in cash, shares of stock or property. Expenses that are not deductible by an 'S' corporation are also charged against this account. This would include payments for shareholder's health and life insurance premiums. This account is closed into Account 3070 — Retained Earnings — Unappropriated at the end of the fiscal year.

3061 Cash Distributions

3062 Estimated Tax Payments

Payment of shareholder's estimated tax payments treated as distributions.

3063 Health Insurance Premiums

Payment of shareholder's health insurance premiums treated as distributions.

3064 Other Payments Treated as Shareholder Distributions

3065 Property Distributions

3070 Retained Earnings — Unappropriated

Net income (or loss) over the life of the corporation minus all distributions to owners and appropriations of retained earnings carried in Account 3075. This account is referred to as the Accumulated Adjustments Account for an 'S' corporation.

3075 Retained Earnings — Appropriated

Restrictions placed on portions of earnings retained in the corporation. These restrictions may temporarily limit the amount of dividends available for distribution to owners. This account should be used to record creation of unfunded reserves required by state HMO laws or regulations.

3080 Current Income/Loss

This account tracks the current year's net earnings/losses. The account is closed out at fiscal year end into Account 3070 — Retained Earnings — Unappropriated.

3090 Treasury Stock

Capital stock repurchased by the corporation that has not been retired. Treasury stock is usually carried at acquisition cost.

EXHIBIT 3.4

Account Number	Description
3000	**STOCKHOLDERS' EQUITY (CORPORATION)**
3010	Preferred Stock
3020	Common Stock
3030	Capital Contributed in Excess of Par
3040	Donated Capital
3050	Allowance for Change in Net Unrealized Gains/Losses on Investments
3060	Dividends and Distributions
3061	Cash Distributions
3062	Estimated Tax Payments
3063	Health Insurance Premiums
3064	Other Payments Treated as Partner Distributions
3065	Property Distributions
3070	Retained Earnings — Unappropriated
3075	Retained Earnings — Appropriated
3080	Current Income/Loss
3090	Treasury Stock

3000 NET ASSETS (NOT-FOR-PROFIT EQUITY)

Excess of the not-for-profit entity's assets over its liabilities. The balances in these accounts are the cumulative results of original investments, grants, gifts, donations, revenues and expenditures.

A not-for-profit organization is a legal entity that has obtained special exemption under Section 501(c) of the Internal Revenue Service code that qualifies the organization to be exempt from federal income taxes. To qualify as a tax-exempt organization, an entity, practice or faculty practice plan would have to provide advance evidence of a planned charitable, educational or research purpose.

3010 Unrestricted Net Assets

Unrestricted equity of the non-for-profit entity. Equity resulting from incurring revenues for providing or agreeing to provide health care services, receiving unrestricted contributions and/or grants, or receiving dividend or interest from investing in income-producing assets. Expenses incurred in providing or agreeing to provide health care services, providing other community benefits and performing administrative functions are deducted from this category.

Further breakdown of this account can be facilitated by the use of Accounts 3011 - 3029. Net assets that have external limits resulting from contractual agreements with suppliers, creditors and others, such as, unfunded reserves required by state HMO laws or regulations, or internal limits such as appropriations of unrestricted fund balance created by board of directors' actions should be credited to these accounts.

3030 Temporarily Restricted Net Assets

Temporarily restricted net assets are those donor-restricted net assets that can be used by the medical organization for their specified purpose once the donor's restriction is met. Generally, these restrictions are met either by the passage of time or by actions taken by the entity, such as the use of funds for the purpose intended.

A further detailed breakdown of this account can be facilitated by the use of 3031 - 3039 for other descriptions at the users' discretion. Temporarily restricted net assets can be further classified into distinct groups that distinguish the nature or purpose of the donor's restriction using these accounts.

3040 Permanently Restricted Net Assets

Permanently restricted net assets are those net assets with donor restrictions that do not expire with the passage of time and cannot be removed by any actions taken by the medical organization. Endowment funds, for example, fit into this category.

A further detailed breakdown of this account can be facilitated by the use of 3041 - 3049 for other descriptions at the users' discretion. Permanently restricted net assets can be further classified into distinct groups that distinguish the nature or purpose of the donor's restrictions using these accounts.

3050 Current Surplus/Deficit

This account tracks the excess of revenues and other inflows over expenses and other outflows (Surplus) or the excess of expenses and other outflows over revenues and other inflows (Deficit) for the current year. The account is closed out at year-end into Account 3010 — Unrestricted Net Assets.

EXHIBIT 3.5

Account Number	Description
3000	**NET ASSETS (NOT-FOR-PROFIT EQUITY)**
3010	Unrestricted Net Assets
3030	Temporarily Restricted Net Assets
3040	Permanently Restricted Net Assets
3050	Current Surplus/Deficit

3000 LIMITED LIABILITY COMPANY/PARTNERSHIP

A legal entity that is a hybrid between a corporation and a partnership. It provides limited liability to owners like a corporation while it passes profits and losses through to owners like a partnership.

3010 Members' Capital/Limited Partners' Interest

Amounts invested by the members. Sub-accounts should be established for each member.

3020 Members' Distributions/Limited Partners' Distributions

Withdrawals made by a member during an operating period, typically one year. This account is closed at year-end into Account 3010 — Members' Capital/ Limited Partners' Interest.

3021 Cash Distributions

3022 Estimated Tax Payments

Partnership payment of partner's estimated tax payments treated as distributions.

3023 Health Insurance Premiums

Partnership payment of partner's health insurance premiums treated as distributions.

3024 Other Payments Treated as Partner Distributions

3030 Current Income/Loss

This account tracks the current year's net earnings/losses. The account is closed out at year-end into Account 3010 — Members' Capital/ Limited Partners' Interest.

EXHIBIT 3.6

Account number	Description
3000	**LIMITED LIABILITY COMPANY/PARTNERSHIP**
3010	Members' Capital/Limited Partners' Interest
3020	Members' Distributions/Limited Partners' Distributions
3021	Cash Distributions
3022	Estimated Tax Payments
3023	Health Insurance Premiums
3024	Other Payments Treated as Partner Distributions
3030	Current Income/Loss

4

Income Statement Account Descriptions

Kathryn P. Glass, M.B.A., M.S.H.A.

Income Statement

The income statement is used to summarize results of business operations for a period of time, not longer than one year, to determine if the organization is operating efficiently. It is a measure of the results of operations representing the difference between revenue and expense for the reported period.

4000 REVENUES

Revenues are inflows of cash and other items of value received or to be received for services rendered. There are different measures of these inflows of cash for Fee-for-Service (FFS) revenues, depending upon whether the organization identifies gross charges, adjustments and allowances; whether the organization uses the cash, modified cash or accrual basis of accounting; and whether an HMO or PPO (Preferred Provider Organization) pays discounted FFS or capitation.

4100 Gross Charges

Accounts 4110 - 4140 are used by organizations recording charges on an accrual basis of accounting. Accounts 4200 - 4269 are used by organizations recording revenues on a cash basis of accounting. Account 4150 (Other Revenue) can be used with either accrual- or cash-basis accounting.

4110 Gross Charges — Fee-For-Service (FFS)

Full dollar value, at the organization's established undiscounted rates, of services provided to FFS patients. Gross charges for services provided to patients covered by managed care and/or prepaid/capitation plans are not included in this account, but rather are included in Account 4120 — Gross Charges — Discounted FFS Contracts or Account 4130 — Gross Charges — FFS Equivalents for Capitation Plan Patients.

Established usual and customary rates are the full price for services before charge restrictions imposed by Medicare or contractual adjustments required by third-party payers, such as commercial insurance carriers or other adjustments. Services to include all medical/surgical services provided by physicians and midlevel providers, as well as professional and technical components of ancillary services, such as radiology and laboratory. If Account 4110 is used, Account 4510 will adjust gross charges to reflect appropriate discounts.

At the organization's discretion, sub-accounts 4111 - 4119 may be used for specific plans, departments and other descriptions.

4120 Gross Charges — Discounted FFS Contracts

Full dollar value, at the organization's established undiscounted rates of all services provided to patients belonging to an HMO or PPO or similar entity that reimburses on a FFS or discounted FFS basis.

Services to include all medical/surgical services provided by physicians and midlevel providers, as well as professional and technical components of ancillary services, such as radiology and laboratory. If Account 4120 is used, Account 4520 will adjust gross charges to reflect appropriate discounts.

The fourth digit may be used to identify the gross charges for a specific HMO, PPO or employer contract. For example, sub-accounts 4121 - 4129 could designate specific payers and sub-accounts 4521 - 4529 could adjust the gross charges to reflect appropriate discounts for each designated account.

4130 Gross Charges — FFS Equivalents For Capitation—Plan Patients

Previous editions of this chart of accounts labeled this account "Gross Payments — Prepaid/Capitation." Gross charges under capitation contracts for assigned enrollees under a patient care contract would be recorded in this account. The 4200 series of accounts should be used to reflect revenues collected on bonuses and risk-pool allocations.

If Account 4130 is used, Account 4530 — Gross Charges — FFS Equivalents for Capitation Plan Patients/Adjustment will adjust gross charges to reflect appropriate adjustments received on contract.

4140 Other Gross Charges (Revenue)

All nonmedical revenues recorded on the accrual basis, such as grant payments, research stipends, honoraria, government support payments, educational subsidies and gross revenue from the sale of products such as pharmaceuticals, hearing aids, optical lenses, orthopedic supplies, medical supplies, etc. If Account 4140 is used, Account 4540 — Other Gross Charges/Adjustment will adjust gross charges to reflect appropriate discounts.

Gross revenue from nonmedical business interests (parking lots, rental property, leased equipment, etc.) should be recorded under Account 9100 (Nonoperating Revenues).

At the organization's discretion, sub-accounts 4141 - 4149 may be used for specific plans, departments, retail operations categories and other descriptions. These accounts will have a corresponding discount/adjustment account using Accounts 4541 - 4549.

4150 Other Revenue

Other revenue that does not fit the specific income categories.

4200 Fees Collected

This account should be used by organizations recording revenues on a cash basis. Fees classified by payer type may be recorded in sub-accounts 4210 - 4289. Account 4200 is the roll-up account for the total fees collected using cash-basis accounting.

4210 Fees Collected — FFS

This account should be used by organizations recording revenues on a cash basis. The actual net payment for all current charges and receivables should be recognized at the time they are received. This eliminates the need for adjustment accounts for any type of discount. Refunds should be recorded in Account 4300 —Patient Refunds. If Account 4200 is used, Accounts 4500 - 4630 and related adjustments and allowances are ***not*** used.

At the organization's discretion, sub-accounts 4211 - 4219 may be used for specific plans and other descriptions.

4220 Fees Collected — FFS For Managed Care

This account should be used by organizations recording revenues on a cash basis. The net payment received from managed-care organizations (such as HMOs, PHOs [Physician Hospital Organizations] and PPOs) should be recognized at the time they are received. This eliminates the need for adjustment accounts for any type of discount. Refunds should be recorded in Account 4300 — Patient Refunds. If Account 4220 is used, Accounts 4500 - 4630 and related adjustments and allowances are ***not*** used.

At the organization's discretion, sub-accounts 4221 - 4229 may be used for specific plans and other descriptions.

4230 Capitated Premium Revenues — Commercial

This account should be used by organizations recording revenues on a cash basis. Net revenue actually collected from capitation payments, risk-sharing revenues and other revenues paid to the organization by an HMO for assigned enrollees under a patient-care contract. This account also should be used to record copayments from HMO enrollees, coordination of benefits income and other revenues associated with a prepaid/capitation contract plan. It may also include global package arrangements such as transplant package price, CABG (Coronary Artery Bypass Graph) package price, etc.

Refunds should be recorded in Account 4300 —Patient Refunds. If Account 4230 is used, Accounts 4500 - 4630 and related adjustments and allowances are ***not*** used.

At the organization's discretion, sub-accounts 4231 - 4239 may be used for specific plans and other descriptions.

4240 Capitated Premium Revenues — Medicare

This account should be used by organizations recording revenues on a cash basis. Net revenue actually collected from capitation payments, risk-sharing revenues and other revenues paid to the organization by an HMO for assigned enrollees under a patient care contract. This account also should be used to record copayments from HMO enrollees, coordination of benefits income and other revenues associated with a prepaid/capitation contract plan. It may also include global package arrangements such as transplant package price, CABG package price, etc.

Refunds should be recorded in Account 4300 — Patient Refunds. If Account 4240 is used, Accounts 4500 - 4630 and related adjustments and allowances are ***not*** used.

At the organization's discretion, sub-accounts 4241 - 4249 may be used for specific plans and other descriptions.

4250 Capitated Premium Revenues—Medicaid

This account should be used by organizations recording revenues on a cash basis. Net revenue actually collected from capitation payments, risk-sharing revenues and other revenues paid to the organization by an HMO for assigned enrollees under a patient care contract. This account also should be used to record copayments from HMO enrollees, coordination of benefits income and other revenues associated with a prepaid/capitation contract plan. It may also include global package arrangements such as transplant package price, CABG package price, etc.

Refunds should be recorded in Account 4300 — Patient Refunds. If Account 4250 is used, Accounts 4500 - 4630 and related adjustments and allowances are ***not*** used.

At the organization's discretion, sub-accounts 4251 - 4259 may be used for specific plans and other descriptions.

4260 Capitated Premium Revenues — Other

This account should be used by organizations recording revenues on a cash basis. Net revenue actually collected from capitation payments, risk-sharing revenues and other revenues paid to the organization by an HMO for assigned enrollees under a patient care contract. This account also should be used to record copayments from HMO enrollees, coordination of benefits income and other revenues associated with a prepaid/capitation contract plan. It may also include global package arrangements such as transplant package price, CABG package price, etc.

Refunds should be recorded in Account 4300 — Patient Refunds. If Account 4260 is used, Accounts 4500 - 4630 and related adjustments and allowances are ***not*** used.

At the organization's discretion, sub-accounts 4261 - 4269 may be used for specific plans and other descriptions.

4270 Risk Sharing Revenue

This account will contain any mechanism that gives incentive to providers to render cost-effective, high-quality hospital care.

4271 *Hospital Risk Sharing — Commercial*

This account should be used to record revenue from risk-sharing arrangements (risk pools) established under commercial contracts to encourage the provider group to utilize inpatient services in an efficient manner. Alternatively, accounts 4271 - 4279 could be categorized by type of service subject to the risk-sharing arrangement (pharmaceutical, ancillary service) or by contract depending upon the entity's needs and reporting requirements.

4272 *Hospital Risk Sharing — Medicare*

This account should be used to record revenue from risk-sharing arrangements (risk pools) established under Medicare contracts to encourage the provider group to utilize inpatient services in an efficient manner.

4273 *Hospital Risk Sharing — Medicaid*

This account should be used to record revenue from risk-sharing arrangements (risk pools) established under Medicaid contracts to encourage the provider group to utilize inpatient services in an efficient manner,

4274 *Hospital Risk Sharing — Pharmacy*

This account should be used to record revenue from risk-sharing arrangements (risk pools) established under contracts to encourage the provider group to utilize pharmacy services in an efficient manner.

4275 *Hospital Risk Sharing — Other*

This account will contain any mechanism that gives incentive to providers to render cost-effective, high-quality outside referrals.

4280 Other Managed Care Collected Revenues

4281 *Copayments*

This account will contain the revenues generated from payment-sharing arrangements between the insurance carriers or federal entity and the patient, which often includes the concept of a specific amount of money per visit.

4282 *Coordination of Benefits*

Use of this account is based on policy guidance within the National Association of Insurance Commissioners (NAIC) to prevent double payment for services when an enrollee has coverage from two or more sources. It is used to ensure that the insured's benefits from all sources do not exceed 100 percent of allowable.

4283 *Other Prepaid Professional Fees Collected*

Other prepaid professional fees collected not recorded elsewhere.

4290 Recoveries

4291 Reinsurance Recoveries

Amounts received as a result of a stop-loss policy issued by an insurance carrier that specializes in underwriting the risks associated with the insurance industry.

4292 Bad Debt Recovery

Recovered revenues from collections that were originally written off as bad debt expense in Account 6700 — Bad Debt Expense, Account 6710 — Accounts Receivable Write-Offs and/or Account 6720 — Collection Agency Write-Offs.

4300 Patient Refunds

Refunds of amounts collected from patients that should not have been collected or need to be returned for some other reason. The corresponding credit is cash or accounts payable. This account should be used only if the specific revenue in which the payment was originally recorded is ***not*** used.

4400 Fees Collected — Other Revenue

This account should be used by organizations recording revenues on a cash basis. Fees charged for transcripts and records for lawyers, insurance companies and others. All nonmedical revenues such as grant payments, research stipends, honoraria, government support payments, educational subsidies used to train residents and gross revenue from the sale of products such as pharmaceuticals, hearing aids, optical lenses, orthopedic supplies, medical supplies, etc. should be recorded in sub-accounts 4410 - 4490.

Gross revenue from nonmedical business interests (parking lots, rental property, leased equipment, etc.) should be recorded under Account 9100. If Account 4400 is used, Accounts 4510 - 4630 are ***not*** used.

4410 Sales — Medical Related

Revenue from pharmaceuticals, medical supplies and equipment sold to patients primarily for use outside the practice, including prescription drugs, hearing aids, optical goods, orthopedic supplies, etc.

4420 Patient Records Copying Reimbursement

Payments received for the reproduction of patients' records.

4430 Fees Collected — Other

Revenue for medical-related activities such as honoraria, educational seminars, expert witness testimonies, etc. Includes:

- Compensation paid by a hospital to a practice physician for services as a medical director
- The hourly wages of physicians working in a hospital emergency room
- Contract Revenue from a hospital for physician services in staffing a hospital indigent care clinic

- Contract revenue from a school district for physician services in conducting physical exams for high school athletes
- Revenue from the preparation of court depositions, expert testimony, postmortem reports and other special reports.

Do ***not*** include capitation revenue used to pay for covered goods and services for capitation patients.

4450 Donations Received (Operating Revenue)

Any endowment or gift revenue received by the organization for use in daily operations.

4460 Research/Clinical Studies Income

Includes research stipends for activities such as pharmaceutical studies and educational subsidies used to train residents. Also includes revenue received from research activities during the fiscal year. Sponsored funding comes from external sources (i.e., grants and contracts) and is awarded for specific research activities. Does not include indirect overhead for your institution (as defined by the federal government). Indirect overhead is the portion of grant or sponsored research applied against the general overhead of the institution.

4470 Grant Revenue

Includes federal, state, or local government or private foundation grants to provide indigent patient care or for case management of the frail and elderly.

4480 Miscellaneous Income

Income from other revenue sources not recorded elsewhere.

4490 Operating Subsidy Income

Medical practices may receive operational support (operating subsidies) from a parent organization such as a hospital, health system, PPMC, MSO or other large integrated system.

EXHIBIT 4.1

Account Number	Description
	INCOME STATEMENT ACCOUNTS
4000	**REVENUES**
4100	GROSS CHARGES
4110	Gross Charges — Fee-for-Service (FFS)
4120	Gross Charges — Discounted FFS Contracts
4130	Gross Charges — FFS Equivalents for Capitation Plan Patients
4140	Other Gross Charges
4150	Other Revenue
4200	Fees Collected
4210	Fees Collected — FFS
4220	Fees Collected — FFS for Managed Care
4230	Capitated Premium Revenues — Commercial
4240	Capitated Premium Revenues — Medicare
4250	Capitated Premium Revenues — Medicaid
4260	Capitated Premium Revenues — Other
4270	Risk Sharing Revenue
4271	Hospital Risk Sharing — Commercial
4272	Hospital Risk Sharing — Medicare
4273	Hospital Risk Sharing — Medicaid
4274	Hospital Risk Sharing — Other
4280	Other Managed Care Collected Revenues
4281	Copayments
4282	Coordination of Benefits
4283	Other Prepaid Professional Fees Collected
4290	Recoveries
4291	Reinsurance Recoveries
4292	Bad Debt Recovery
4300	Patient Refunds
4400	Fees Collected — Other Revenue
4410	Sales — Medical Related
4420	Patient Records Copying Reimbursement
4430	Fees Collected — Other
4450	Donations Received (Operating Revenue)
4460	Research/Clinical Studies Income
4470	Grant Revenue
4480	Miscellaneous Income
4490	Grant Operating Subsidy Income

4500 ADJUSTMENTS

Adjustments are the differences between the Gross Charges FFS Accounts 4110 - 4140 and the amounts actually received from patients or third-party agencies. Adjustments include charge restrictions imposed by Medicare, charitable adjustments, contractual adjustments required by third-party payers, courtesy adjustments, employee discounts, etc. Most adjustments apply only to organizations using *accrual-basis accounting.*

Adjustments represent the value of services performed for which payment is not expected to be received.

4510 Gross Charges — FFS Discount/Adjustment

This is the contra-account for Account 4110 — Gross Charges — FFS.

Difference between revenue Account 4110 and the amounts actually paid by patients or third-party payers. Adjustments represent the value of services performed for which payment is not expected.

At the organization's discretion, sub-accounts 4511 - 4519 may be used for specific plans, departments and other descriptions.

4520 Gross Charges — Discounted FFS Contracts Discount/Adjustment

This is the contra-account for Account 4120 — Gross Charges — Discounted FFS Contracts.

Difference between revenue Account 4120 and the amounts actually paid by patients or third-party payers. Adjustments represent the value of services performed for which payment is not expected.

At the organization's discretion, sub-accounts 4521 - 4529 may be used for specific plans, departments and other descriptions.

4530 Gross Charges — FFS Equivalents For Cap Plan Patients/Adjustment

This is the contra-account for Account 4130 — Gross Charges — FFS Equivalents for Capitation Plan Patients.

An organization may use these accounts (4130 and 4530) in different ways. Most would reflect the fee-for-services equivalent charges under capitated contracts under Account 4130 and reflect all revenues actually received under the 4200 Account series. Account 4530 would then be used as a contra-account to eliminate all Fee-for-Service charges originally posted as a contractual adjustment in the accounts receivable.

Using the accounts in this manner allows the user to compare cash revenues received on capitated contracts to the Fee-for-Service equivalents for a barometer of how the entity is performing under these contracts.

This account reflects the difference between revenue Account 4130 and the amounts actually paid by patients, third-party payers or package price cases. Adjustments represent the value of services such as: copayments from HMO enrollees, coordination of benefits income and other revenues associated with a prepaid/capitation contract with an HMO for which payment is not expected.

At the organization's discretion, sub-accounts 4531 - 4539 may be used for specific plans, departments and other descriptions.

4540 Other Gross Charges/Adjustments

This is the contra-account for Account 4140 — Other Gross Charges.

Difference between revenue Account 4140 and the amounts actually paid by patients or third-party payers. Adjustments represent the value of services performed for which payment is not expected.

At the organization's discretion, sub-accounts 4541 - 4549 may be used for specific plans, departments and other descriptions.

4550 Other Revenue Discount/Adjustment

This is the contra-account for Account 4150 — Other Revenue.

Difference between revenue Account 4150 and the amounts actually paid by patients or third-party payers. Adjustments represent the value of services performed for which payment is not expected.

At the organization's discretion, sub-accounts 4551 - 4559 may be used for specific plans, departments and other descriptions.

4600 Financial Hardship Care Discount/Adjustment

This is the contra-account to Account 1324 — Allowance for Charity Care. Differences between the full dollar value of services provided (gross charges) to charity patients and the amount (if any) to be received in payment for these services. These debits and the corresponding credits to the appropriate accounts receivable account should be recorded at the same time the gross charges are recorded. Charity patients should be identified at the time service is provided. Any write-offs for charitable services should ***not*** be made to Account 6700 — Bad Debt Expense.

At the organization's discretion, sub-accounts 4601 - 4609 may be used for specific plans, departments and other descriptions.

4610 Courtesy Discount/Adjustment

Differences between the gross charges for services rendered and the amounts actually charged for such services. This account is used for "policy adjustments," such as discounts to clergy and nonorganization physicians and may also be debited for adjustments made at the specific request of organization physicians on behalf of patients who would not otherwise qualify for an adjustment.

At the organization's discretion, sub-accounts 4611 - 4619 may be used for specific plans, departments and other descriptions.

4620 Employee Discount/Adjustment

Differences between the gross charges for services rendered to employees and their immediate families and the amounts (if any) to be received in payment for these services. As with charity patients, the entry to this account should be made at the time of service.

At the organization's discretion, sub-accounts 4621 - 4629 may be used for specific plans, departments and other descriptions.

4630 Charity Care Discount/Adjustment

Differences between the gross charges for services rendered to individuals and organizations considered charity cases and the amounts (if any) to be received in payment for these services.

4700 Third-Party Settlements

This account should be used with accrual, modified cash and cash-basis accounting. Under a retrospective rate-setting system, third parties usually determine an interim payment rate and, during the rate period, pay the medical organization for services rendered using the rate. After the rate period has ended, the medical organization may be entitled to receive additional payments or may be required to refund amounts received in excess of amounts earned under the system. An example of this type of arrangement is an interim billing for reimbursement under Part A of Medicare for a rural health clinic or a certified Mental Health Center.

Under prospective rate setting, third parties set payment rates in advance of the delivery of health care services. Prospective rate setting may result from a contractual agreement with a third party, such as a Blue Cross plan, or it may be mandated through legislation. Some rate setting methods described as prospective may include provisions for retrospective adjustments and some third parties pay prospective rates for certain services and retrospective rates for other services.

Any year-end cost reimbursement settlement to a third-party agency is charged to the respective 4701 - 4709 sub-account (which the organization would set up and define) and a corresponding credit is recorded in the appropriate accounts payable. If an organization receives more than its established rates or its anticipated adjusted gross charges from the third-party agency, the difference should be credited to the settlements accounts and debited to the appropriate accounts receivable.

4800 Provision For Cash-Basis Conversion

Used to convert revenues recorded on the accrual basis to collections recorded on the cash basis. This adjustment is optional and is provided for the organization that may wish to compute revenues on both the cash and accrual bases. This account is used in conjunction with Account 2371 — Deferred Revenue — Fee-For-Service.

EXHIBIT 4.2

Account Number	Description
4500	ADJUSTMENTS
4510	Gross Charges — FFS Discount/Adjustment
4520	Gross Charges — FFS for Managed Care Discount/Adjustment
4530	Gross Charges — FFS Equivalents for Cap Plan Patients/Adjustment
4540	Other Gross Charges/Adjustments
4550	Other Revenue Discount/Adjustment
4600	Financial Hardship Care Discount/Adjustment
4610	Courtesy Discount/Adjustment
4620	Employee Discount/Adjustment
4630	Charity Care Discount/Adjustment
4700	Third-Party Settlements
4800	Provision for Cash Basis Conversion

5000 OPERATING EXPENSES — SALARY AND FRINGE BENEFITS

On the accrual basis, expenses are resources consumed in the process of generating revenue, regardless of when payment for the resources occurs. Conversely, on a cash basis of accounting, expenses are realized when paid regardless of when a service was provided or a resource consumed.

Operating expenses are expired costs incurred in the process of providing medical services to the organization's patients and exclude all costs pertaining to nonoperating activities such as general investments, endowments, etc.

This chart of accounts has been revised from those previously issued by moving physician and midlevel provider salaries and their related direct payroll costs to a separate series of accounts in the 8000 series. This has been done to make the MGMA chart of accounts more useful in performing benchmarking comparisons of overhead and physician earnings among practices. For those organizations (such as not-for-profits) that prefer to use the more traditional approach of grouping all human resources costs in their chart of accounts, Account Series 5100, 5200, 5300 and 5400 have been left open for that purpose. The same account titles and descriptions from 8100, 8200, 8300 and 8400 may be used and moved into the open slots. (For additional explanation and examples, please refer to Chapter 7 about not-for-profit.)

Account Series 5000 includes all forms of nonphysician employee compensation, including salaries regularly paid or stipulated to be paid (before deductions), to individuals for services performed while on the payroll of the medical organization. For the purpose of comparisons with peer medical organizations or comparative data services, salaries also may include the fair market value of services donated to the organization by persons performing in an employee capacity. The credit for the donated services should be made to Account 4450 — Donations Received.

Payments to independent contractors, including consulting physicians or an outside laboratory, are not employee costs. Accordingly, they should be *excluded* from Accounts 5000 - 5920 as well as from Accounts 8100 - 8200. They should be recorded in Account 7800 — Purchased Services for HMO/PPO Patients — Professional and Medical for services provided to nonprepaid patients of the organization or in Account 7850 — Sub-capitation Payments for services provided to prepaid patients of the organization.

5500 ANCILLARY STAFF — SALARIES

Salaries and incentives of all employees of ancillary departments. At the organization's discretion, sub-accounts 5510 - 5550 may be used to record individual staff category salaries.

5510 Salaries — Radiology

5520 Salaries — Laboratory

5530 Salaries — Optical

5540 Salaries — Physical Therapy

5550 SALARIES — OTHER ANCILLARY SERVICES

5600 ANCILLARY STAFF — EMPLOYEE RELATED EXPENSES

5610 Payroll Taxes (Ancillary)

Employer's share of the ancillary staff payroll taxes. At the organization's discretion, sub-accounts 5611 - 5614 may be used to record individual payroll tax categories for ancillary staff.

5611 Payroll Taxes — FICA/Medicare (Ancillary)

5612 Payroll Taxes — Federal Unemployment Insurance (Ancillary)

5613 Payroll Taxes — State Unemployment Insurance (Ancillary)

5614 Payroll Taxes — Other (Ancillary)

5620 Insurance (Ancillary)

Employer's share of the insurance premiums paid for the benefit of ancillary staff excluding professional liability insurance, which is recorded in Account 6188. At the organization's discretion, sub-accounts 5621 - 5629 may be used to record individual insurance categories for ancillary staff.

5621 Insurance — Health (Ancillary)

5622 Insurance — Dental (Ancillary)

5623 Insurance — Life (Ancillary)

5624 Insurance — Disability (Ancillary)

5625 Insurance — Workers' Compensation (Ancillary)

5626 Insurance — Other (Ancillary)

5630 Pension and Retirement Benefits (Ancillary)

Payments by the organization to the pension plan or other retirement program established for the ancillary staff in the organization. If an organization offers a 401(k), 403(b) or similar pension/retirement plan, only include the employer contribution, not the employee contribution.

5631 Pension (Ancillary)

Payments by the organization to the pension plan established for the ancillary staff.

5632 Deferred Compensation (Ancillary)

Deferred compensation of the organization's ancillary staff paid or expensed during the period. On cash-basis accounting, this account would appear on the statements only when paid, not as it is accrued.

5633 Severance Plan (Ancillary)

Costs paid or expensed by the organization for the ancillary staff's severance plan during the year. Typically amounts earned on assets set aside, if funded, are also recorded in this account. On cash-basis accounting, this account would appear on the statements only when paid, not as it is accrued.

5635 Professional Development (Ancillary)

Costs paid by the organization for ancillary staff's continuing education, including costs of study materials. Sub-accounts 5636 - 5639 may be used to identify continuing education, degree-awarding institutions, etc.

5640 Books and Subscriptions (Ancillary)

Costs paid by the organization for ancillary staff books and subscriptions to professional journals and magazines.

5645 Dues and Memberships (Ancillary)

Costs paid by the organization for ancillary staff's dues and memberships in professional organizations. Consideration should be given to properly documenting the nondeductible "political contributions" of dues, memberships, contributions and donations paid and charged under an expense sub-account.

5650 Licenses (Ancillary)

Costs paid by the organization for ancillary staff's state and local licenses.

5655 Meetings (Ancillary)

Costs paid by the organization for ancillary staff's meetings.

5660 Travel (Ancillary)

Costs paid by the organization for ancillary staff's travel.

5665 Medical Reimbursement Plan (Ancillary)

Medical- and dental-related expenses incurred by ancillary staff, and typically their families, which are paid for or reimbursed to the ancillary staff in accordance with a formal plan. Account 7800 — Purchased Services for HMO/PPO Patients — Professional and Medical should ***not*** be used for these services. Any free medical or dental services provided within the organization to ancillary staff should be treated as an adjustment to revenue and debited to Account 4620 — Employee Discount/Adjustment.

5670 Vehicles (Ancillary)

Lease and operating costs of a vehicle acquired for the exclusive use of ancillary staff.

5675 Parking (Ancillary)

Costs paid by the organization for ancillary staff's parking.

5680 Telephones (Ancillary)

Costs paid by the organization for telephones (and cell phones) acquired for the exclusive use of ancillary staff.

5685 Beepers (Ancillary)

Costs paid by the organization for beepers and pagers acquired for the exclusive use of ancillary staff.

5690 Meals and Entertainment (Ancillary)

Costs paid by the organization for ancillary staff's business-related meals and entertainment.

5695 Other Benefits (Ancillary)

Other ancillary staff benefits not recorded elsewhere, such as travel for spouse, etc.

EXHIBIT 4.3

Account Number	Description
5000	**OPERATING EXPENSES — Salary and Fringe Benefits**
5500	ANCILLARY STAFF — SALARIES
5510	Salaries — Radiology
5520	Salaries — Laboratory
5530	Salaries — Optical
5540	Salaries — Physical Therapy
5550	Salaries — Other Ancillary Services
5600	ANCILLARY STAFF — EMPLOYEE-RELATED EXPENSES
5610	Payroll Taxes (Ancillary)
5611	Payroll Taxes — FICA/Medicare (Ancillary)
5612	Payroll Taxes — Federal Unemployment Insurance (Ancillary)
5613	Payroll Taxes — State Unemployment Insurance (Ancillary)
5614	Payroll Taxes — Other (Ancillary)
5620	Insurance (Ancillary)
5621	Insurance — Health (Ancillary)
5622	Insurance — Dental (Ancillary)
5623	Insurance — Life (Ancillary)
5624	Insurance — Disability (Ancillary)
5625	Insurance — Workers' Compensation (Ancillary)
5626	Insurance — Other (Ancillary)
5630	Pension and Retirement Benefits (Ancillary)
5631	Pension (Ancillary)
5632	Deferred Compensation (Ancillary)
5633	Severance Plan (Ancillary)
5635	Professional Development (Ancillary)
5640	Books and Subscriptions (Ancillary)
5645	Dues and Memberships (Ancillary)
5650	Licenses (Ancillary)
5655	Meetings (Ancillary)
5660	Travel (Ancillary)
5665	Medical Reimbursement Plan (Ancillary)
5670	Vehicles (Ancillary)
5675	Parking (Ancillary)
5680	Telephones (Ancillary)
5685	Beepers (Ancillary)
5690	Meals and Entertainment (Ancillary)
5695	Other Benefits (Ancillary)

5700 EMPLOYEES — SALARIES

Salaries and incentives of all other employees not listed in other categories. At the organization's discretion, sub-accounts 5710 - 5795 may be used to record individual categories of other employees.

5710 Salaries — General Administrative

Salaries and incentives of all general administrative and practice management staff and their direct support staff employees. General administrative support staff includes executive personnel such as the administrator, assistant administrator, chief financial officer, medical director, other directors, human resources employees, marketing employees, administrative secretaries and purchasing department employees.

5715 Salaries — Business Office

Salaries and incentives of all business office staff, such as business office manager and secretaries and all insurance, billing, credit, accounting, cashiering, collections, bookkeeping and accounting data input employees. Business office activity includes data input of physician charges.

5720 Salaries — Managed Care Administrative

Salaries and incentives of all managed care administrative staff and their direct support staff employees such as secretaries, administrative assistants, etc. The managed care administrative support staff employees include HMO/PPO contract administrators, case management staff, actuaries, managed care medical directors and managed care marketing, quality assurance and utilization review staff.

5725 Salaries — Information Services

Salaries and incentives of data processing, computer programming and telecommunications staff. This would include the systems administrator.

5730 Salaries — Housekeeping/Maintenance/Security

Salaries and incentives for all housekeeping, maintenance and security personnel employed by the organization. Housekeeping is responsible for all care and cleaning of the interior of facilities. Maintenance includes all exterior care and cleaning as well as renovation and repair of all furniture, fixtures and equipment (for example, painting, elevator repair, vehicle maintenance, groundskeeping, minor construction projects). Security is responsible for the protection of personnel and facilities.

Do ***not*** include salaries for parking attendants if the parking area generates revenue, since parking-area revenue should be reported in Account 4430 — Fees Collected — Other Revenue and the salaries of the parking attendants should be reported in Account 6440 — Other Office and Administrative Expense.

5735 Salaries — Medical Receptionists

Salaries and incentives of all medical receptionists, switchboard operators, schedulers and appointment staff.

5735 Salaries — Medical Receptionists

Salaries and incentives of all medical receptionists, switchboard operators, schedulers and appointment staff.

5740 Salaries — Medical Secretaries/Transcribers

Salaries and incentives of all medical secretaries and transcribers employed by the organization.

5745 Salaries — Medical Records

Salaries and incentives of all medical records and coding staff employed by the organization.

5750 Salaries — Other Administrative Support

Salaries and incentives of all other administrative staff employed by the organization, such as mailroom, cafe[illegible] laundry personnel.

5755 Salaries — Registered Nurses

Salaries and incentives of all regist[illegible]egistered nurses working as front-line managers or lea[illegible] the organization. Do ***not*** include midlevel provider s[illegible] which should be reported in Account 8300 — Midleve[illegible]d Account 8400 — Midlevel Provider Employee-Relate[illegible]

5760 Salaries — Licensed Practical [illegible]

Salaries and incentives of all lice[illegible]s employed by the organization.

5765 Salaries — Medical Assistants/Nurses' Aids

Salaries and incentives of all medical assistants, nurses' aids and other nursing support staff.

5800 EMPLOYEES — EMPLOYEE RELATED EXPENSES

5810 Payroll Taxes (Other)

Employer's share of other staff payroll taxes. At the organization's discretion, sub-accounts 5811 - 5814 may be used to record individual tax categories.

5811 ***Payroll Taxes — FICA/Medicare (Other)***

5812 ***Payroll Taxes — Federal Unemployment Insurance (Other)***

5813 ***Payroll Taxes — State Unemployment Insurance (Other)***

5814 ***Payroll Taxes — Other (Other)***

5820 Insurance (Other)

Employer's share of the insurance premiums paid for the benefit of other employees. At the organization's discretion, sub-accounts 5821 - 5829 may be used to record individual insurance categories.

5821 ***Insurance — Health (Other)***

5822 ***Insurance — Dental (Other)***

5823 ***Insurance — Life (Other)***

5824 ***Insurance — Disability (Other)***

5825 ***Insurance — Workers' Compensation (Other)***

5826 ***Insurance — Other (Other)***

5830 Pension and Retirement Benefits (Other)

Payments by the organization to the pension plan or other retirement program established for other employees in the organization. If an organization offers a 401(k), 403(b) or similar pension/retirement plan, only include the employer contribution, not the employee contribution.

5831 ***Pension (Other)***

Payments by the organization to the pension plan established for other employees.

5832 ***Deferred Compensation (Other)***

Deferred compensation of the organization's other employees paid or expensed during the period. On cash-basis accounting, this account would appear on the statements only when paid, not as it is accrued.

8333 ***Severance Plan (Other)***

Costs paid or expensed by the organization for other employees' severance plan during the year. Typically amounts earned on assets set aside, if funded, are also recorded in this account. On cash-basis accounting, this account would appear on the statements only when paid, not as it is accrued.

5835 Professional Development (Other)

Costs paid by the organization for other employees' continuing education, including costs of study materials. Sub-accounts 5836 - 5839 may be used to identify continuing education, degree awarding institutions, etc.

5840 Books and Subscriptions (Other)

Costs paid by the organization for other employees' books and subscriptions to professional journals and magazines.

5845 Dues and Memberships (Other)

Costs paid by the organization for other employees' dues and memberships in professional organizations. Consideration should be given to properly documenting the nondeductible "political contributions" of dues, memberships, contributions and donations paid and charged under an expense sub-account.

5850 Licenses (Other)

Costs paid by the organization for other employees' state and local license fees.

5855 Meetings (Other)

Costs paid by the organization for other employees' meetings.

5860 Travel (Other)

Costs paid by the organization for other employees' travel.

5865 Medical Reimbursement Plan (Other)

Medical- and dental-related expenses incurred by other employees, and typically their families, which are paid for or reimbursed to the employees in accordance with a formal plan. Account 7800 — Purchased Services for HMO/PPO Patients — Professional and Medical should ***not*** be used for these services. Any free medical or dental services provided within the organization to other employees should be treated as an adjustment to revenue and debited to Account 4620 — Employee Discount/Adjustment.

5870 Vehicles (Other)

Operating costs of a vehicle acquired for the exclusive or business use by other employees.

5875 Parking (Other)

Costs paid by the organization for other employees' parking expenses.

5880 Telephones (Other)

Costs paid by the organization for telephones (including cell phones) acquired for the exclusive use of other employees.

5885 Beepers (Other)

Costs paid by the organization for beepers and pagers acquired for the exclusive use of other employees.

5890 Meals and Entertainment (Other)

Costs paid by the organization for other employees' business-related meals and entertainment.

5895 Other Benefits (Other)

Other employee benefits not included elsewhere.

5900 Temporary Employee Salaries

Costs incurred by the organization for employees on a temporary basis to support short-term needs. At the organization's discretion, sub-accounts 5901 - 5909 may be used to record individual provider and other employee categories.

5901 ***Physician Salaries***

5902 ***Midlevel Provider Salaries***

5903 ***Ancillary Staff Salaries***

5904 ***Administrative and Other Staff***

5910 Temporary Employee Benefits

Fringe benefit costs incurred by the organization for employees on a temporary basis to support short-term needs. At the organization's discretion, sub-accounts 5911 - 5919 may be used to record individual insurance categories.

5911 ***Physician Benefits***

5912 ***Midlevel Provider Benefits***

5913 ***Ancillary Staff Benefits***

EXHIBIT 4.4

Account Number	Description
5700	EMPLOYEES — SALARIES
5710	Salaries — General Administrative
5715	Salaries — Business Office
5720	Salaries — Managed Care Administration
5725	Salaries — Information Services
5730	Salaries — Housekeeping/Maintenance/Security
5735	Salaries — Medical Receptionist
5740	Salaries — Medical Secretaries/Transcribers
5745	Salaries — Medical Records
5750	Salaries — Other Administrative Support
5755	Salaries — Registered Nurses
5760	Salaries — Licensed Practical Nurses
5765	Salaries — Medical Assistants/Nurses' Aids
5766	Personnel Services
5800	EMPLOYEE — EMPLOYEE-RELATED EXPENSES (OTHER)
5810	Payroll Taxes (Other)
5811	Payroll Taxes — FICA/Medicare (Other)
5812	Payroll Taxes — Federal Unemployment Insurance (Other)
5813	Payroll Taxes — State Unemployment Insurance (Other)
5814	Payroll Taxes — Other (Other)
5820	Insurance (Other)
5821	Insurance — Health (Other)
5822	Insurance — Dental (Other)
5823	Insurance — Life (Other)
5824	Insurance — Disability (Other)
5825	Insurance — Workers' Compensation (Other)
5826	Insurance — Other (Other)
5830	Pension and Retirement Benefits (Other)
5831	Pension (Other)
5832	Deferred Compensation (Other)
5833	Severance Plan (Other)
5835	Professional Development (Other)
5840	Books and Subscriptions (Other)
5845	Dues and Memberships (other)
5850	Licenses (Other)
5855	Meetings (Other)
5860	Travel (Other)
5865	Medical Reimbursement Plan (Other)
5870	Vehicles (Other)
5875	Parking (Other)
5880	Telephones (Other)
5885	Beepers (Other)
5890	Meals and Entertainment (Other)
5895	Other Benefits (Other)
5900	Temporary Employee Salaries
5901	Physician Salaries
5902	Midlevel Provider Salaries
5903	Ancillary Staff Salaries
5904	Administrative and Other Staff
5910	Temporary Employee Salaries
5911	Physician Benefits
5912	Midlevel Provider Benefits
5913	Ancillary Staff Benefits
5914	Administrative and Other Staff

6000 SERVICES AND GENERAL EXPENSE

Services and general expenses that are not considered purchased services. Purchased services belong under Account 7700. Accounts are broken out according to whether they are associated with Accounts 6100 — Office and Administrative Expense, Accounts 6500 — Billing Expense, Accounts 7000 — Clinical Expense, or Accounts 7500 — Occupancy Expense.

6100 Office and Administrative Expense

Expenses related to the administration department. At the organization's discretion, sub-accounts 6110 - 6499 may be used to individually categorize various expenses.

6110 Equipment Rentals (Admin)

Costs associated with equipment rental or leasing for the administration department.

6115 Equipment Maintenance (Admin)

Costs associated with equipment maintenance within the administration department.

6120 Telephones (Admin)

Costs of all telephone and other communication services or equipment purchased or leased by the organization for the administration department.

6130 Postage (Admin)

Costs of all postage and other charges for shipping and mailing associated with the administration department.

6140 Courier and Overnight Delivery (Admin)

Costs of all courier, overnight deliver and airfreight and other charges for shipping and mailing associated with the administration department.

6150 Security

Expenses, other than salaries, associated with the protection of personnel and property. Includes the cost of contracted security services and systems.

6160 Library/Books and Subscriptions

Costs of operating a technical library, including technical books and subscriptions not acquired for a specific employee.

6170 Advertising and Marketing

Costs of marketing services and advertising media used to promote the health care services provided by the organization. Includes the costs of listings such as the yellow pages or inclusion in similar health care directories, patient newsletters, information booklets, fliers and brochures.

6180 General Business and Other Insurance

Cost of general business and casualty policies such as fire, flood, theft, casualty, general liability, officers' and directors' liability, reinsurance, etc. At the organization's discretion, sub-accounts 6181 - 6184 may be used to record expenses by insurance type.

6181 Officers' and Directors' Liability

Premiums for coverage of officers' and directors' liability insurance.

6182 Other Liability

Premiums paid or self-insurance costs for general liability not recorded elsewhere.

6183 Reinsurance for Capitation Contracts

Cost incurred for stop-loss insurance (reinsurance) coverage of catastrophic claims, emergency care outside the contract parameters and insolvency.

6184 Keyman and Overhead Insurance

Cost incurred for insurance premiums on contracts that insure the lives of certain owners or management of the organization and that insure against certain business risks.

6185 Malpractice Insurance

Premiums or self-insurance cost for coverage of professional liability claims. At the organization's discretion, sub-accounts 6186 - 6189 may be used to record expenses by provider type.

6186 Physicians

6187 Midlevel Providers

6188 Ancillary and Clinical Staff

6189 Global Coverage

6190 Printing (Admin)

Costs of printing services used by the administration department, excluding forms that are recorded in Account 6210 — Medical Forms.

6200 Copying (Admin)

Costs of copying services used by the administration department.

6210 Medical Forms

Costs of printing medical forms used by the organization.

6220 Answering Service

Costs associated with an answering service used outside normal business hours.

6230 Meals and Entertainment

Corporate expenses associated with visitors or similar expenses associated with the organization as a whole. Individual expenses for specific physicians, midlevel providers, ancillary staff or other staff should be expensed under Accounts 8260, 8460, 5660 or 5860 respectively.

6240 Cafeteria

Amount of loss (total operating expenses minus revenues) from operating cafeteria for the organization's employees.

6250 Employee Relations

Corporate costs of employee coffee room, employee picnics, dinners and other entertainment.

6260 Physician Recruitment

Costs associated with recruiting and hiring physicians, including the costs of advertising, screening, testing, entertainment and travel for the recruiting process.

6270 Nonphysician Recruitment

Costs associated with recruiting and hiring midlevel providers, ancillary staff and other employees, including the costs of advertising, screening, testing, entertainment and travel for the recruiting process.

6300 Depreciation/Amortization

As a general rule, depreciation is used to record the consumption/utilization over time of *tangible* property. Amortization is used to record the consumption/utilization over time of *intangible* property.

At the organization's discretion, sub-accounts 6301 - 6307 may be used to record individual categories of depreciation/amortization.

6301 ***Furniture and Fixtures***

6302 ***Capital Leases***

6303 ***Equipment***

6304 ***Computers***

6305 ***Vehicles***

6306 ***Amortization***

6307 ***Other Depreciation***

6310 Accounting Services

Costs related to accounting services provided by outside accountants, including an audit by a certified public accountant (CPA).

6320 Legal Services

Costs related to legal services paid to attorneys who are not employees of the organization.

6330 Actuarial Services

Cost of actuarial services purchased from outside actuaries or consultants. Actuary services may be purchased to predict managed care utilization, defined benefit retirement plan contributions, etc.

6340 Pension Administration Expense

Costs related to management of a retirement plan by an outside administrator.

6350 Consulting Services

Costs related to outside consulting services.

6360 Other Professional Services

Costs related to other professional services purchased and not recorded elsewhere.

6370 Medical Transcription

Costs related to medical transcription services purchased outside the organization.

6380 Payroll Services

Costs related to payroll services purchased outside the organization.

6390 Business Transportation

Costs of organization-related travel including trips to satellite clinics, errands, and etc.

6400 General Supplies

Supplies and minor equipment purchased for day-to-day use in the organization. Includes expenses for items used in providing medical/surgical services. The administrator should decide the degree of detail required in the supply accounts.

6410 Taxes — Excise and Other Business Taxes

6410 - SBT
6411 - Personal Property Tax

Sales, excise and other taxes not recorded elsewhere. This account also includes business, occupation, use and corporate franchise taxes paid by the group.

6420 Computer Supplies

Costs related to computer supplies for the organization.

6430 Computer Software

Costs related to computer software for the organization.

6440 Other Office and Administrative Expense

Other office and administrative expenses not recorded elsewhere.

EXHIBIT 4.5

Account Number	Description
6000	**SERVICES AND GENERAL EXPENSE**
6100	Office and Administrative Expense
6110	Equipment Rentals (Admin)
6115	Equipment Maintenance (Admin)
6120	Telephones (Admin)
6130	Postage (Admin)
6140	Courier and Overnight Delivery (Admin)
6150	Security
6160	Library/Books and Subscriptions
6170	Advertising and Marketing
6180	General Business and Other Insurance
6181	Officers' and Directors' Liability
6182	Other Liability
6183	Reinsurance for Capitation Contracts
6184	Keyman and Overhead Insurance
6185	Malpractice Insurance
6186	Physicians
6187	Midlevel Providers
6188	Ancillary and Clinical Staff
6189	Global Coverage
6190	Printing (Admin)
6200	Copying (Admin)
6210	Medical Forms
6220	Answering Service
6230	Meals and Entertainment
6240	Cafeteria
6250	Employee Relations
6260	Physician Recruitment
6270	Nonphysician Recruitment
6300	Depreciation/Amortization
6301	Furniture and Fixtures
6302	Capital Leases
6303	Equipment
6404	Computers
6305	Vehicles
6306	Amortization
6307	Other Depreciation
6310	Accounting Services
6320	Legal Services
6330	Actuarial Services
6340	Pension Administration Expense
6350	Consulting Services
6360	Other Professional Services
6370	Medical Transcription
6380	Payroll Services
6390	Business Transportation
6400	General Supplies
6410	Taxes — Excise and Other Business Taxes
6420	Computer Supplies
6430	Computer Software
6440	Other Office and Administrative Expense

6401 Office Paper Supplies
6441 License & Fees

6446 Professional Relations
6447 Contributions
6429 Computer Software Maintenance

6500 Billing Expense

6510 Equipment Rentals (Billing)

Costs associated with equipment rental or leasing for the billing department.

6515 Equipment Maintenance (Billing)

Costs associated with equipment maintenance within the billing department.

6520 Electronic Data Processing

Costs related to outside service bureaus providing electronic data processing services purchased by the organization.

6530 Telephones (Billing)

Costs of all telephone and other communication services or equipment purchased or leased by the organization for the billing department.

6540 Postage (Billing)

Costs of all postage charges for shipping and mailing associated with the billing department.

6550 Courier and Overnight Delivery (Billing)

Costs of all courier, overnight delivery and airfreight associated with the billing department.

6560 Printing (Billing)

Costs of printing services used by the billing department, excluding forms that are recorded in Account 6210 - Medical Forms.

6570 Copying (Billing)

Costs of copying services used by the billing department.

6580 Depreciation (Billing)

Depreciation of billing-related equipment and billing department furniture.

6600 General Services

Fees and charges for services not recorded elsewhere.

6650 Other Billing Expense

Other billing department expenses not recorded elsewhere.

6700 Bad Debt Expense

This account is used for uncollectable accounts receivable and notes receivable. A historical analysis of bad debt write-offs is usually required to determine periodic credits to this account. Other methods may be used, but a consistent and justifiable method of estimating the periodic charge to provision for bad debts (and the corresponding credit to Account 1320 — Allowance for Estimated uncollectable Receivables or Account 1321 —Allowance for Bad Debts — Patient Accounts) should be applied systematically. At the organization's discretion, bad debts may be individually categorized using sub-accounts 6701 - 6709.

6710 Accounts Receivable Write-Offs

Differences between adjusted gross charges and the amount actually collected as settlements for particular accounts. These write-offs may be the result of negotiating a payment less than adjusted gross charges with an individual patient or third-party agency. At the organization's discretion, write-offs of individual private-pay patients may be recorded in sub-account 6711 and write-offs with individual third-party agencies may be recorded in sub-accounts 6712 - 6719.

6720 Collection Agency Write-Offs

Any accounts turned over to a collection agency. The corresponding accounts receivable should be credited. At the organization's discretion, sub-accounts 6721 - 6729 may be used to identify separately private-pay accounts turned over to collection agencies or different collection agencies.

6730 Collection Expenses

Amounts incurred in connection with using outside parties to assist in collection process including collection agency fees, commissions or discounts.

EXHIBIT 4.6

Account Number	Description
6500	Billing Expense
6510	Equipment Rentals (Billing)
6515	Equipment Maintenance (Billing)
6520	Electronic Data Processing
6530	Telephones (Billing)
6540	Postage (Billing)
6550	Courier and Overnight Delivery (Billing)
6560	Printing (Billing)
6570	Copying (Billing)
6580	Depreciation
6600	General Services
6650	Other Billing Expense
6700	Bad Debt Expense
6710	Accounts Receivable Write-Offs
6720	Collection Agency Write-Offs
6730	Collection Expenses

7000 Clinical Expense

7010 Drugs and Medications

Costs of pharmaceutical supplies used in providing medical services. Does ***not*** include the costs of medical supplies sold to patients, which should be reported in Account 7600 — Cost of Goods Sold — Medical Related.

7020 Medical Supplies

Medical supplies, minor equipment and instrument costs. Does ***not*** include the costs of medical supplies sold to patients, which should be reported in Account 7600 — Cost of Goods Sold — Medical Related. At the organization's discretion, sub-accounts 7021 - 7029 may be used to record ancillary department medical supplies.

7021 Radiology

Medical supplies, minor equipment and instrument costs for the radiology department. Does ***not*** include the costs of medical supplies sold to patients, which should be reported in Account 7600 — Cost of Goods Sold — Medical Related.

7022 Laboratory

Medical supplies, minor equipment and instrument costs for the laboratory department. Does ***not*** include the costs of medical supplies sold to patients, which should be reported in Account 7600 — Cost of Goods Sold — Medical Related.

7023 Other Ancillary Supplies

Other ancillary department supplies not recorded elsewhere.

7030 Linen Supplies

Cost of linen and other fabric supplies for clinical-related activities.

7040 Uniforms and Laundry

Cost of uniforms and laundry for clinical-related activities.

7050 Patient Education

Costs of patient education, excluding salaries, dealing with preventive medicine and better use of the group's facilities. This would include patient education brochures and pamphlets provided to patients at no charge. Use this account only if the patient is not charged for the service.

7060 Photography

Costs of medical photography or medical illustrations used to document clinical services.

7070 Biohazardous Waste Removal

Costs related to the removal of biohazardous waste.

7100 Equipment Rentals (Clinical)

Costs related to clinical equipment rentals or leases.

7110 Equipment Maintenance (Clinical)

Costs related to clinical equipment maintenance.

7120 Telephone (Clinical)

Costs of all telephone and other communication services or equipment purchased or leased by the organization for the clinical department.

7130 Postage (Clinical)

Costs of all postage, UPS, airfreight and other charges for shipping and mailing associated with the clinical department.

7140 Medical Record Supplies

Costs related to medical record maintenance and storage.

7150 Other Clinical Expense

Other clinical expenses not recorded elsewhere.

7160 Depreciation (Clinical)

7161 ***General Clinical***

7162 ***Radiology***

7163 ***Laboratory***

EXHIBIT 4.7

Account Number			Description
7000			Clinical Expense
	7010		Drugs and Medications
	7020		Medical Supplies
		7021	Radiology
		7022	Laboratory
		7023	Other Ancillary Supplies
	7030		Linen Supplies
	7040		Uniforms and Laundry
	7050		Patient Education
	7060		Photography
	7070		Biohazardous Waste Removal
	7100		Equipment Rentals (Clinical)
	7110		Equipment Maintenance (Clinical)
	7120		Telephone (Clinical)
	7130		Postage (Clinical)
	7140		Medical Record Supplies
	7150		Other Clinical Expense
	7160		Depreciation (Clinical)
		7161	General Clinical
		7162	Radiology
		7163	Laboratory

7500 Occupancy Expense

Expenses related to the occupancy and use of land and buildings. In the event that another legal entity owns the land or buildings, any rental fees, commissions or charges paid to the other entity are charged to this account. For the purpose of peer comparison (for example, a comparative data or cost survey), a fair market rental value may be charged to this account even if no rent is otherwise charged to the organization by the owning entity.

7510 Rent/Lease

Rent/lease for building (building and land if not identified separately) used for operations of the organization. Facilities leased for nonoperating purposes should not be included in this account. At the organization's discretion, sub-account 7515 may be set up exclusively for recording rent/lease expenses for land.

7520 Condominium Assessments and Monthly Maintenance Fees

Costs incurred typically on a monthly basis to record commonly charged rental property expenses. Include one-time assessments charged to owners for periodic maintenance, repairs and renovations.

7530 General Maintenance

Costs not recorded in other specific accounts.

7540 Utilities

Cost of utilities, such as water, electric power, space heating fuels, and waste disposal used in organization operations. At the organization's discretion, sub-accounts 7541 - 7544 may be used to record individual categories of utilities.

7541 Utilities — Water

7542 Utilities — Electricity

7543 Utilities — Waste Disposal

7544 Other Utilities

7550 Property Taxes

City, county and state taxes related to occupancy.

7560 Housekeeping/Maintenance Services

Cost of supplies and materials used in the housekeeping and maintenance of buildings, grounds and parking facilities. Include the costs for contracted support services such as janitorial services, grounds maintenance, snow removal, etc.

7570 Other Occupancy Expense

Any occupancy expenses not recorded elsewhere, such as contracted building repairs.

7580 Insurance (Occupancy)

Fire, theft, flood and other casualty insurance related to occupancy.

7590 Depreciation (Occupancy)

Systematic periodic allocation of the cost of land improvements included in asset Account 1712.

7595 Amortization — Leasehold Improvements (Occupancy)

Systematic periodic amortization of the cost of leasehold improvements included in asset Account 1715.

7600 Cost of Goods Sold — Medical Related

Cost of goods sold to patients. This account is used in those areas where items are sold to patients on a retail basis.

EXHIBIT 4.8

Account Number	Description
7500	Occupancy Expense
7510	Rent/Lease
7520	Condominium Assessments/Monthly Maintenance Fees
7530	General Maintenance
7540	Utilties
7541	Utilities — Water
7542	Utilities — Electricity
7543	Utilities — Waste Disposal
7544	Other Utilities
7550	Property Taxes
7560	Housekeeping/Maintenance Services
7570	Other Occupancy Expense
7580	Insurance (Occupancy)
7590	Depreciation (Occupancy)
7595	Amortization — Leasehold Improvements (Occupancy)
7600	Cost of Goods Sold — Medical Related

7700 PURCHASED SERVICES/MANAGEMENT FEES

The 7700 series of accounts are used to record services acquired by the organization on a fee-for-service contract basis. Hospital-owned medical groups should give consideration within the 7700 account series to the "assessments" payable to hospitals.

7710 Medical Directorships

Payments to physicians for services related to acting as medical directors in an administrative or executive capacity. Accounts 7711 - 7719 could actually be used to record various Medical Director expense categories for the organization with more than one type of directorship.

7720 General and Administrative Expense—Purchased Services

Costs of all services of a general and administrative nature purchased on a one-time or short-term basis from outside vendors. At the organization's discretion, sub-accounts may include costs associated with accounting services, accounting audits, legal services, management consultants, transcription services, collection services, clerical services, electronic data processing, actuarial services and other general and administrative purchased services.

7730 Management Fees — MSO/PPMC

Amounts paid in accordance with managed service organization, physician practice management company, hospital or other parent organization agreements for covered services including management, administrative, and/or related support services. Includes other services from management or parent organizations that are reflected in the accounting system as an expense by a journal entry, particularly in the circumstance where such services would otherwise need to be purchased in order to operate the medical practice. Does not include other services from management or parent organizations that are not reflected in the accounting system as an expense by a journal entry.

7731	***Management fees — Commercial***
7732	***Management fees — Medicare***
7733	***Management fees — Medicaid***
7734	***Management fees — Other***

7740 Management Company Incentive

Management companies are increasingly becoming encouraged to be better performers by entering into contracts in which they get paid a bonus based on performance. This account can be used to reflect the incentive portion of that management fee.

7800 Purchased Services for HMO/PPO Patients — Professional and Medical

These accounts will usually come into play for an organization that accepts full risk contracts. Such contracts require the organization to accept risk for and therefore pay claims for all professional services rendered to a specific population.

7810 FFS Purchased Services for HMO/PPO Patients

Fees and other charges paid to health care providers and organizations outside the organization (such as referrals to specialists) for services provided to prepaid patients of the organization where the organization is responsible for referrals under a prepaid contract and those services are contracted on a Fee-for-Service basis.

Accounts 7811 - 7819 can actually be adapted at the discretion of the user to the entity's reporting requirements. The example reflected here categorizes these expenses by type of contract (commercial, Medicare, Medicaid). They could just as appropriately be categorized by type of service purchased, by contract or on some other basis.

7811	***FFS Purchased Services — Commercial***
7812	***FFS Purchased Services — Medicare***
7813	***FFS Purchased Services — Medicaid***
7814	***FFS Purchased Services — Other***

7850 Sub-capitation Payments — Primary Care

The 7850 series of accounts are used to record purchased services acquired by the organization on a sub-capitated contract basis with outside organizations. The categorization proposed here reflects expense by type of care provided, i.e., primary vs. specialty and by contract type within those groupings. This series of accounts can also be adapted to the reporting entity's needs and categorized in some other manner such as by service type or contract.

7851	***Sub-capitation payments — Primary Care — Commercial***
7852	***Sub-capitation payments — Primary Care — Medicare***

7853 ***Sub-capitation payments — Primary Care — Medicaid***

7854 ***Sub-capitation payments — Primary Care — Other***

7860 Sub-capitation payments — Specialty Care

7861 ***Sub-capitation payments — Specialty Care — Commercial***

7862 ***Sub-capitation payments — Specialty Care — Medicare***

7863 ***Sub-capitation payments — Specialty Care — Medicaid***

7864 ***Sub-capitation payments — Specialty Care — Other***

7870 Sub-capitation payments — Hospital

7880 – 7890 Sub-Capitation Payments — Other

EXHIBIT 4.9

Account Number	Description
7700	**PURCHASED SERVICES/MANAGEMENT FEES**
7710	Medical Directorships
7720	General and Administrative Expense — Purchased Services
7730	Management Fees — MSO/PPMC
7731	Management Fees — Commercial
7732	Management Fees — Medicare
7733	Management Fees — Medicaid
7734	Management Fees — Other
7740	Management Company Incentive
7800	Purchased Services for HMO/PPO Patients — Professional and Medical
7810	FFS Purchased Services for HMO/PPO Patients
7811	FFS Purchased Services — Commercial
7812	FFS Purchased Services — Medicare
7813	FFS Purchased Services — Medicaid
7814	FFS Purchased Services — Other
7850	Sub-Capitation Payments — Primary Care
7851	Sub-Capitation Payments — Primary Care — Commercial
7852	Sub-Capitation Payments — Primary Care — Medicare
7853	Sub-Capitation Payments — Primary Care — Medicaid
7854	Sub-Capitation Payments — Primary Care —Other
7860	Sub-Capitation Payments — Specialty Care
7861	Sub-Capitation Payments — Specialty Care — Commercial
7862	Sub-Capitation Payments — Specialty Care — Medicare
7863	Sub-Capitation Payments — Specialty Care — Medicaid
7864	Sub-Capitation Payments — Specialty Care — Other
7870	Sub-Capitation Payments — Hospitals
7880	Sub-Capitation Payments — Other

8000 PROVIDER-RELATED EXPENSES

This chart of accounts has been revised from those previously issued by moving physician and midlevel provider salaries and their related direct payroll costs to a separate series of accounts in the 8000 series. This has been done to make the MGMA chart of accounts more useful in performing benchmarking comparisons of overhead and physician earnings among practices. For those organizations (such as not-for-profits) that prefer to use the more traditional approach of grouping all human resources costs in their chart of accounts, Account Series 5100, 5200, 5300 and 5400 have been left open for just that purpose. The same account titles and descriptions from 8100, 8200, 8300 and 8400 may be used and moved into the open slots. (For additional explanation and examples, please refer to the not-for-profit chapter in this publication.)

8100 PHYSICIANS — SALARIES

Accounts 8120 - 8170 may be combined into Account 8110 if no distinction is made between physician employees and physician owners or if salaries, distributions and incentives are not recorded separately within your organization. Indeed, smaller organizations may not need this level of detail whereas larger, integrated systems may require even greater delineation. If greater detail is needed, sub-accounts may be established under the 8110 - 8170 accounts.

8110 Salaries, Distributions and Incentives (Physician)

All payments to physician-owners and physician-employees, including salaries, bonuses, incentives and other distributions to physicians.

8120 Salaries — Owner/Stockholder (Physician)

Salaries paid to physician-owners. A separate Account 8130 may be used to record bonuses, incentives and other distributions to physician-owners if the additional level of detail is needed. If the organization would rather combine all physician-owner compensation, Account 8120 should be used.

8130 Distributions and Incentives (Physician)

Compensation other than salaries paid to physician-owners.

8140 Global/Capitation Distributions (Physician)

Payments made to physicians related to amounts received under global/capitation arrangements and paid out in a manner determined by the organization.

8150 Employee Salaries (Physician)

Salaries paid to physician-employees. A separate Account 8160 may be used to record bonuses, incentives and other distributions to physician-employees if the additional level of detail is needed. If the organization would rather combine all physician-employee compensation, Account 8150 should be used.

8160 Employee Incentives (Physician)

Compensation other than salaries paid to physician-employees.

8170 Administrative Salaries (Physician)

Salaries or fees paid to physicians for services in an administrative capacity, such as medical director, corporate officer or member of the board or executive committee.

8180 – 8190 Other Compensation (Physician)

Other compensation not listed above paid to physicians.

8200 PHYSICIAN — EMPLOYEE RELATED EXPENSES

These accounts track the expenses related to physicians. Expenses include those of physician-owners as well as physician-employees.

8210 Payroll Taxes (Physician)

Employer's share of the physicians' payroll taxes. At the organization's discretion, sub-accounts 8211 - 8214 may be used to record individual payroll tax categories.

8211 Payroll Taxes — FICA/Medicare (Physician)

8212 Payroll Taxes — Federal Unemployment Insurance (Physician)

8213 Payroll Taxes — State Unemployment Insurance (Physician)

8214 Payroll Taxes — Other (Physician)

8220 Insurance (Physician)

Employer's share of the insurance premiums paid for the benefit of an individual physician excluding professional liability insurance that is recorded in Account 6186. At the organization's discretion, sub-accounts 8221 - 8229 may be used to record individual insurance categories.

8221 Insurance — Health (Physician)

8222 Insurance — Dental (Physician)

8223 Insurance — Life (Physician)

8224 Insurance — Disability (Physician)

8225 Insurance — Workers' Compensation (Physician)

8226 Insurance — Other (Physician)

8227 Insurance — Officers' Life (Physician)

8230 Pension and Retirement Benefits (Physician)

Payments by the organization to the pension plan or other retirement program established for the organization's physicians. If an organization offers a 401(k), 403(b) or similar pension/retirement plan, only include the employer contribution, not the employee contribution.

8231 Pension (Physician)

Payments by the organization to the pension plan established for the physicians.

8232 Deferred Compensation (Physician)

Deferred compensation of the organization's physicians paid or expensed during the period. On cash-basis accounting, this account would appear on the statements only when paid, not as it is accrued.

8233 Severance Plan (Physician)

Costs paid or expensed by the organization for a physician's severance plan during the year. Typically amounts earned on assets set aside, if funded, are also recorded in this account. On cash-basis accounting, this account would appear on the statements only when paid, not as it is accrued.

8235 Professional Development (Physician)

Costs paid by the organization for physicians' continuing education, including costs of study materials. Sub-accounts 8236 - 8239 may be used to identify continuing education, degree awarding institutions, etc.

8240 Books and Subscriptions (Physician)

Costs paid by the organization for the physicians' books and subscriptions to professional journals and magazines.

8245 Dues and Memberships (Physician)

Costs paid by the organization for physicians' dues and memberships in professional organizations. Consideration should be given to properly documenting the nondeductible "political contributions" of dues, memberships, contributions and donations paid and charged under an expense sub-account.

8250 Licenses (Physician)

Costs paid by the organization for physicians' state and local license fees.

8255 Meetings (Physician)

Costs paid by the organization for physicians' meetings.

8260 Travel (Physician)

Costs paid by the organization for physicians' travel.

8265 Medical Reimbursement Plan (Physician)

Medical- and dental-related expenses incurred by physicians, and typically their families, which are paid for or reimbursed to the physician in accordance with a formal plan. Account 7800 — Purchased Services for HMO/PPO Patients — Professional and Medical should ***not*** be used for these services. Any free medical or dental services provided within the organization to physicians should be treated as an adjustment to revenue and debited to Account 4620 — Employee Discount/Adjustment.

8270 Vehicles (Physician)

Operating costs of a vehicle acquired for the exclusive use of a physician. At the discretion of the user, Account 8271 may be used to cover the costs of motor vehicle leases.

8271 Leased Motor Vehicles (Physician)

Costs associated with leased motor vehicles acquired for the exclusive use of a physician.

8275 Parking (Physician)

Costs paid by the organization for the physicians' parking expenses.

8280 Telephones (Physician)

Costs paid by the organization for telephones (including cell phones) acquired for the exclusive use of physicians.

8285 Beepers (Physician)

Costs paid by the organization for beepers and pagers acquired for the exclusive use of physicians.

8290 Meals and Entertainment (Physician)

Costs paid by the organization for the physicians' business-related meals and entertainment.

8295 Other Benefits (Physician)

Physician benefits not included elsewhere, such as country/athletic club membership, travel for spouse, etc.

8300 MIDLEVEL PROVIDERS — SALARIES

Salaries and incentives for physician extenders (midlevel providers) who can provide medical care and bill for services without continuous supervision by a physician.

Includes all payments to midlevel provider owners and midlevel provider employees, including salaries, bonuses, incentives and other distributions to midlevels. Accounts 8320 - 8390 may be combined into Account 8310 if no distinction is made between midlevel provider employees and midlevel provider owners or if salaries, distributions and incentives are not recorded separately within your organization. Indeed smaller organizations may not need this level of detail whereas larger, integrated systems may require even greater detail. If greater detail is needed, sub-accounts may be established under the 8310 - 8390 accounts.

Examples of midlevel providers include:

- Audiologist
- Certified Registered Nurse Anesthetist (CRNA)
- Dental Hygienists/Oral Therapists
- Dietitian/Nutritionist
- Midwife
- Nurse Practitioner (NP)
- Occupational Therapist
- Optometrist
- Perfusionist — Surgery
- Pharmacist
- Physician's Assistant
- Physical Therapist

- Psychologist
- Social Worker
- Speech Therapist
- Surgeon's Assistant

8310 Salaries, Distributions and Incentives (Midlevel)

All payments to midlevel provider-owners and midlevel provider-employees, including salaries, bonuses, incentives and other distributions to midlevels.

8320 Salaries — Owner/Stockholder (Midlevel)

Salaries paid to midlevel provider-owners. A separate Account 8330 may be used to record bonuses, incentives and other distributions to midlevel provider-owners if the additional level of detail is needed. If the organization would rather combine all midlevel provider-owner compensation, Account 8320 should be used.

8330 Distributions and Incentives (Midlevel)

Compensation other than salaries paid to midlevel provider-owners.

8340 Global/Capitation Distributions (Midlevel)

Payments made to midlevel providers related to amounts received under global/capitation arrangements and paid out in a manner determined by the organization.

8350 Employee Salaries (Midlevel)

Salaries paid to midlevel provider-employees. A separate Account 8360 may be used to record bonuses, incentives and other distributions to midlevel provider-employees if the additional level of detail is needed. If the organization would rather combine all midlevel provider-employee compensation, Account 8350 should be used.

8360 Employee Incentives (Midlevel)

Compensation other than salaries paid to midlevel provider-employees.

8370 Administrative Salaries (Midlevel)

Salaries or fees paid to midlevel providers for services in an administrative capacity, such as medical director, corporate officer, or member of the board or executive committee.

8380 – 8390 Other Compensation (Midlevel)

Other compensation not listed above paid to midlevel providers.

8400 MIDLEVEL PROVIDERS — EMPLOYEE RELATED EXPENSES

8410 Payroll Taxes (Midlevel)

Employer's share of the midlevel providers' payroll taxes. At the organization's discretion, sub-accounts 8411 - 8414 may be used to record individual tax categories.

8411 ***Payroll Taxes — FICA/Medicare (Midlevel)***

8412 ***Payroll Taxes — Federal Unemployment Insurance (Midlevel)***

8413 ***Payroll Taxes — State Unemployment Insurance (Midlevel)***

8414 ***Payroll Taxes — Other (Midlevel)***

8420 Insurance (Midlevel)

Employer's share of the insurance premiums paid for the benefit of an individual midlevel provider excluding professional liability insurance, which is recorded in Account 6187. At the organization's discretion, sub-accounts 8421 - 8429 may be used to record individual insurance categories.

8421 ***Insurance — Health (Midlevel)***

8422 ***Insurance — Dental (Midlevel)***

8423 ***Insurance — Life (Midlevel)***

8424 ***Insurance — Disability (Midlevel)***

8425 ***Insurance — Workers' Compensation (Midlevel)***

8426 ***Insurance — Other (Midlevel)***

8430 Pension and Retirement Benefits (Midlevel)

Payments by the organization to the pension plan or other retirement program established for the midlevel providers in the organization. If an organization offers a 401(k), 403(b) or similar pension/retirement plan, only include the employer contribution, not the employee contribution.

8431 ***Pension (Midlevel)***

Payments by the organization to the pension plan established for the midlevel providers.

8432 ***Deferred Compensation (Midlevel)***

Deferred compensation of the organization's midlevel providers paid or expensed during the period. On cash-basis accounting, this account would appear on the statements only when paid, not as it is accrued.

8433 ***Severance Plan (Midlevel)***

Costs paid or expensed by the organization for a midlevel provider's severance plan during the year. Typically amounts earned on assets set aside, if funded, are also recorded in this account. On cash-basis accounting, this account would appear on the statements only when paid, not as it is accrued.

8435 Professional Development (Midlevel)

Costs paid by the organization for midlevel providers' formal and/or continuing education, including costs of study materials, which benefit the employees' long-term professional career. Sub-accounts 8436 - 8439 may be used to identify continuing education, degree awarding institutions, etc.

8440 Books and Subscriptions (Midlevel)

Costs paid by the organization for midlevel providers' books and subscriptions to professional journals and magazines.

8445 Dues and Memberships (Midlevel)

Costs paid by the organization for midlevel providers' dues and memberships in professional organizations. Consideration should be given to properly documenting the nondeductible "political contributions" of dues, memberships, contributions and donations paid and charged under an expense sub-account.

8450 Licenses (Midlevel)

Costs paid by the organization for midlevel providers' state and local license fees.

8455 Meetings (Midlevel)

Costs paid by the organization for midlevel providers' meetings.

8460 Travel (Midlevel)

Costs paid by the organization for midlevel providers' travel.

8465 Medical Reimbursement Plan (Midlevel)

Medical- and dental-related expenses incurred by midlevel providers, and typically their families, which are paid for or reimbursed to the midlevel providers in accordance with a formal plan. Account 7800 — Purchased Services for HMO/PPO Patients — Professional and Medical should not be used for these services. Any free medical or dental services provided within the organization to midlevel providers should be treated as an adjustment to revenue and debited to Account 4620 — Employee Discount/Adjustment.

8470 Vehicles (Midlevel)

Lease and operating costs of a vehicle acquired for the exclusive use of a midlevel provider.

8475 Parking (Midlevel)

Costs paid by the organization for midlevel providers' parking fees.

8480 Telephones (Midlevel)

Costs paid by the organization for telephones (including cell phones) acquired for the exclusive use of midlevel providers.

8485 Beepers (Midlevel)

Costs paid by the organization for beepers and pagers acquired for the exclusive use of midlevel providers.

8490 Meals and Entertainment (Midlevel)

Costs paid by the organization for midlevel providers' business-related meals and entertainment.

8495 Other Benefits (Midlevel)

Midlevel provider benefits not included elsewhere, such as travel for spouse, etc.

EXHIBIT 4.10

Account Number	Description
8000	**PROVIDER-RELATED EXPENSES**
8100	PHYSICIANS — SALARIES
8110	Salaries, Distributions and Incentives (Physician)
8120	Salaries — Owner/Stockholder (Physician)
8130	Distributions and Incentives (Physician)
8140	Global/Capitation Distributions (Physician)
8150	Employee Salaries (Physician)
8160	Employee Incentives (Physician)
8170	Administrative Salaries (Physician)
8180	Other Compensation (Physician)
8200	PHYSICIAN — EMPLOYEE-RELATED EXPENSES
8210	Payroll Taxes (Physician)
8211	Payroll Taxes — FICA/Medicare (Physician)
8212	Payroll Taxes — Federal Unemployment Insurance (Physician)
8213	Payroll Taxes — State Unemployment Insurance (Physician)
8214	Payroll Taxes — Other (Physician)
8220	Insurance (Physician)
8221	Insurance — Health (Physician)
8222	Insurance — Dental (Physician)
8223	Insurance — Life (Physician)
8224	Insurance — Disability (Physician)
8225	Insurance — Workers' Compensation (Physician)
8226	Insurance — Other (Physician)
8227	Insurance — Officers' Life (Physician)
8230	Pension and Retirement Benefits (Physician)
8231	Pension (Physician)
8232	Deferred Compensation (Physician)
8233	Severance Plan (Physician)
8235	Professional Development (Physician)
8240	Books and Subscriptions (Physician)
8245	Dues and Memberships (Physician)
8250	Licenses (Physician)
8255	Meetings (Physician)
8260	Travel (Physician)
8265	Medical Reimbursement Plan (Physician)
8270	Vehicles (Physician)
8271	Leased Motor Vehicles (Physician)
8275	Parking (Physician)
8280	Telephones (Physician)
8285	Beepers (Physician)
8290	Meals and Entertainment (Physician)
8295	Other Benefits (Physician)
8300	MIDLEVEL PROVIDERS — SALARIES
8310	Salaries, Distributions and Incentives (Midlevel)
8320	Salaries — Owner/Stockholder (Midlevel)
8330	Distributions and Incentives (Midlevel)
8340	Global/Capitation Distributions (Midlevel)
8350	Employee Salaries (Midlevel)
8360	Employee Incentives (Midlevel)
8370	Administrative Salaries (Midlevel)
8380	Other Compensation (Midlevel)

Exhibit 4.10 continued

Account Number	Description
8400	MIDLEVEL PROVIDERS — EMPLOYEE-RELATED EXPENSES
8410	Payroll Taxes (Midlevel)
8411	Payroll Taxes — FICA/Medicare (Midlevel)
8412	Payroll Taxes — Federal Unemployment Insurance (Midlevel)
8413	Payroll Taxes — State Unemployment Insurance (Midlevel)
8414	Payroll Taxes — Other (Midlevel)
8420	Insurance (Midlevel)
8421	Insurance — Health (Midlevel)
8422	Insurance — Dental (Midlevel)
8423	Insurance — Life (Midlevel)
8424	Insurance — Disability (Midlevel)
8425	Insurance — Workers' Compensation (Midlevel)
8426	Insurance — Other (Midlevel)
8430	Pension and Retirement Benefits (Midlevel)
8431	Pension (Midlevel)
8432	Deferred Compensation (Midlevel)
8433	Severance Plan (Midlevel)
8435	Professional Development (Midlevel)
8440	Books and Subscriptions (Midlevel)
8445	Dues and Memberships (Midlevel)
8450	Licenses (Midlevel)
8455	Meetings (Midlevel)
8460	Travel (Midlevel)
8465	Medical Reimbursement Plan (Midlevel)
8470	Vehicles (Midlevel)
8475	Parking (Midlevel)
8480	Telephones (Midlevel)
8485	Beepers (Midlevel)
8490	Meals and Entertainment (Midlevel)
8495	Other Benefits (Midlevel)

9000 NONOP REVENUE & EXP; INCOME TAXES & OTHER EXP

9100 Nonoperating Revenues

Revenues not directly related to patient care of the provision of medical services. Sub-accounts 9110 - 9170 are not intended to be definitive but only to show the general nature of nonoperating revenues. The nature of nonoperating revenues will vary greatly from organization to organization. Each entity should determine the accounts that will best serve its own needs.

9110 Interest Income

Interest earned on marketable securities, certificates of deposit, savings accounts and/or other short-term investments.

9120 Income from Long-Term Investments

Income from securities and other long-term investments not currently used in the organization's operations. Includes interest, dividends and/or capital gains earned on certificates of deposit, securities, stocks, bonds and/or other long-term investments.

9130 Property Rentals

Rent/lease revenue received from property owned by the organization but not used in organization operations.

9140 Unrealized Gains and Losses — Investments

The accounting recognition of the difference between the fair market value of carried investments and the adjusted cost (current "book" value) of those investments for the period.

9150 Realized Gains and Losses — Investments

Gains or losses recognized on closed and sold securities during the period.

9160 Donations Received (Nonoperating Revenue)

Any endowment or gift revenue received by the organization for nonoperational activities such as facility construction.

9170 Nonoperating Subsidy Income

Medical practices may receive nonoperational support from a parent organization for capitalization projects such as facility construction.

9200 Nonoperating Expenses

Expenses not directly related to patient care or the provision of medical services. Sub-accounts 9210 - 9240 are not intended to be definitive but only to show the general nature of nonoperating expenses. The nature of nonoperating expenses will vary greatly from organization to organization. Each entity should determine the accounts that will best serve its own needs.

9210 Interest Expense

Interest incurred on borrowings not related to organization operations.

9220 Contributions Expense

Amounts paid out by the organization to recognized nonprofit entities or to charitable causes.

9230 Current Income Tax Expense (Recovery)

Taxes, based on net profit, paid to federal, state or local government. Sub-accounts 9231 - 9233 may be used to facilitate individual tax reporting.

For cash-basis accounting, income taxes equal the cash payment or refund for the previous tax year paid or received during the current tax year plus all periodic estimates paid for current year taxes during the current year.

For accrual accounting, the income tax equals the total tax liability for the current year regardless of when the tax was paid or refunds received.

9231 Current Income Taxes — Federal

9232 Current Income Taxes — State

9233 Current Income Taxes — Other

9240 Deferred Income Tax Expense (Recovery)

Taxes, based on net profit, paid to federal, state or local government. Sub-accounts 9241 - 9243 may be used to facilitate individual tax reporting.

9241 Current Income Taxes — Federal

9242 Current Income Taxes — State

9243 Current Income Taxes — Other

9300 Other Income/Expense

Amounts of a nonoperating nature not recorded elsewhere including extraordinary gains/losses.

EXHIBIT 4.11

Account Number	Description
9000	**NONOP REVENUE & EXP; INCOME TAXES & OTHER EXP**
9100	Nonoperating revenues
9110	Interest Income
9120	Income from Long-Term — Investments
9130	Property Rentals
9140	Unrealized Gains and Losses — Investments
9150	Realized Gains and Losses — Investments
9160	Donations Received (Nonoperating Revenue)
9170	Nonoperating Subsidy Income
9200	Nonoperating Expenses
9210	Interest Expense
9220	Contributions/Donations Expense
9230	Current Income Tax Expense (Recovery)
9231	Current Income Taxes — Federal
9232	Current Income Taxes — State
9233	Current Income Taxes — Other
9240	Deferred Income Tax Expense (Recovery)
9241	Deferred Income Taxes — Federal
9242	Deferred Income Taxes — State
9243	Deferred Income Taxes — Other
9300	Other Income/Expense

5

Adapting the Chart of Accounts to Activity-Based Costing

Beverly H. Donehoo, M.Ed., CMPE and Leanne C. Travers

Today's Need for More Sophisticated Tools

Traditional financial management accounting and reporting processes are simply not adequate in a managed-care environment. The traditional accounting approach to financial reporting has historically focused on total revenue collected and total expenses incurred. The financial management and reporting needs of today's physician organizations (PO) are far more abundant and complex. For example, is your physician organization currently able to answer the following questions?

1. What is the actual Resource-Based Relative Value Scale (RBRVS) unit cost for each provider, clinical program and member practice within your physician organization?

2. What is the variance between the monthly payment of each capitation contract and the actual utilization costs per-provider, per-clinical program and per-member practice?

3. What is the cost of services for a particular bundled procedure, diagnosis related group (DRG) or clinical protocol?

Focusing on Costs

In today's managed-care environment, successful financial management must focus on cost of services and not on income received. Detailed cost information is necessary for conducting payer negotiations, strategic business planning and clinical pathways review. To obtain detailed expense information, every aspect of PO operations, both clinical and administrative, has to be delineated and costed. This can only be achieved by implementing Activity-Based Cost (ABC) accounting. In doing so, conventional accounting practices are in no way hindered or compromised.

Financial systems that are structured with a bottom-up versus a top-down approach allow users to combine relevant building blocks of information to produce the specific data needed for a particular task. The information must be current if a PO is to be prepared to respond to the unknown and the unexpected. If not, the practice loses control of the operation.

Preparing for the Unexpected

Too often, POs are unprepared for sudden cash-flow crises. To prepare the PO to respond to the unexpected, ABC accounting systems can be set up to routinely provide data for the purpose of dissecting the viability of every aspect of PO operations. Once in place, the series of reports and analyses serves as an early alarm system. Deviations in accounts receivable (A/R), expenditures or operations activity are quickly identified and an appropriate response can prevent a crises. Examples of such situations include the following:

1. A major payer withholds or delays claims payments, resulting in a devastating blow to the provider's cash flow.

2. Without notification, a payer changes the regulations for claims submission or procedure authorization — even for services that have already been provided. Claims are initially denied and paid only after a lengthy review process. Cash flow to the PO is severely compromised at the same time that overhead costs increase because of additional administrative effort spent to resolve the contract and claims issues with the payer.

Having an in-depth knowledge of all aspects of the organization allows PO management to develop contingency financial management and operations plans as a hedge against the unexpected. A PO can implement carefully conceived contingency plans instead of panicking when managed care erects another barrier to smooth operations and prompt payment. These plans can prevent debt accrual and a crisis-management approach that may result in inappropriate and dangerous decisions during the financial crisis.

Dealing with Tricky Reimbursement Scenarios

Financial management is an ever-increasing challenge for practice organizations because of the payment schemes devised by payers. Conventional financial management does not provide the means to determine an accurate accounting of outstanding receivables and maintain a steady cash flow while struggling with today's tricky reimbursement scenarios. Examples of these reimbursement plans are as follows:

1. Capitation risk contracts replete with withhold and bonus/penalty formulations of staggering complexity.

2. Contractual requirements that increase staff and overhead costs (e.g., the need to purchase new medical equipment or outfit a space for a new clinical procedure).

3. Network bundled procedure contracts that cause the PO to receive considerably less per CPT-4 *(Current Procedural Terminology, 4th Edition,* copyright American Medical Association) code.

4. Network claims submission processes that are disorganized and do not pay in a timely fashion. The PO reimbursement portion is apt to be delayed in the network's hospital financial office for weeks, negatively impacting PO cash flow.

5. Reduced Fee-for-Service (FFS) contracts with payers that don't provide the PO with a fee schedule. Every Explanation of Benefits (EOB) is a big surprise.

An ABC accounting system with its associated reporting and analysis structure provides precise data for determining the effect of any individual contract:

1. ABC facilitates the determination of cost of services. At the end of each month, clinical utilization costs can be calculated and compared against per-member per-month (PMPM) income. If costs consistently exceed income, a review to identify the cause and subsequent remedial action will be necessary. This methodology is valid for all types of contractual models.

2. ABC supports contract negotiations. Entering network contract or bundled procedure negotiations without detailed cost information is a formula for disaster. Armed with accurate cost-per-procedure data, payer claims data, and historical data derived from the PO's cost analysis-reporting system, the PO representative is ready to be an informed participant, a strong advocate for the organization and a formidable negotiator.

3. ABC accounting allows the PO to cost clinical services at every level of the organization. Costs can be calculated by CPT-4 code, by ambulatory patient classification (APC) or by DRG.

Managed care is continuing to evolve at almost warp speed. The greatest challenge of the health care industry in general and physician organizations in particular is the ability to convert financial, administrative, and clinical data into the timely and accurate reports and analyses necessary to compete in a dynamic environment.

Activity-Based Cost Accounting Explained

ABC accounting is a type of cost accounting. Unlike conventional financial accounting, cost accounting is a tool primarily used by management to measure internal operations. When management wants to develop cost and performance measures, ABC accounting is the methodology of choice.

ABC accounting was developed in the early 1980s to assist manufacturing companies in determining product cost. Since then, the methodology has proven to be useful in all aspects of a company's operations. ABC is widely accepted as transferable to many other types of businesses. To quote Dr. Robert S. Kaplan, the developer of ABC accounting, "ABC reveals the links between performing particular activities and the demands those activities make on the organization's resources. It can give managers a clear picture of how products, brands, customers, facilities, regions or distribution channels both generate revenue and consume resources." To understand how applicable ABC accounting is to physician organization management, simply substitute health care phrases into Dr. Kaplan's quote: "...clear picture of how patient services, clinical service lines/programs, patients, sites, practices, or payer contracts both generate revenue and consume resources."[1]

As was the objective in manufacturing, ABC analysis can assist a PO in identifying which activities in the organization are viable and which are not. Management then has the ability to set priorities and spend time and money on those efforts that will be most beneficial to improving and protecting the financial viability of the organization.

Getting Started: The Planning Process

To compete successfully in a managed-care environment, physician organizations can no longer run clinical, administrative and financial operations as separate and autonomous entities. The demands of managed-care payers force all parts of a PO to work together if success is to be achieved in each of the operations. This is especially true of a cost-based financial system. The cost data and financial reports and analyses generated by an ABC format are useful for each type of operation: clinical, administrative and financial.

- The physician staff and the ancillary clinical professionals want to be able to determine the cost per CPT-4 code, as well as calculate the cost of a clinical pathway, a bundled procedure, a DRG or an APG. In time, clinicians will be able to document when best practices disease management results in a reduction in patient service costs.
- In order to be an informed and articulate negotiator of payer and provider network contracts, the marketing director wants all of the above but also needs the costs specific to each of the organization's patient sites and affiliated hospitals (locations).
- The administrative director wants the most accurate expense detail possible to conduct financial and operational feasibility studies and analyses for:
    - New clinical program development
    - Short/long range corporate strategic planning
    - Physician compensation plan formulations
    - Staff utilization modeling
    - The ability to respond to ad hoc analysis requests in a timely manner which saves administrative effort

- The reimbursement director needs to know the cost of bundled/global CPT-4 codes so that these costs can be monitored and compared by payer and against contractual allowances and actual reimbursements.

It is the challenge of the administrative director to lead the management team in discussing and planning the system. It is the challenge of the financial director to compile the information requirements of all the teams and work to meet each of these needs when building the final design of the cost-based financial system.

Financial Costing Format Design

The easiest way to initiate discussion about the format of a cost-based chart of accounts is to create a schematic representation of the organization. The schematic should reflect the levels within the organization at which the PO wants to capture expense detail.

The descriptive terms suggested below are fairly generic to every type of physician organization. Do not hesitate to adapt the terms and to re-sort their priority in your design so the final format is specific to your physician organization.

Descriptive Term	Definition
CORPORATE:	Corporation/Partnership/LLC/Foundation — Legal Entity Form
PRACTICE:	Physician group entities within corporation
COST CENTERS:	Categories of income/expenses to be tracked that typically support an organization's clinical "points of service." Examples include overhead departments such as billing, administration and occupancy, often-termed "centers of activity."
ACCOUNT NUMBER:	Basic field of natural expense categories
SITES:	Practice patient service and administration offices
CLINICAL SPECIALTIES:	Practice Medical/Surgical clinical specialties
PROVIDER:	Physician and/or ancillary clinical staff (personnel who provide billable, CPT-coded services)
LOCATIONS:	Non-practice patient care sites: hospitals, ambulatory centers, nursing homes, clinics
SUB-SPECIALTIES/ ANCILLARY SERVICES/ CLINICS/ PROGRAMS:	Further delineation of practice's clinical services

After finalizing the group's list of account number categories, create a map (Exhibit 5.1) of the account number structure of the group's accounting system. Now see how the number of categories and the number of account number segments match up. (For this example, the account number is 20 digits long with no segment restrictions.)

EXHIBIT 5. 1 Northeast Medical Associates

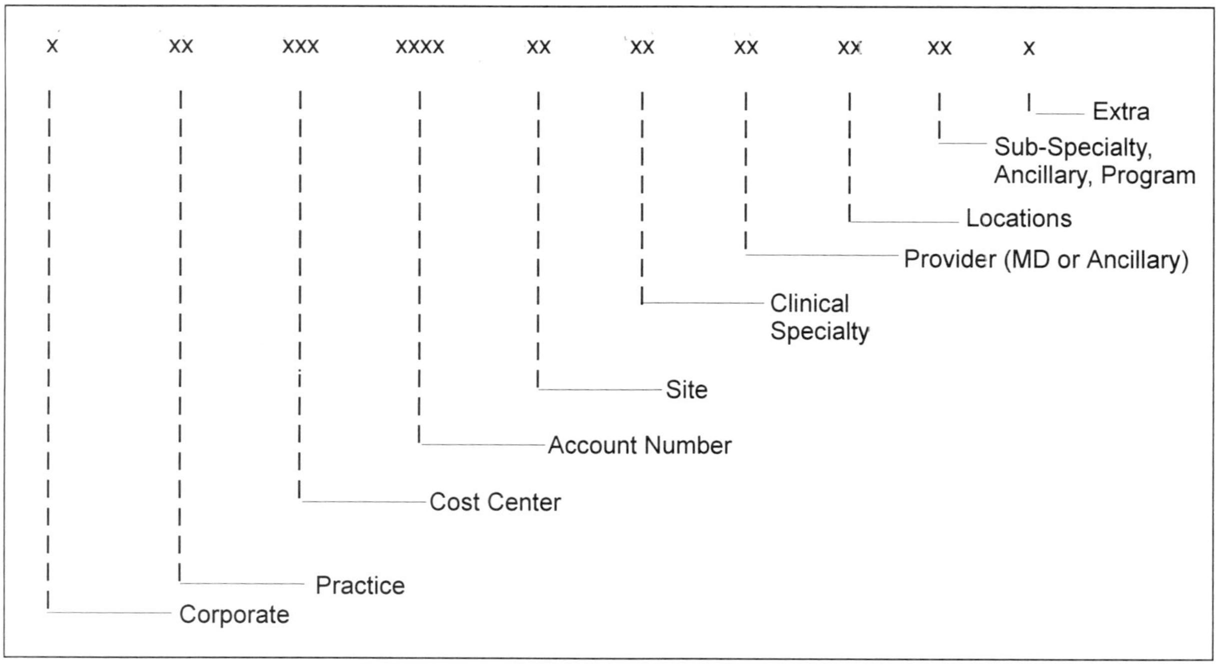

Given that in a cost-based chart of account format four digits are reserved for the basic account number and another two digits are reserved for the cost centers, how many digits remain in the PO accounting system? How many digits does the physician organization require to capture the level of cost detail it desires? Remember that the cost-basis system being created must be adequate not only for today but also capable of growing with the PO for some years to come. Provide enough digits per category segment in anticipation of future growth. Some physician organizations will not need to utilize every digit available in their accounting system. Others will find they currently have a system that cannot provide the range of flexibility required by a cost-based system.

It is at this point that some physician organizations will come to the realization that they must upgrade and/or invest in a more powerful and sophisticated financial system if they are to gain the level of financial, managerial and information resource capability they are seeking. One option is to invest in an "add-on" allocation system. Expense information is exported from the accounting system into the add-on module, and all of the organization's multilayered ABC allocation distribution is managed within the add-on system. Buying the add-on system eliminates the cost, time lost, and stress of a financial system conversion while providing a physician organization with the sophisticated allocation distribution, reporting, analysis and costing capabilities required.

Once an organization's chart of accounts has been expanded and upgraded, the financial management system is ready to be converted into a multifaceted informational resource capable of providing a wide variety of reports and analyses.

Prior to initiating the costing system, the capabilities of the organization's financial software must be assessed. If the accounting system does not have an internal allocation capability (e.g., distribution of direct salary expense to points of service using percentages, ratios or a set dollar amount), expense data can be collected over the course of a month in the general ledger. At the end of the month, export the expense information into a financial system report writer module. The majority of top-level direct expense distributions and indirect allocations can be conducted in the more sophisticated financial system report writer modules. Most likely, the next level of cost breakdown to provider, specialty and program levels will need to be done in a spreadsheet or database. Implementation of the ABC system will be facilitated by determining beforehand which systems will best support the organization's needs.

Converting Plan into Design

ABC is a management tool that provides the ability to determine not only the cost of clinical services but also the supporting administrative operations, both top to bottom and from the bottom to the top. As an analysis tool, ABC is unique in its ability to identify each individual patient service or program and attribute to the service ***only*** those direct and indirect costs required to produce the service. Management can "drill down" and scrutinize the components that contribute to the cost of each service or program within the organization. The degree of benefit derived from an ABC accounting model is directly related to the amount of effort spent planning and designing the system.

The first step in designing the system is to determine and define the points of service and the centers of activity specific to the organization (Exhibit 5.2). In ABC accounting, expenses are captured at either a "point of service" or a "center of activity." Clinical services are delivered at a point of service. Centers of activity are activities that support the delivery of services.

If you install an allocation add-on system, the development of the ABC allocation process is somewhat different, but the ABC concepts remain the same. The following information explains how to adapt a conventional accounting system to one with ABC costing capability. However, this information is relevant when implementing an add-on system, as well as when designing and setting up a system.

EXHIBIT 5. 2 Defining Points of Service and Centers of Activity

Northeast Medical Associates

INCOME	No. Site*		So. Site*		Occup.	Admin.	Clinical	Billing		TOTAL
Fee-For-Service										
Capitation										
EXPENSES										
Salaries/Benefits										
Physicians										
Salary										
Fringe Benefits										
Clinical Staff										
Salary										
Fringe Benefits										
Administrative Staff										
Salary										
Fringe Benefits										
Billing Staff										
Salary										
Fringe Benefits										
Temp. Staff										
Facility Expenses										
Rent										
Property Ins.										
Building Maint.										
Utilities										
Office Equipment										
Maint. Agreement										
Lease Payments										
Supplies										
Service Contracts										
Purchases										
Office Expenses										
Postage										
Federal Express										
Courier										
Printing										
Photography										
Telephone										
Coffee Service										
General Supplies										
Business Expenses										
Workers Comp. Ins.										
Legal										
Accounting										
Prof. Jour/Books										
Stop Loss Ins.										
Clinical Expenses										
Beepers										
Medical Supplies										
Outside Labs										
Equipment Supp.										
Equip. Maint.										
Equip. Lease										
Transcription										
Cellular Phones										
TOTALS										

*Physician; Program; Site and Detail

Direct costs are so named because they are assigned directly to the point of service, while indirect costs are assigned to the appropriate center of activity. The next step is a careful determination of those expenses to assign directly to a point of service and those to assign to a center of activity (Exhibit 5.3). It is worth emphasizing that there is no right or wrong way to set up an ABC system. The objective is to custom design an organization-specific system. The resulting cost data, unique to the organization, is the source of power behind this resource tool.

Assigning direct costs to points of service sounds fairly straightforward but requires more effort than may be initially obvious. An example of this is a PO with multiple practices and with multiple sites. If the physicians and ancillary and administrative staff have an established site rotation schedule, salary and benefit expenses can be directly applied to the various sites using a percentage breakdown that reflects full-time equivalent (FTE) status at each site. However, if rotation schedules change frequently, these expenses can be allocated to the points of service using formulas that reflect the previous month's actual physician and staff site rotations between the various centers of activity.

To implement the ABC system, each expense line item must be categorized, assigned and/or allocated. This is a one-time, albeit extremely critical task. To maximize the usefulness of the cost data produced, all expenses must be detailed to the fullest extent possible.

EXHIBIT 5.3 Assigning Direct Costs

Northeast Medical Associates

INCOME	No. Site*	So. Site*	Occup.	Admin.	Clinical	Billing	TOTAL
Fee-for-Service							
Capitation							
EXPENSES							
Salaries/Benefits							
Physicians							
Salary	646692	448931					**1095623**
Fringe Benefits	220450	156350					**376800**
Clinical Staff							
Salary	151250	96250					**247500**
Fringe Benefits	38000	24400					**62400**
Administration Staff							
Salary				218400			**218400**
Fringe Benefits				79100			**79100**
Billing Staff							
Salary						71500	**71500**
Fringe Benefits						23800	**23800**
Temp. Staff				5000			**5000**
Facility Expense							
Rent			127000				**127000**
Property Ins.			2500				**2500**
Building Maint.			7480				**7480**
Utilities			8000				**8000**
Office Equipment							
Maint. Agreement				2500			**2500**
Lease Payments				3000		7000	**10000**
Supplies				4000		2000	**6000**
Service Contracts				750		750	**1500**
Purchases				2000		3000	**5000**
Office Expenses							
Postage				4000		6000	**10000**
Federal Express				1500			**1500**
Courier				500			**500**
Printing				5000			**5000**
Photography				300			**300**
Telephone				6600		10000	**16600**
Coffee Service				1200			**1200**
General Supplies				10000			**10000**
Business Expenses							
Workers' Comp. Ins.				1250			**1250**
Legal				3500			**3500**
Accounting				10000			**10000**
Prof. Jour./Books				500			**500**
Stop Loss Inc.						10000	**10000**
Clinical Expenses							
Beepers					600		**600**
Medical Supplies					16160		**16160**
Outside Labs					38632		**38632**
Equipment Supp.					2000		**2000**
Equip. Maint.					2000		**2000**
Equip. Lease					2700		**2700**
Transcription					25000		**25000**
Cellular Phones					6000		**6000**
TOTALS	**1056392**	**725931**	**144980**	**359100**	**93082**	**134050**	**2513545**

*Physician; Program; Site and Detail

The "art" of ABC accounting is the allocation of expenses to the centers of activity (Exhibit 5.4). Indirect costs are distributed to each of the points of service using allocation formulas. Expense allocation formulas should accurately reflect the actual utilization of resources by each center of activity. When first implementing the ABC system, actual usage breakdown of all overhead expenses by each of the points of service may not be available. This lack of information should not be allowed to delay the project. Initial best-guess distribution formulas can be updated as actual usage information is obtained.

NOTE: Always document the date, the formula and any changes made to each allocation. This prevents confusion when comparing financial reports from one fiscal period to another.

Before beginning the process of allocating costs associated with centers of activity to the points of service, costs associated with certain centers of activity may need to be allocated to other centers of activity. For example, occupancy costs must be allocated to both the administration and billing centers of activity, as well as to the various points of service.

EXHIBIT 5.4 Allocating Indirect Costs

Northeast Medical Associates

INCOME	No. Site*	So. Site*	Occup.	Admin.	Clinical	Billing	TOTALS
Fee-For-Service							
Capitation							
EXPENSES							
Salaries/Benefits							
Physicians	867142	605281					**1472423**
Salary							
Fringe Benefits							
Clinical Staff	189250	120650					**309900**
Salary							
Fringe Benefits							
Administrative Staff				297500			**297500**
Salary							
Fringe Benefits							
Billing Staff						95300	**95300**
Salary							
Fringe Benefits							
Temp. Staff				5000			**5000**
Facility Expenses			144980				**144980**
Office Equipment				12250		12750	**25000**
Office Expenses				29100		16000	**45100**
Business Expenses				15250		10000	**25250**
Clinical Expense					93092		**93092**
Sub-Totals	**1056392**	**725931**	**144980**	**359100**	**93092**	**134050**	**2513545**
Occupancy	97137		(97137)				
		47843	(47843)				
Administration	240597			(240597)			
		118503		(118503)			
Clinical	62372				(62372)		
		30720			(30720)		
Billing	89814					(89814)	
		44236				(44236)	
Sub-Totals	489920	241302					
TOTAL	**1546312**	**967233**	**0**	**0**	**0**	**0**	**2513545**

*Physician; Program; Site and Detail

Allocation of indirect expenses (Exhibit 5.4) represents the first layer of ABC costing. After determining site costs, it is now possible to determine individual provider costs by following the same steps: Determine each provider's direct costs (Exhibit 5.5) and then use appropriate allocation formulas to attribute indirect costs. This same process can be used for costing clinical specialties, ancillary programs, etc., by simply determining the direct costs and then distributing indirect costs using relevant and accurate allocation formulas.

EXHIBIT 5.5 Provider Expense Allocation

Direct Compensation Expense (as defined in EXHIBIT 5.8)

Salary
Pension Plan
Dental Insurance
Health Insurance
Life Insurance
Disability Insurance
FICA & Medicare
Travel
Books/Journals
Licenses
Professional Dues/Memberships
Other

Direct Overhead Expense

Malpractice Insurance Expense
Percentage FTE of Dedicated/Assigned Clinical Staff Costs
Percentage FTE of Dedicated/Assigned Clerical Staff Costs
Other

Indirect Overhead Expense (as percentage of pRVUs [practice expense RVUs] or other allocation methodology)

Occupancy
Administration
Clinical
Billing
Other

Developing Cost Analysis Capability

After designing a complete ABC costing program and installing it into the financial system, match the cost data with claims utilization data so that the myriad of reports and analyses the PO requires can be generated. This is where the management team will reap the rewards of its system design planning efforts. The team should reconvene to discuss what standard reports and analysis capabilities it requires now and those that it anticipates needing in the future. One of the most powerful attributes of ABC is the ability to create customized analyses.

The onset of managed care with its unending demands for information has far outstripped the capability of the majority of PO information systems. Before going further, review some of the basics of your practice management system.

1. Is the PO capturing all patient utilization information? As obvious as it seems the answer to this question should be, it is often the case that not all information is captured. A case in point:

   An OB/GYN group has large global OB payer contracts. The group only enters OB patient data during the first patient visit and then one more time months later after the patient delivers. At that point, a bill is produced to send to the payer. None of the clinical utilization information from the intervening nine months is recorded. The clinical care is recorded in detail in the medical record, but in order to perform utilization and cost analyses, all patient clinical utilization activity must be recorded in the practice management system. This is true for all managed care payer plans whether they are FFS, global, bundled or capitated contracts. Without this information, it is impossible to determine if the cost of services (capitation utilization, global procedures, bundled procedures) exceeds or falls below payments.

2. How is the practice management system configured? To what degree have the identifying location categories been delineated? The objective is to match as closely as possible the data categories of the financial system to those of the reimbursement system.

Financial System	***Reimbursement System***
Practice	**Practice**
Sites	**Sites**
Provider	**Provider**
Location	**Location**

3. How detailed are the payer category files in the reimbursement system? Did the PO reimbursement staff establish generic payer categories, or did they list all payer plans with accompanying details? If the system has this capability, ensure that the capability is operational. Capturing utilization information specific to each payer and plan is imperative. This information is essential for a number of reasons but is particularly indispensable in contract renegotiations.

4. Has the current list of the RBRVS relative value units (RVUs) been entered onto the practice management system?

ABC costing can be accomplished using a variety of relative value systems, but the Health Care Financing Administration's (HCFA's) RBRVS is increasingly becoming the standard throughout the payer industry. Using RBRVS as the basis for your cost calculations ensures your results will correspond to those of the majority of payers.

The financial office needs a full rendering of the current RVUs in spreadsheet or database format. Most practice management system vendors provide RBRVS updates to users. However, a copy of the annually updated RVUs can be purchased on disk from the U.S. Government Printing Office (GPO).

The Printing Office disk version contains the format needed:

CPT	DESCRIPTION	wRVU	pRVU	mRVU	Total
99212	Office/OP visit, established patient	.45	.32	.02	.79

Once a year, it is necessary to update the RVUs in your system. The annual updates are published by HCFA after the RBRVS Update Committee tweaks the RVUs at the end of each calendar year for the next calendar year.

To determine actual internal costs and establish internal financial benchmarks, do not use Geographic Practice Cost Indices (GPCIs). GPCIs are used to determine Medicare reimbursements and adjusted costs. Adjusted costs per RVU, both aggregate and component, are useful for comparing internal costs with those from another region of the country. To use the GPCIs, use the spreadsheet format shown above, but insert three additional columns after the malpractice column. Multiply the three RBRVS components by their respective GPCI components (also on the GPO disk). Insert another column after the total RVUs column and label it *Total Adjusted RVUs*.

Choose a timeframe. If an annual timeframe is chosen, use the annual production data (all CPT codes generated by the practice and their frequencies), and apply the corresponding RVUs to determine unit cost (Exhibit 5.6).

PO Unit Cost	**=**	**Total PO Expense**	**÷**	**Total PO RVUs**

EXHIBIT 5.6 Total Production Units

NORTHEAST MEDICAL ASSOCIATES				
				TOTAL
CPT	Procedure Description	RBRVs	QTY.	RBRVs
36410	Drawing blood	0.4	5588	2235.20
86580	TB intradermal test	0.26	128	33.28
93272	Ecg/review, interpret only	0.97	1340	1299.80
99204	Office/outpatient. new	2.86	336	960.96
99205	Office/outpatient, new	3.61	400	1444.00
99211	Office/outpatient, est	0.38	1344	510.72
99212	Office/outpatient, est	0.75	228	171.00
99213	Office/outpatient, est	1.08	2772	2993.76
99214	Office/outpatient, est	1.64	7996	13113.44
99215	Office/outpatient, est	2.6	1908	4960.80
99217	Observation care discharge	1.84	4	7.36
99219	Observation care	3.28	8	26.24
99220	Observation care	4.22	8	33.76
99223	Initial hospital care	4.2	216	907.20
99232	Subsequent hospital care	1.55	356	551.80
99233	Subsequent hospital care	2.16	612	1321.92
99238	Hospital discharge day	1.83	260	475.80
99243	Office consultation	2.79	4	11.16
99244	Office consultation	3.92	48	188.16
99245	Office consultation	5.28	8	42.24
99253	Initial inpatient consult	2.87	12	34.44
99254	Initial inpatient consult	3.95	64	252.80
99255	Initial inpatient consult	5.36	4	21.44
99262	Follow up inpatient consult	1.35	28	37.80
99263	Follow up inpatient consult	1.98	28	55.44
99282	Emergency dept visit	0.96	8	7.68
99283	Emergency dept visit	1.77	32	56.64
99303	Nursing facility care	3.03	76	230.28
99312	Nursing facility care, subseq	1.44	44	63.36
99313	Nursing facility care, subseq	1.92	416	798.72
99342	Home visit, new patient	2.17	4	8.68
99395	Preventive visit, est, 18 - 39	2.69	12	32.28
99396	Preventive visit, est, 40 - 64	3.02	468	1413.36
TOTAL				**34301.52**

Because time has been taken to detail expenses at the various sub-levels within the organization, they can now be retrieved and entered into this formula, thereby providing unit costs per site, per provider, per specialty, and per ancillary service. Be sure that the time frame for the expenses coincides with the time frame for the production data.

Once the unit cost has been calculated, return to the Total Production Units worksheet (Exhibit 5.6). Add an additional column on the right side, and title it "CPT Cost" (Exhibit 5.7). For the sake of illustration, use $64.60 as the unit cost. To calculate the cost per code, multiply the unit cost by the total relative value units for each code.

CPT Code	RVU x Unit Code	Cost per Code
99211	.38 x $64.60	$24.55

Continue the calculation down the length of the spreadsheet to determine the cost of providing each clinical service.

EXHIBIT 5.7 Cost Per CPT Code

NORTHEAST MEDICAL ASSOCIATES

CPT	PROCEDURE DESCRIPTION	RBRVs	QTY.	TOTAL RBRVs	TOTAL COST
36410	Drawing Blood	0.4	5588	2235.20	25.84
86580	TB Intradermal test	0.26	128	33.28	16.80
93272	Ecg/review, interpret only	0.97	1340	1299.80	62.66
99204	Office/outpatient, new	2.86	336	960.96	184.76
99205	Office/outpatient, new	3.61	400	1444.00	233.21
99211	Office/outpatient, est	0.38	1344	510.72	24.55
99212	Office/outpatient, est	0.75	228	171.00	48.45
99213	Office/outpatient, est	1.08	2772	2993.76	69.77
99214	Office/outpatient, est	1.64	7996	13113.44	105.94
99215	Office/outpatient, est	2.6	1908	4960.80	167.96
99217	Observation care discharge	1.84	4	7.36	118.86
99219	Observation care	3.28	8	26.24	211.89
99220	Observation care	4.22	8	33.76	272.61
99223	Initial hospital care	4.2	216	907.20	271.32
99232	Subsequent hospital care	1.55	356	551.80	100.13
99233	Subsequent hospital care	2.16	612	1321.92	139.54
99238	Hospital discharge day	1.83	260	475.80	118.22
99243	Office consultation	2.79	4	11.16	180.23
99244	Office consultation	3.92	48	188.16	253.23
99245	Office consultation	5.28	8	42.24	341.09
99253	Initial inpatient consult	2.87	12	34.44	185.40
99254	Initial inpatient consult	3.95	64	252.80	255.17
99255	Initial inpatient consult	5.36	4	21.44	346.26
99262	Follow up inpatient consult	1.35	28	37.80	87.21
99263	Follow up inpatient consult	1.98	28	55.44	127.91
99282	Emergency dept visit	0.96	8	7.68	62.02
99283	Emergency dept visit	1.77	32	56.64	114.34
99303	Nursing facility care	3.03	76	230.28	195.74
99312	Nursing facility care, subseq	1.44	44	63.36	93.02
99313	Nursing facility care, subseq	1.92	416	798.72	140.18
99342	Home visit, new patient	2.17	4	8.68	173.77
99395	Preventive visit, est, 18 - 39	2.69	12	32.28	195.09
99396	Preventive visit, est, 40 - 64	3.02	468	1413.36	
TOTAL				34301.52	

For ease of explanation, the example depicts total RVUs and total expenses. To increase the usefulness of the cost data, especially for comparison with national cost surveys, expenses should be tracked by component RVU, breaking expenses down to match the three RVU component categories: Provider Compensation or Work, Practice Expense (i.e., overhead) and Malpractice.

Provider Compensation Expenses:	wRVU
Overhead Expenses:	pRVU
Malpractice Insurance Expense:	mRVU

EXHIBIT 5.8

COMPONENT EXPENSE WORKSHEET

	Details	Subtotals	Totals
Total Practice Expense			$2,703,672
Provider Compensation Expense (see details column)		1,229,250	- 1,226,550
(Include all personnel who provide medical services [billable CPT codes] for the practice, such as nurse practitioners, physician assistants, dietitians, physical therapists, etc. If any provider plays a dual role, i.e., clinical and managerial, include only the percentage of expenses that apply to compensation for clinical services. For example, if a provider is slated to spend 60 percent of her time providing clinical services and 40 percent providing administrative services, multiply all compensation figures for that provider by 60 percent. Include expenses for salaried staff and for providers working under contract, whether permanent, temporary or PRN.)			
Salaries	1,060,395		
Pension Plan Contribution	48,000		
Health Insurance	54,539		
Dental Insurance	10,000		
Life Insurance	4,354		
Disability Insurance (include if, in case of disability, benefits will be paid to provider and not to practice)	7,651		
FICA & Medicare (employer portion)	41,311		
Travel	1,000		
Books/Journals	500		
Licenses	1,000		
Professional Dues/Memberships	500		
Other	0		
Malpractice insurance expense		32,514	- 32,514
Overhead expenses (the remainder)			**$1,441,908**

After calculating cost per component RVU, multiply these component costs by the corresponding component RVU for each CPT code. Add these three figures for each CPT code to calculate the total cost per CPT code.[2]

Because ABC formats and delineates expenses at the various sub-levels within the organization, expenses can be readily retrieved and entered into the appropriate categories. The inclusion of bonuses is discretionary but not recommended.

This is one of many informative and multifaceted reports that can now be produced using an ABC accounting system. The report takes on great significance when an additional column is added to the report for each of the PO's payer contracts. Under each payer column, fill in the current allowable for each CPT procedure. The cost of providing care can now be compared against the payer allowable per procedure.

Implementing the Design

The final step to creating a costing capability is to begin developing a package of cost reports and a set of cost data spreadsheets or files that feed information into the cost reports. The number and types of reports and data files will be determined over time. The frequency of updates to the various reports will depend on the makeup of the PO. However, every PO will require certain standard reports.

For instance, POs with capitation contracts of any size will generally want to create an end-of-month utilization report template for each capitation plan:

CPT Code/RVUs	X	CPT COST	X	UTIL. TOT.	=	TOTAL COST

Remember to update the variables in the worksheet when appropriate. **(Always document any changes made on the respective report.)** The CPT Cost will change from month to month as group expenses fluctuate. The per-CPT utilization figure will be unique each month.

The intent is to determine if the group's Total Utilization Cost exceeds the PMPM payment amount for that month. If it does, the PO now has the information and capability necessary to drill down and determine underlying causes. Is it over utilization by a particular physician or site? Has the number of covered lives for a contract changed, and the payer has not notified or paid the PO accordingly? Once the cause is determined, informed decisions can be made concerning remedial actions to take.

One of the most effective uses of costing data is the ability to readily respond to ad hoc requests. To facilitate this ad hoc ability, establish data files or spreadsheets, and ensure that the data is current and accurate.

For example, set up an Expense Sheet for each of the providers. Update the sheets regularly as compensation, direct and indirect expenses change. **(Always document changes with a description and date.)** Set up similar expense sheets for each entity delineated in the costing schematic. Maintaining current and accurate data files or spreadsheets will greatly facilitate unexpected ad hoc analysis requests.

An example of an ad hoc analysis request is the following. Upcoming fiscal year departmental budgets have been submitted in a large academic medical center. The chief financial officer demands that 10 percent across-the-board cuts be made in each clinical department. Departments with detailed cost information are prepared for such a situation. Due to the accurate and current cost information on every segment of the department's operation, the physicians, staff and the medical center realize that the cost-cutting decisions made by the department are based on sound and substantiated administrative judgement.

Another type of ad hoc report and analysis request is generated in response to new or renewal of payer contracts. If the contract is a new one, the cost of services data can be compared with the proposed fee schedule. Often, new contracts impact group clinical and patient management operations. Does the payer require longer patient hours? Will the contract considerably increase the patient load? Does the payer require that certain medical procedures be performed in the physician office instead of an ambulatory setting? Will that mean the PO has to outfit a new treatment room just for the procedure? What will be the impact on overhead expenses? Staff utilization? Physician schedules? All of these variables can be entered into a "what if" model of current expense detail and new contract requirements.

Additionally, when preparing for contract renewal negotiations, the PO now has months of utilization and cost reports providing a very detailed rendering per CPT code and evidence of the success of this contract during the previous years. The marketing director can enter negotiations fully informed, equipped to initiate tactics and respond appropriately. The marketing director is also prepared for bundled fee negotiations with the physicians and hospital representatives of the health care network. Most POs enter network global and bundled fee discussions with payment requests based on Medicare and other payable allowables. **The question is, however, does the allowable cover the cost of providing the service?** If not, the PO will lose money consistently. Since reimbursements will in all likelihood not increase, the PO's challenge is to reduce cost so that service costs do not exceed payer allowables.

By establishing an ABC costing capability, all of the necessary detailed building blocks of information are available to compile an analysis or report of almost any kind. The organization now has the tools necessary for controlling costs and utilization, the indispensable keys to flourishing within a capitation framework. The organization leadership can rest easy knowing that the group is prepared to respond to the continuing waves of change in the managed-care market. The organization now fully possesses the data necessary for successfully navigating the turbulent managed care waters.

References

[1] Cooper, Robin and Kaplan, Robert S., "Profit Priorities frcm Activity-Based Costing," *Harvard Business Review* (May - June 1991): 130–135.

[2] Berlin, Mark, "Using Cost Accounting in a Medical Group Practice," *MGM Journal,* Vol. 42, No. 3, (May - June 1995): 22–30.

6

Adapting the Chart of Accounts to Small Group Practices

Hal Prink, FHFMA

Dedication: This chapter is dedicated to an MGMA member who had a great influence on my health care career. Bob Hall, past president of MGMA and administrator of the Diagnostic Clinic of Houston worked with me on a number of financial management issues; we served on MGMA committees and both worked as consultants on the MGMA accounting system in the late 1970s. Bob passed away in 1995; he is greatly missed by his family and friends.

Introduction

This chapter will address chart of account issues for small groups (physician practices with 10 or fewer physicians). These practices face many of the same challenges of larger practices but not at the same level of complexity. For this reason, the chart of accounts can be scaled down from the examples shown in the "General Detailed Chart of Accounts" shown in a table in the Appendix.

In this section of the book we will address the following issues:

- Accounting methods
- Uses of accounting data for small group practices and adaptability for expansion based on operational changes
- Account structure
- Application to MGMA Surveys

Accounting Methods

A determination of the method of accounting needs to be made before developing an accounting system and structure. Although many accountants recommend accrual-basis accounting, a small medical group may have limitations that make the modified cash basis of accounting more practical. Considerations include:

1. **Physicians' understanding of the accounting process.** The more knowledgeable physicians in the group are of business practices, the more likely they will understand the accrual method.

2. **Skills of a bookkeeping staff.** Many times small offices cannot afford to hire trained accountants or bookkeepers who can accurately keep accrual-based accounting records.

3. **Your accountant's recommendations.** Work with your accountant to help you decide what method will be most beneficial to your medical group.

The accrual basis of accounting allows expenses to be recorded during the time period they benefit and the income during the period it is earned. The rationale for using accrual basis is that you need to know accurate, current financial information. The practice owners, potential investors, banking institutions, and many others require the financial reports to reflect the organization's value at a given point in time.

The modified cash basis of accounting focuses on the collection of revenues or receipts rather than gross production and contractual adjustments. Revenue is recorded at the time cash is received, and expenses are recorded at the time they are paid. Since most small medical groups pay all of their expenses on a monthly basis, recording accounts payable on the balance sheet becomes less important. Neither receivables nor prepaid expenses are recorded in the modified cash method. This may cause some to think it does not provide accurate data because it may inflate expenses and not show income in the period it was earned instead of in the period income was received.

The major argument in the past for using modified cash-basis accounting was that physicians did not want to pay income taxes on money they had not received. This can still be a valid reason for using the modified cash basis. If a group chooses to use the accrual method, they can keep their financial records on the accrual basis and tax records on the cash basis. Using the accrual method for monthly financial statements and the cash method for tax purposes is a legal and common practice. When the original text "Financial Management for Medical Groups" was written in 1978, the health care environment was not as complex and small groups, at that time, were referred to "as groups with limited objectives." Today, no matter what size the medical group, the complexity with managed care, mergers, acquisitions and buyouts, to name a few, makes all groups much more complex than 20 years ago.

For information on the need for accrual accounting in medical groups refer to the paper, "The Need For Accrual Accounting in Physician Owned Medical Groups" by Bruce C. Steinhardt, FACMPE, March 24, 1994, MGMA Library Resource Center.

Use of Accounting Data for Small Groups

Accounting information in medical groups has numerous users and purposes. Grouped into two major areas of internal and external, some of these are listed below:

Internal

- Physician owners
- Management information
- Planning and control
- Short- and long-term decision making
- Pricing of services
- Determination and analysis of managed care contracts
- Use in surveys conducted by MGMA
- Use on a comparative basis for groups of similar size and/or type
- Benchmarking purposes
- Cost reporting

External

- Potential investors
- Lending institutions
- Tax reporting
- Financial statement audits
- Potential buyers

For these and many more reasons, accounting records must be accurate, timely, provide the necessary financial information and be easily understood by the reader. This is where the development of the chart of accounts comes into effect. There are certain steps you must go through in developing any chart of accounts, regardless of the size or type of organization. The steps are as follows:

1. Obtain the current chart of accounts being used.
2. Identify the needs of your accounting information using the list above and others that may be appropriate for your medical group.
3. Determine the goals and objectives of your accounting system.
4. Review the current chart of accounts and determine if revisions can be made or if a totally new chart of accounts needs to be implemented.
5. Implement the new chart of accounts and tie its structure into your financial statements.
6. Prepare a list of the new chart of accounts with a detailed description of what is included in each account and provide to all staff for their use.
7. Develop a reporting format for your financial statements to reflect which account numbers are included in each line item of the financial statements.
8. Consider the accounting software package that you will use and any limitations it may have.

Account Structure

As discussed in Chapter 2, which outlines the chart of accounts, the structure is in a format that allows for minimum or maximum detail. This is done through the process of summarizing categories (of assets, liabilities, equity, revenues and expenses) using the last digit of the account (zero) as the summary number and 1 - 9 in the last digit rolling up to the zero account so data can be summarized without extensive detail. An example follows:

EXHIBIT 6. 1

Account Number	Description
7540	Utilities
7541	Utilities — Water
7542	Utilities — Electricity
7543	Utilities — Waste Disposal
7544	Other Utilities

In this example the last digits 1 - 4 can be rolled up into the overall utilities Account 7540 for reporting purposes. You will find a similar pattern throughout this chart of accounts that will allow you to expand and collapse the accounts to meet your practice's accounting requirements. In this book are both summary and detailed versions of the same chart of accounts. Smaller medical group practices (with fewer than 10 full-time equivalent providers) may find that the summary version of the accounts suits their needs. Sometimes you may have to utilize additional accounts that are included in the detailed version of this chart of accounts. The key is to start with the basic templates of account structure and external financial information users. This chart of accounts is very comprehensive and for purposes of small group practices, there are some brief examples in the categories below.

Assets

Assets are the property or economic resources owned by a business. They are usually classified in terms of current or short-term assets that are expected to be used or consumed in the normal course of business operations in a year or less. Noncurrent or long-term assets are expected to last longer than a year.

Some assets, such as furniture, fixtures and equipment, are depreciated each year. That is, a portion of the cost of the asset is assigned as an expense to a certain period. Accounts for furniture, fixture and equipment in the 1700 series in the example on the next page have corresponding depreciation accounts in the 1800 series. The 1700 series accounts can be expanded into great detail (see detailed chart of accounts in the Appendix) or summed into the major account categories ending in zero depending on the accounting needs of your organization. Matching accumulated depreciation accounts (1800 series) should be used for any 1700 account utilized.

EXHIBIT 6. 2 Assets (In an accrual-based system)

Account Number	Description	Accrual	Modified Cash	Cash
1100	Cash	X	X	X
1110	Cash — Banks	X	X	X
1111	General Checking Accounts	X	X	X
1112	Payroll Checking Accounts	X	X	X
1113	Other Checking Accounts	X	X	X
1120	Cash — On Hand	X	X	X
1121	Change Fund	X	X	X
1122	Petty Cash	X	X	X
1130	Cash — Restricted	X	X	X
1200	Marketable Securities & Short -Term Investments	X	X	X
1210	Valuation Allowance — Short-Term Investments	X	X	X
1300	Accounts Receivable [1]	X	X	
1301	Accounts Receivable — Fee-for-Service Amounts	X	X	
1302	Accounts Receivable — Prepaid Contracts	X	X	
1320	Allowance for Estimated uncollectable Receivables	X	X	
1321	Allowance for Bad Debts — Patient Amounts	X	X	
1322	Allowance for Contractual Adjustments	X	X	
1323	Allowance for Bad Debts — Third-Party Payers	X	X	
1324	Allowance for Charity Care	X	X	
1340	Notes Receivable — Short Term	X	X	X
1345	Managed Care Contract — Bonus/Withhold	X	X	
1350	Other Short-Term Receivables [2]	X	X	X
1351	Interest Receivables	X	X	
1352	Intercompany Receivables	X	X	X
1353	Due from Employees	X	X	X
1354	Due from Related Parties	X	X	X
1400	Supply Inventories	X	X	
1401	Drugs and Medications	X	X	
1402	Medical Supplies	X	X	
1403	Administrative Supplies	X	X	
1404	Forms	X	X	
1405	Housekeeping and Maintenance	X	X	
1406	Linen Supplies	X	X	
1407	Other Supplies	X	X	
1420	Ancillary Department Supplies	X	X	
1500	Prepaid Expenses	X	X	
1510	Other Current Assets	X	X	X
1600	**INVESTMENTS — LONG-TERM RECEIVABLES**	X	X	X
1610	Long-Term Receivables	X	X	X
1630	Long-Term Investments	X	X	X
1635	Valuation Allowance — Long-Term Investments	X	X	X
1700	**PROPERTY, FURNITURE, FIXTURES & EQUIPMENT**	X	X	
1710	REAL PROPERTY	X	X	
1750	FURNITURE, FIXTURES & EQUIPMENT	X	X	
1760	Computer	X	X	

Account Number	Description	Accrual	Modified Cash	Cash
1770	Capital Leases — Computer	X	X	
1780	Vehicles	X	X	
1790	Ancillary Service Equipment	X	X	
1795	Capital Leases — Ancillary Service Equipment	X	X	

Exhibit 6.2 continued

[1] You may want to break down your Accounts Receivable in further detail to keep track of individual contracts. This can be done by using Account numbers 1303 - 1319 for the receivables and Account numbers 1325 - 1339 for the allowances.

[2] This level of detail may not be required in your organization. Remember that the sub-accounts 1351-1354 will roll up into the 1350 Account if this level of detail is not needed. The sub-accounts will give you an idea of the types of assets that belong in the 1350 Account, therefore they do serve a purpose if only informational. The same can be said for Accounts 1350, 1400 and 1500.

EXHIBIT 6. 3

Account Number	Description	Accrual	Modified Cash	Cash
1800	**ACCUMULATED DEPRECIATION — PROPERTY, FURNITURE, ETC.**	X	X	
1810	ACCUMULATED DEPRECIATION — REAL PROPERTY	X	X	
1760	Computer	X	X	
1850	ACCUMULATED DEPRECIATION — FURNITURE, FIXTURES & EQUIPMENT	X	X	
1860	Accum Depreciation — Computer	X	X	
1870	Accum Depreciation — Capital Leases — Computer	X	X	
1880	Accum Depreciation — Vehicles	X	X	
1890	Other Accum Depreciation — Ancillary Service Equipment	X	X	
1895	Accum Depreciation — Capital Leases — Ancillary Service Equipment	X	X	

Liabilities

Liabilities, like assets, are considered either current or long term. Current liabilities are obligations that need to be paid within one year and long-term liabilities will mature in a time period of greater than one year. The following is an example of how the current liability accounts are used to record payroll liability on an accrual basis.

With Account 2210—Payroll Tax Withholdings Payable—use detail accounts 2211 - 2215 for specific sub-accounts. Detailed sub-accounts (2221 - 2224) under 2220 — Insurance Withholdings Payable — may be used for specific insurance withholding accounts. Under 2250 — Accrued Payroll Liabilities —

detail sub-accounts 2251 - 2257 allow you to keep track of individual payroll accruals that are due to employees based on benefits or tax withholdings. Not all sub-accounts may be required under Accounts 2310 - 2370; use only the sub-accounts for those expenses appropriate to your practice. As for Account 2400 — Long-Term Liabilities — use Accounts 2410 - 2480 as appropriate.

EXHIBIT 6. 4

Account Number	Description	Accrual	Modified Cash	Cash
2000	**LIABILITIES**			
2100	**CURRENT LIABILITIES — PAYABLES**	X		
2110	Accounts Payable	X		
2120	Bank Overdrafts Payable	X		
2130	Other Current Liabilities Payable	X		
2200	**CURRENT LIABILITIES — PAYROLL**	X	X	X
2210	Payroll Tax Withholdings Payable	X	X	X
2220	Insurance Withholdings Payable	X	X	X
2250	Accrued Payroll Liabilities	X	X	X
2300	**CURRENT LIABILITIES — OTHER**	X		
2310	Accrued Liabilities — Nonpayroll	X		
2320	Notes and Loans Payable	X	X	X
2330	Long-Term Debt — Current Portion	X	X	X
2340	Advances from Settlements Due to Third-Party Agencies	X	X	X
2350	Patient Deposits	X	X	
2360	Claims Payable Incurred But Not Reported	X		
2370	Deferred Revenue	X		
2400	**LONG-TERM LIABILITIES**	X	X	X

Owners' Equity

Equity is the excess of an entity's assets over its liabilities, or the owners' residual interest in assets. Depending on the type of entity the organization is (partnership or corporation), equity may be called "Partners' Equity" or "Owners' Equity." Exhibit 6. 5 displays the accounts that could be used for a partnership; Exhibit 6. 6 shows the corporate account structure for owners' equity.

EXHIBIT 6. 5

Account Number	Description	Accrual	Modified Cash	Cash
3000	**PARTNERS' EQUITY (PARTNERSHIP)**			
3010	Contributed Capital (Each Partner)	X	X	X
3020	Undistributed Earnings	X	X	X
3030	Partners' Drawing Accounts (Each Partner)	X	X	X
3031	Cash Distributions	X	X	X
3032	Estimated Tax Payments	X	X	X
3033	Health Insurance Premiums	X	X	X
3034	Other Payments Treated as Partner Distributions	X	X	X
3035	Property Distributions	X	X	X
3040	Current Income/Loss	X	X	X

EXHIBIT 6. 6

Account Number	Description	Accrual	Modified Cash	Cash
3000	**STOCKHOLDERS' EQUITY (CORPORATION)**	X	X	X
3010	Preferred Stock	X	X	X
3020	Common Stock	X	X	X
3030	Capital Contributed in Excess of Par	X	X	X
3040	Donated Capital	X	X	X
3050	Allowance for Change in Net Unrealized Gains/Losses on Investments	X	X	
3060	Dividends and Distributions	X	X	X
3061	Cash Distributions	X	X	X
3062	Estimated Tax Payments	X	X	X
3063	Health Insurance Premiums	X	X	X
3064	Other Payments Treated as Partner Distributions	X	X	X
3065	Property Distributions	X	X	X
3070	Retained Earnings — Unappropriated	X	X	X
3075	Retained Earnings — Appropriated	X	X	X
3080	Current Income/Loss	X	X	X
3090	Treasury Stock			

Income Statement Accounts

Revenue

Revenue is an inflow of assets, not necessarily cash, in exchange for goods or services provided. A medical group using the modified cash basis of accounting will consider its collections as revenue, while a group using the accrual basis will consider its gross billings or production as revenue on its income statement. In the accrual method, contractual adjustments, taken as a result of providing services for a discounted rate, are also recorded. Contractual adjustments are not recorded on the modified cash basis income statement.

Exhibit 6.7 on the following page identifies the revenue categories a medical group using the accrual method of accounting would use. The modified cash basis would not use the 4100 series of accounts but would start with the 4200 series.

EXHIBIT 6. 7

Account Number	Description	Accrual	Modified Cash	Cash
4100	Gross Charges	X		
4110	Gross Charges — Fee-for-Service (FFS)	X		
4120	Gross Charges — Discounted FFS Contracts	X		
4130	Gross Charges — FFS Equivalents for Capitation Plan Patients	X		
4140	Other Gross Charges	X		
4150	Other Revenue	X	X	X
4200	Fees Collected		X	X
4210	Fees Collected — FFS		X	X
4220	Fees Collected — FFS for Managed Care		X	X
4230	Capitated Premium Revenues — Commercial		X	X
4240	Capitated Premium Revenues — Medicare		X	X
4250	Capitated Premium Revenues — Medicaid		X	X
4260	Capitated Premium Revenues — Other		X	X
4270	Risk Sharing Revenue		X	X
4271	Hospital Risk Sharing — Commercial		X	X
4272	Hospital Risk Sharing — Medicare		X	X
4273	Hospital Risk Sharing — Medicaid		X	X
4274	Hospital Risk Sharing — Pharmacy		X	X
4275	Hospital Risk Sharing — Other		X	X
4280	Other Managed Care Collected Revenues		X	X
4281	Copayments	X	X	X
4283	Other Prepaid Professional Fees Collected	X	X	X
4290	Recoveries	X	X	X
4300	Patient Refunds	X	X	X
4400	Fees Collected — Other Revenue	X	X	X

All income statement Accounts 4110 through 4400 are appropriate for small group practices using the accrual method. In today's complex health care environment small groups in most parts of the country will deal with discounted Fee-for-Service arrangements, capitation, prepaid contracts and possibly direct contracting for health services.

Use the appropriate adjustment accounts to offset the gross charges accounts you used in the revenue category. Only use Account 4800 if converting accounting records from accrual basis to cash basis; it is to be used in conjunction with Account 2371 — Deferred Revenue — FFS.

Notice that the 4600 series accounts reference various types of discounts. In the event that questions arise regarding the criteria for financial hardship care or charity care, refer to Chapter 7, page 160 in Charity Care section. That section provides a good description of the process for determining patient eligibility in these special cases.

EXHIBIT 6. 8

Account Number	Description	Accrual	Modified Cash	Cash
4500	**ADJUSTMENTS**	X		
4510	Gross Charges — FFS Discount/Adjustment	X		
4520	Gross Charges — FFS Managed Care Discount/Adjustment	X		
4530	Gross Charges — FFS Equivalents for Capitation Plan Patients/Adjustment	X		
4540	Other Gross Charges/Adjustments	X		
4550	Other Revenue Discount/Adjustment	X		
4600	Financial Hardship Care Discount/Adjustment	X		
4610	Courtesy Discount/Adjustment	X		
4620	Employee Discount/Adjustment	X		
4630	Charity Care Discount/Adjustment	X		
4800	Provision for Cash Basis Conversion		X	X

Professional Courtesy Discounts — To Use or Not to Use

(Editorial Comment — Marilyn Happold-Latham)

In the development of the *Chart of Accounts for Health Care Organizations,* there has been controversy about the inclusion of courtesy discounts.One can see that Accounts 4610 for "courtesy discount/ adjustments" and 4620 for "employee discount/adjustment" remain in the chart. This editor of the book attempts to educate the reader on the issues surrounding these discounts and convince the reader not to utilize them.

Professional courtesy, employee discounts or courtesy discounts cover a wide variety of reasons physicians provide services to patients for discounted prices. Professional courtesy discounts are often used when caring for the families of other physicians without charge. Employee discounts are used when providing services to employees of the medical practice, and courtesy discounts can be used for any reason an individual physician deems appropriate.

Although once considered a generous gesture, professional and other courtesy discounts are now surrounded by a number of legal issues. Physicians who give such write-offs may find they are liable for fraud and abuse charges from Medicare, Medicaid and private insurers.

A provision of the Health Insurance Portability and Accountability Act (HIPAA) makes it possible to consider actions such as waiving copay- ments and deductibles for reasons other than documented financial hardship as health care fraud. When a doctor bills "insurance only" for services provided to a colleague, it can be considered as unlawfully inducing referrals and unlawfully charging a fee less than the doctor's normal fee. Some legal experts consider that even the complete waiving of a fee is a risky practice since the services provided have value and could be considered a kickback for referrals.

Penalties for violating laws governing fraud and abuse or antikickbacks include not only denial of claims but also substantial fines and possible imprisonment.

When Accounts 4610 and 4620 appear in the chart of accounts for a medical group, it gives the use of these discounts an air of acceptability and appropriateness. One may ask, "Why would CRAHCA include these accounts if they shouldn't be used?" For the reasons noted above the use of courtesy discounts should be reviewed by the executive management of the medical group, and the decision to use them should be based on a thorough understanding of the legal risks involved. When dollars are posted to these accounts, it provides a "red flag" to an auditor that could result in a more in-depth review of the medical group's billing and accounting practices.

Some physicians may be outraged or upset when their medical group administrator informs them of the legal risks they take by giving professional courtesy discounts. To help them further understand the arguments against these discounts, the following reference list is offered as a resource:

- "Professional courtesy can be okay at times, but advice is to abandon it altogether," *Part B News*, Vol. 13, No. 8, April 12, 1999.
- "Is Professional Courtesy Dead?" *The Physician's Advisory*, June 1998.
- Gianelli, Dianne. "Rethinking Professional Courtesy," *American Medical News*, March 8, 1999.
- Konow, Dan, M.B.A., PA-C, and Resener, Mike, J.D. "Avoiding the Pitfalls of Courtesy Write-Offs," *Group Practice Journal*, November/December 1997.
- Long, Robert S., M.D. "Professional Courtesy — Ethics and the Law In The Medical Treatment of Physicians and their Families," *Nebraska Medical Journal*, February 1994.
- Rathbun, Katharine C., M.D. and Richards, Edward P. III, J.D. "Professional Courtesy — Legal issues in offering discounted Services," *CPA Health Niche Advisor*, Harcourt Brace, Volume 1998, Issue 2, February 1998.
- Winkler, Alan, FACMPE. "Welcome to professional courtesy discounts: The medical community's Pandora's box," *College Review*, American College of Medical Practice Executives, Vol. 15, No. 2, Fall 1998.

Operating Expenses

The most notable change from the previous chart of accounts published by CRAHCA is the restructuring of the operating expense accounts to remove the physicians and midlevels from this category and create a new category for them under the 8000 series. This will be discussed in more detail later in the chapter.

Operating expenses are generally considered the overhead or practice expense. Your practice may need more detail than these summary accounts. If so, please refer to the detailed chart of accounts in the Appendix. As always, if you do not require this level of detail in the expenses, roll them into the next higher category such as 5600 for all ancillary staff employee-related expenses.

EXHIBIT 6. 9

Account Number	Description	Accrual	Modified Cash	Cash
5000	**OPERATING EXPENSES — Salary And Fringe Benefits**	X	X	X
5500	ANCILLARY STAFF — SALARIES	X	X	X
5600	ANCILLARY STAFF — EMPLOYEE-RELATED EXPENSES	X	X	X
5610	Payroll Taxes (Ancillary)	X	X	X
5620	Insurance (Ancillary)	X	X	X
5630	Pension and Retirement Benefits (Ancillary)	X	X	X
5635	Professional Development (Ancillary)	X	X	X
5640	Books and Subscriptions (Ancillary)	X	X	X
5645	Dues and Memberships (Ancillary)	X	X	X
5650	Licenses (Ancillary)	X	X	X
5655	Meetings (Ancillary)	X	X	X
5660	Travel (Ancillary)	X	X	X
5665	Medical Reimbursement Plan (Ancillary)	X	X	X
5670	Vehicles (Ancillary)	X	X	X
5675	Parking (Ancillary)	X	X	X
5680	Telephones (Ancillary)	X	X	X
5685	Beepers (Ancillary)	X	X	X
5690	Meals and Entertainment (Ancillary)	X	X	X
5695	Other Benefits (Ancillary)	X	X	X
5700	EMPLOYEES — SALARIES	X	X	X
5800	EMPLOYEES — EMPLOYEE-RELATED EXPENSES	X	X	X
5810	Payroll Taxes (Other)	X	X	X
5820	Insurance (Other)	X	X	X
5830	Pension and Retirement Benefits (Other)	X	X	X
5835	Professional Development (Other)	X	X	X
5840	Books and Subscriptions (Other)	X	X	X
5845	Dues and Memberships (Other)	X	X	X
5850	Licenses (Other)	X	X	X
5855	Meetings (Other)	X	X	X
5860	Travel (Other)	X	X	X
5865	Medical Reimbursement Plan (Other)	X	X	X
5870	Vehicles (Other)	X	X	X
5875	Parking (Other)	X	X	X
5880	Telephones (Other)	X	X	X
5885	Beepers (Other)	X	X	X
5890	Meals and Entertainment (Other)	X	X	X
5895	Other Benefits (Other)	X	X	X
5900	Temporary Employee Salaries — Professional	X	X	X
5910	Temporary Employee Benefits — Professional	X	X	X

Services and General Expenses

The general expenses for your particular practice may not need to be reported in such detail, therefore remember you may pick and choose which of these accounts are applicable to your practice. The office and administrative expense sub-accounts under 6100 will roll up into Account 6100 so do not concern yourself with using each and every account regardless of whether or not it currently applies to your practice. As your practice grows, you may require the addition of new account categories; this chart of accounts can be easily expanded to accommodate your needs.

EXHIBIT 6. 10

Account Number	Description	Accrual	Modified Cash	Cash
6000	**SERVICES AND GENERAL EXPENSE**	X	X	X
6100	Office and Administrative Expense	X	X	X
6110	Equipment Rentals (Admin.)	X	X	X
6115	Equipment Maintenance (Admin.)	X	X	X
6120	Telephone (Admin.)	X	X	X
6130	Postage (Admin.)	X	X	X
6180	General Business and Other Insurance	X	X	X
6185	Malpractice Insurance	X	X	X
6240	Cafeteria	X	X	X
6250	Employee Relations	X	X	X
6300	Depreciation/Amortization	X	X	
6310	Accounting Services	X	X	X
6320	Legal Services	X	X	X
6340	Pension Administration Expense	X	X	X
6370	Medical Transcription	X	X	X
6380	Payroll Services	X	X	X
6410	Taxes — Excise and Other Business Taxes	X	X	X
6700	Bad Debt Expense	X	X	X
7500	Occupancy Expense	X	X	X
7510	Rent/Lease	X	X	X
7530	General Maintenance	X	X	X
7540	Utilities	X	X	X
7550	Property Taxes	X	X	X
7560	Housekeeping/Maintenance Services	X	X	X
7580	Insurance (Occupancy)	X	X	X
7590	Depreciation (Occupancy)	X	X	
7595	Amortization — Leasehold Improvements (Occupancy)	X	X	
7600	Cost of Goods Sold — Medical Related	X		
7700	**PURCHASED SERVICES/MANAGEMENT FEES**	X	X	X

Provider Expenses

In prior CRAHCA charts of accounts physician and midlevel provider expenses could be found under the 5000 series of operating expense accounts. In this particular chart of accounts, the structure has changed to carve out these providers. This is to follow current industry trends that view these providers as a category other than general overhead. It also mirrors the logic of the MGMA surveys thus making it easier to complete the surveys with the correct information. The 8000 series of provider-related expense accounts is broken down into four major categories (that can be used for account roll ups): 8100 — Physician compensation, 8200 — Physician expenses, 8300 — Midlevel provider compensation and 8400 — Midlevel provider expenses. Smaller practices may need only a few sub-accounts under each of these categories. Note that these accounts mirror those set up for the ancillary and other staff.

EXHIBIT 6. 11

Account Number	Description	Accrual	Modified Cash	Cash
8000	**PROVIDER-RELATED EXPENSES**	X	X	X
8100	PHYSICIAN — SALARIES	X	X	X
8110	Salaries, Distributions and Incentives (Physician)	X	X	X
8200	PHYSICIAN — EMPLOYEE-RELATED EXPENSES	X	X	X
8210	Payroll Taxes (Physician)	X	X	X
8220	Insurance (Physician)	X	X	X
8230	Pension and Retirement Benefits (Physician)	X	X	X
8235	Professional Development (Physician)	X	X	X
8240	Books and Subscriptions (Physician)	X	X	X
8245	Dues and Memberships (Physician)	X	X	X
8250	Licenses (Physician)	X	X	X
8255	Meetings (Physician)	X	X	X
8260	Travel (Physician)	X	X	X
8265	Medical Reimbursement Plan (Physician)	X	X	X
8270	Vehicles (Physician)	X	X	X
8275	Parking (Physician)	X	X	X
8280	Telephones (Physician)	X	X	X
8285	Beepers (Physician)	X	X	X
8290	Meals and Entertainment (Physician)	X	X	X
8295	Other Benefits (Physician)	X	X	X
8300	MIDLEVEL PROVIDER**S** — SALARIES	X	X	X
8310	Salaries, Distributions and Incentives (Midlevel)	X	X	X
8400	PROVIDERS — EMPLOYEE-RELATE MIDLEVEL EXPENSES	X	X	X
8410	Payroll Taxes (Midlevel)	X	X	X
8420	Insurance (Midlevel)	X	X	X
8430	Pension and Retirement Benefits (Midlevel)	X	X	X
8435	Professional Development (Midlevel)	X	X	X
8440	Books and Subscriptions (Midlevel)	X	X	X
8445	Dues and Memberships (Midlevel)	X	X	X
8450	Licenses (Midlevel)	x	X	X
8455	Meetings (Midlevel)	X	X	X
8460	Travel (Midlevel)	X	X	X
8465	Medical Reimbursement (Midlevel)	X	X	X
8470	Vehicles (Midlevel)	X	X	X
8475	Parking (Midlevel)	X	X	X
8480	Telephones (Midlevel)	X	X	X
8485	Beepers (Midlevel)	X	X	X
8490	Meals and Entertainment (Midlevel)	X	X	X
8495	Other Benefits (Midlevel)	X	X	X

Nonoperating Revenues and Expenses

The subtotal representing revenues, less operating expenses and provider expense is titled income from operations. Generally Accepted Accounting Principles define this concept very broadly and include most all income and expense items. The only things excluded would be extraordinary items and nonrecurring charges and recoveries. The MGMA chart of accounts categorizes certain income and expenses, such as interest, contributions and donations as nonoperating in order to make financial studies and benchmark comparisons more consistent.

Additionally, federal income tax expense accounts are included in this category. The following represents a sample chart of accounts layout for nonoperating revenue and expense to be used by a small group:

EXHIBIT 6. 12

Account Number	Description	Accrual	Modified Cash	Cash
9000	**NONOPERATING REVENUE & EXPENSE; INCOME TAXES & OTHER EXPENSES**	X	X	X
9100	Nonoperating Revenues	X	X	X
9110	Interest Income	X	X	X
9200	Nonoperating Expenses	X	X	X
9210	Interest Expense	X	X	X
9220	Contributions/Donations Expense	X	X	X
9230	Current Income Tax Expense (Recovery)	X	X	X
9240	Deferred Income Tax Expense (Recovery)	X	X	X
9300	Other Income Expense	X	X	X

Application to MGMA Surveys

MGMA conducts numerous surveys that are beneficial to group practices. If you follow this chart of accounts numbering system it will simplify completion of the surveys and allow comparison of your data to that of other survey participants. Smaller organizations do not have the luxury of a lot of staff and time to complete external surveys. With this system in place, you will be able to complete numerous surveys quickly and accurately so you will have comparable data at your fingertips to make informed decisions.

Summary

These account categories are for groups of 10 or fewer physicians. You may find that, to meet your individual needs, you will need to expand or contract from what is provided here. That is the flexibility of the chart of accounts system and how it is designed to meet your individual needs. No matter how you use it, it will give you the ability to more easily connect with other medical groups if you acquire them, are acquired by them, or if you participate in a merger. There should be no need to start from the beginning as you have a system in place that is adaptable to similar type of organizations. It cannot be stressed enough how important it is that you adapt this chart of accounts to your group, both for internal and external users of your financial information.

7

Adapting the Chart of Accounts to Not-For-Profit Health Care Organizations

Richard L. Gundling, FHFMA, CMA

Introduction

No matter what type of ownership health care organizations (HCOs) may have — investor-owned, not-for-profit (NFP) or governmental — all HCOs need to have clear information provided by the accounting process. Clear communication of financial data is imperative to the decision making of internal and external users. While there are different concepts guiding the financial reporting of HCOs under different types of ownership, users need the same information. Even among HCOs with various types of ownership, it is important that a chart of accounts achieve comparability, whenever permissible, through Generally Accepted Accounting Principles (GAAP). Although the chart of accounts is designed to meet the information needs of the HCO management, the requirements of investors, creditors, donors, taxing and regulatory agencies also influence the design of your chart of accounts. The discussion in this chapter is based on the assumption that the NFP entity is using the accrual basis of accounting. If a particular organization is a NFP using cash-basis accounting, particular attention should be given to which accounts listed in the tables at the back of this publication are applicable for strictly cash versus accrual.

Defining the Ownership Types

The Financial Accounting Standards Board (FASB) in its Statement of Financial Accounting Standards (SFAS) No. 117 says a not-for-profit organization has these characteristics:

- Resources, significant contributions, come from providers who do not expect commensurate or proportionate pecuniary (i.e., monetary) return.
- Business purposes do not include providing goods or services at a profit.

- There are no ownership interests like those of other business enterprises.

In investor-owned HCOs owners are entitled to a return on their investments made in the organization. The key characteristics of a governmental HCO include the manner in which the governing board is selected, the government's residual interest in the HCO, or the HCO's ability to levy taxes or to issue tax-exempt debt. Governmental HCOs are beyond the scope of this chapter.

Financial statements for both managerial and external use should be prepared in conformity with GAAP — a term that encompasses the conventions, rules and procedures necessary to define acceptable accounting practices at a particular time. The highest authoritative source of GAAP is the FASB for investor-owned and not-for-profit entities. The American Institute of Certified Public Accountants (AICPA) issues guides and statements that apply FASB Statements of SFAS to specific entities and transactions. Governmental HCOs are subject to the Governmental Accounting Standards Board (GASB). Many times accounting issues do arise and may not be covered adequately by any of these sources, and one must look to other sources for guidance. The Healthcare Financial Management Association's (HFMA's) Principles and Practices (P&P) Board is one such source on the applicability of GAAP to HCOs.

FASB has said that "its goal is to develop an integrated conceptual framework that has relevance to all entities ..." and the "line between not-for-profit organizations and business enterprises (or investor-owned) is not always sharp..." Many FASB statements apply to both not-for-profit and investor-owned. However, some FASB rules are applicable to only certain not-for-profit entities but not investor-owned or even between different not-for-profit types. The AICPA Audit and Accounting Guide, *Health Care Organizations*, takes away some of the ambiguity between the types of not-for-profit entities created by FASB and applies the same rules to all entities. This guide is the highest GAAP authority dealing specifically with health care accounting and financial reporting issues.

The following summarizes the concepts that are applicable to HCOs of different ownership types. The Statement of Financial Accounting Concepts (SFAC) No. 1, *Objectives of Financial Reporting by Business Enterprises*, which includes investor-owned HCOs, outlines three objectives:

- Provide information that is useful to present to potential investors and others making rational business decisions
- Provide information to be able to assess cash flows
- Provide information about the economic resources of the HCO

SFAC No. 4, *Objectives of Financial Reporting by Nonbusiness Organizations*, established the financial reporting for not-for-profit HCOs. The objectives include providing information that:

- Helps people make decisions
- Explains services

- Tells how managers discharge their stewardship
- Describes economic resources
- Explains the organization's performance
- Clarifies the financial data

Key Areas for Not-For-Profit HCOs

Charity Care

The provision of charity service is an important indicator of the fulfillment of a not-for-profit HCO's charitable mission. Since charity service will not result in cash inflows, it does not meet the definition of revenues or receivables. However, financial statement users have a high level of interest in information about how much charity service is provided. The charity service policy and amount should be disclosed in a note to the financial statements.

HCOs must differentiate bad debts from charity services. Bad debt is an amount some party has an obligation to pay but is uncollectible. Bad debts are not deductions from charges but rather are treated as expenses. HFMA's P&P Board Statement No. 15, *Valuation & Financial Statement Presentation of Charity Service & Bad Debts by Institutional Healthcare Providers* includes guidelines concerning the valuation and disclosure of charity service. The statement also provides guidelines regarding an HCO's charity service policy and format for disclosure. Section II of P&P Board Statement No. 15 outlines criteria for charity service along with guidelines for all HCOs to use in their charity determinations:

"2.1 Each institutional provider of health care services[1] must establish criteria for charity service consistent with the organization's mission and financial ability. Some providers have financial resources designated for the provision of charity service, while other providers must recover the cost of charity service from the amounts paid by or for other patients. Some communities provide financial support to specific organizations to ensure that charity service is available, while other communities prefer that each health care provider arrange for charity service based on demand. For these reasons, no single set of criteria is universally applicable, and each provider must develop and administer its own criteria.

"2.2 Some government regulations identify criteria for charity service for specific purposes, such as eligibility for certain types of financial assistance. While these external criteria may influence the provider's criteria, and the provider must be able to identify patients who fulfill these externally determined criteria, such external criteria do not supersede the organization's own criteria, which may be more or less stringent.

"2.3 Criteria for determining the amount of charity service for which a patient is eligible at the time of an occasion of service could include some of the following factors as well as others. (The following factors are discussed in the indicated paragraphs of this statement.)

- *Individual or family income (see 2.4)*
- *Individual or family net worth (see 2.5)*
- *Employment status and earning capacity (see 2.6)*
- *Family size (see 2.7)*
- *Other financial obligations (see 2.8)*
- *The amount and frequency of bills for health care services (see 2.9)*
- *Other sources of payment for the services rendered (see 2.10)*

"2.4 Individual or family income may recognize standards for determination of poverty with consideration of family size, geographic area and other pertinent factors. Individual or family incomes generally are not the exclusive criteria for determining the appropriate amount of charity service.

"2.5 Individual or family net worth considers all liquid and nonliquid assets owned, less liabilities and claims against those assets. Eligibility for Medicaid if some assets are depleted can be considered.

"2.6 Employment status should consider the likelihood of future earnings sufficient to meet the health care-related obligation within a reasonable period of time.

"2.7 Implications of family size in addition to adequacy of individual or family income are appropriate considerations.

"2.8 Other financial obligations include living expenses and other items of a reasonable and necessary nature.

"2.9 The amount and frequency of bills for health care services must be considered in relation to all the other factors outlined above. While eligibility relates to meeting criteria at the time service is rendered, the history of service and the need for future service may be considered. A separate determination of the amount of charity service for which a patient is eligible is made on each occasion of service, or regular confirmation of eligibility is made during extended programs of service.

"2.10 The appropriate amount of charity service is determined in relation to amounts due after applying all other resources. Criteria may be more detailed and call for more specific evidence of eligibility for large amounts than for small amounts.

"2.11 A number of factors must be considered, all of which require judgment. Thus, adoption of rigid criteria is undesirable.

"2.12 Different providers may apply similar criteria differently. For example, a patient with catastrophic hospitalization costs but with substantial net worth may be eligible for charity service by one provider, but another provider may require that net worth in excess of a threshold be used to pay for health care services before the patient is eligible for charity

service. Some providers may be able to establish automatic criteria for certain classes of patients (such as for noncovered services to Medicaid patients), and other providers may require case-by-case determination.

"2.13 Application of these factors by individual providers involves several considerations, including:

- *Availability of information (see 2.14)*
- *Verification of information (see 2.15)*

"2.14 Determining the amount of charity service for which a patient is eligible is based in large part on information supplied by the patient or someone acting on the patient's behalf. The charity service policy needs to address eligibility for charity service when there is insufficient information to fully evaluate all the criteria and the ability to pay cannot be reliably determined.

"2.15 Data used in making a determination concerning eligibility for charity service should be verified to the extent practical in relation to the amount involved and the significance of an element of information in the overall determination. For example, extensive investigation in relation to a small balance due would not be cost effective. Similarly, a single element of information may provide all the information necessary to make a reasonable determination, and additional investigation would not be cost effective. The procedures implementing the charity service policy should address the extent of verification and any modification of a determination already made if subsequent information indicates that information relied upon was in error."

P&P Board Statement No. 15 also states that charity service is not to be reported in revenue or receivables. However, it is generally not known whether services will meet charity service criteria at the time the services are rendered, so there is no alternative to keeping records for charity service the same as for any other service. Use of a charity service provision and allowance is usually necessary. Appropriate record keeping for charity service consists of:

- **Recording Services** at the full established charges amount in revenue and receivables as services are rendered
- **Adjusting Revenue** and receivables to the amount that a payer has an obligation to pay (Note: It is desirable to identify charity service as soon as possible to minimize collection effort and deal with patients more equitably.)
- **Estimating the Amount** of the remaining receivables that will eventually be written off as charity service. This amount is recorded as a provision for charity services (a revenue contra account) and an allowance for charity service (a receivable contra account)
- **Writing Off Receivables** as they are determined to meet charity service criteria against the allowance for charity service. Documentation concerning the eligibility for charity service should be retained

- **Regularly Evaluating** the adequacy of the allowance for charity service with adjustments to increase or decrease the allowance offset by adjustments in the provision for charity service

The accounts used to record the reduction of accounts receivable for charity services are in the 1320 series. The accounts used to record the deduction from charges for charity service are in the 4600 series.

EXHIBIT 7.1 Accounts Receivable Detail

Account Number	Description
1300	Accounts Receivable
1301	Accounts Receivable — Fee-for-Service Amounts
1302	Accounts Receivable — Prepaid Contracts
1320	Allowance for Estimated uncollectible Receivables
1321	Allowance for Bad Debts — Patient Accounts
1322	Allowance for Contractual Adjustments
1323	Allowance for Bad Debts — Third-Party Payers
1324	**Allowance for Charity Care**
1340	Notes Receivable — Short Term
1345	Managed Care Contract — Bonus/Withhold
1350	Other Short-Term Receivables
1351	Interest Receivables
1352	Intercompany Receivables
1353	Due from Employees
1354	Due from Related Parties
	Adjustments Detail
4500	**ADJUSTMENTS**
4600	Financial Hardship Care Discount/Adjustment
4610	Courtesy Discount/Adjustment
4620	Employee Discount/Adjustment
4630	**Charity Care Discount/Adjustment**

Investment In Securities

HCOs record changes in the value of securities in different ways depending on the organization type. Not-for-profit HCOs record changes in value restricted by donors or by law according to those restrictions. SFAS No. 124, *Accounting for Certain Investments Held by Not-for-Profit Organizations*, establishes requirements concerning recording changes in value of securities by not-for-profit HCOs. GASB Statement No. 31, *Accounting and Financial Reporting for Certain Investments,* sets the requirements for governmental hospitals. Investor-owned HCOs would follow SFAS No. 115, *Accounting for Certain Investments in Debt and Equity Securities*. Not-for-profit HCOs record unrealized changes in value of these securities in the account series 9140.

EXHIBIT 7.2

Account Number	Description
Balance Sheet — Assets Detail	
1200	Marketable Securities & Short-Term Investments
1210	**Valuation Allowance — Short-Term Investments**
1600	INVESTMENTS — LONG-TERM RECEIVABLES
1630	Long-Term Investments
1635	**Valuation Allowance — Long-Term Investments**
Income Statement — Nonoperating Revenue Detail	
9000	**NONOP REVENUE & EXP; INCOME TAXES & OTHER EXP**
9100	Nonoperating Revenues
9110	Interest Income
9120	Income from Long-Term Investments
9130	Property Rentals
9140	**Unrealized Gains and Losses — Investments**
9150	Realized Gains and Losses — Investments
9160	Donations Received (Nonoperating Revenue)
9170	Nonoperating Subsidy Income

Accounting for Contributions

Fund raising and contributions may be a large source of revenue for many not-for-profit HCOs. Generally, contributions received are measured at their fair market value and recognized as revenues in the fiscal year received. A contribution means an unconditional transfer of cash or other assets to an entity, or a settlement or cancellation of its liabilities in a voluntary nonreciprocal transfer by another entity acting other than as an owner. HCOs may either account for contributions as revenues or gains, depending on the mission of the recipient HCO. Contributions may be unrestricted or donor restricted (i.e., there is a stipulation by a donor concerning how or when a contribution may be used). A restriction may be temporary or permanent. Contributions include contributed services, materials, utilities and property. SFAS No. 116, *Accounting For Contributions Received and Contributions Made*, is the authoritative source for the proper accounting treatment for contributions.

An endowment is a contribution that is permanently donor restricted. While the principle of an endowment may not be used, return on investment of the principle may be used according to the stipulations of the donor or by applicable law. The HCO's governing board may set aside funds in a board-designated endowment. Such a designation is classified as unrestricted.

A fund-raising entity known as a foundation is often formed to help not-for-profit HCOs fulfill their missions. Rules for recording and reporting contributions or donations are quite complex and are beyond the scope of this book. More detail is provided by the *Association for Healthcare Philanthropy Chart of Accounts for Healthcare Fund Raising.*

The Chart of Accounts for Health Care Organizations contains several variations on inflows and outflows of donations. Exhibit 7.3 displays an accounting option (Account 9160) for *nonoperating* (revenue) donations received. This is not to be confused with Account 9220 which is cash outflow (expense) for contributions made by your organization to a charitable entity or cause. Likewise, do not confuse the *nonoperating* donations received with Account 4450, which is for *operating* revenue received in the form of donations.

EXHIBIT 7.3 Nonoperating Revenue Detail

Account Number	Description
9000	**NONOP REVENUE & EXP; INCOME TAXES & OTHER EXP**
9100	Nonoperating Revenues
9110	Interest Income
9120	Income from Long-Term Investments
9130	Property Rentals
9140	Unrealized Gains and Losses — Investments
9150	Realized Gains and Losses — Investments
9160	**Donations Received (Nonoperating Revenue)**
9170	Nonoperating Subsidy Income

Equity

Equity is the difference between total assets and total liabilities. Equity is increased by an excess of revenues over expenses (profit) and, all entities, including not-for-profit and government HCOs, must earn a profit to maintain capital. The term "not-for-profit" or "nonprofit" often leaves the incorrect impression that such organizations may not earn a profit, therefore, the term "tax-exempt" is used many times. Equity of investor-owned HCOs is also increased by investments by owners and is decreased by distribution to owners.

The equity accounts of a not-for-profit are considerably different from an investor-owned HCO. The equity of an investor-owned HCO is substantially the same as any other investor-owned business. The equity of a not-for-profit differs from the equity of an investor-owned HCO because there are no owners who invest in or receive ownership returns (dividends). The equity of a not-for-profit HCO is divided into three classes: unrestricted, temporarily restricted and permanently restricted. Each of these classes may be subdivided into separate accounts to be used to identify specific purposes of unrestricted equity. The unrestricted resources of an HCO may be used in any manner deemed appropriate by the governing board and within the broad limits established by the mission of the HCO. Amounts with donor restrictions should be recorded in either a temporarily or permanently restricted equity account. Donor restrictions related to plant replacement and expansions are quite prevalent in the health care industry. Only donors may create equity restrictions. Donor temporary restrictions may specify the time when contributed funds may be used and the purpose for which they must be used.

EXHIBIT 7.4 Net Assets (Not-for-Profit Equity) Detail

Account Number	Description
3000	**NET ASSETS (NOT-FOR-PROFIT EQUITY)**
3010	Unrestricted Net Assets
3030	Temporarily Restricted Net Assets
3040	Permanently Restricted Net Assets
3050	Current Surplus/Deficit

Reporting Requirements for the Internal Revenue Service

Most health care organizations exempt from federal income tax must annually file Form 990, "Return of Organization Exempt from Income Tax." Form 990 is an information-only return; therefore no tax liability is computed. Form 990 is composed of a revenue and expense statement, balance sheet, analysis of fund balances and questions regarding the organization's structure and activities. The Internal Revenue Service (IRS) mandates that Form 990 be made available for public inspection and copying. HCOs should be aware that Form 990 is more than an IRS reporting requirement, it is also a communication document to the public of the organization's charitable activities. An HCO's chart of accounts should be able to accumulate the appropriate data for the completion of Form 990 in accordance with IRS instructions. A Form 990-T, "Exempt Organization Business Income Tax Return," may have to be filed by a not-for-profit HCO to report its unrelated business income. Public review requirements do not apply to Form 990-T. Although Form 990 is an informational return, penalties apply to those HCOs that fail to file a complete return. Care should be taken to accurately report all information.

Chart of Accounts

The account numbers and descriptions referred to in the not-for-profit category in the spreadsheets included with this text should be used to the extent necessary to produce financial statements for not-for-profit organizations discussed in this chapter.

There is one major change to the overall structure of this chart of accounts that can easily be modified by not-for-profits. This chart of accounts has been revised from those previously issued by CRAHCA in that physician and midlevel provider salaries and their related direct payroll costs have been moved to a separate series of accounts in the 8000 series. This has been done to make the *Chart of Accounts for Health Care Organizations* more useful in performing benchmarking comparisons of overhead and physician earnings among practices. This new structure follows the logic of the MGMA Cost Survey and other surveys that focus on benchmarking.

For those organizations (such as not-for-profits) that prefer to use or need to use the more traditional approach in their chart of accounts, account series 5100,

5200, 5300 and 5400 have been left open for that purpose. The same account titles and descriptions from 8100, 8200, 8300 and 8400 may be used and moved into the open slots. Exhibit 7.5 clarifies how those accounts can be modified for use.

EXHIBIT 7.5

Modified Account #	Description	Current Account #
5000	**OPERATING EXPENSES — SALARY AND FRINGE BENEFITS**	8000
5100	**PHYSICIANS — SALARIES**	8100
5110	Salaries, Distributions and Incentives (Physician)	8110
5120	Salaries — Owner/Stockholder (Physician)	8120
5130	Distributions and Incentives (Physician)	8130
5140	Global/Capitation Distributions (Physician)	8140
5150	Employee Salaries (Physician)	8150
5160	Employee Incentives (Physician)	8160
5170	Administrative Salaries (Physician)	8170
5200	**PHYSICIAN — EMPLOYEE RELATED EXPENSES**	8200
5210	Payroll Taxes (Physician)	8210
5211	Payroll Taxes — FICA/Medicare (Physician)	8211
5212	Payroll Taxes — Federal Unemployment Insurance (Physician)	8212
5213	Payroll Taxes — State Unemployment Insurance (Physician)	8213
5214	Payroll Taxes — Other (Physician)	8214
5220	Insurance (Physician)	8220
5221	Insurance — Health (Physician)	8221
5222	Insurance — Dental (Physician)	8222
5223	Insurance — Life (Physician)	8223
5224	Insurance — Disability (Physician)	8224
5225	Insurance — Workers' Compensation (Physician)	8225
5226	Insurance — Other (Physician)	8226
5227	Insurance — Officers' Life (Physician)	8227
5230	Pension and Retirement Benefits (Physician)	8230
5231	Deferred Compensation (Physician)	8231
5232	Severance Plan (Physician)	8232
5235	Professional Development (Physician)	8235
5240	Books and Subscriptions (Physician)	8240
5245	Dues and Memberships (Physician)	8245
5250	Licenses (Physician)	8250
5255	Meetings (Physician)	8255
5260	Travel (Physician)	8260
5265	Medical Reimbursement Plan (Physician)	8265
5270	Vehicles (Physician)	8270
5271	Leased Motor Vehicles (Physician)	8276
5275	Parking (Physician)	8275
5280	Telephones (Physician)	8280
5285	Beepers (Physician)	8285
5290	Meals and Entertainment (Physician)	8290
5295	Other Benefits (Physician)	8295

Exhibit 7.5 continued

Modified Account #	Description	Current Account #
5300	MIDLEVEL PROVIDERS — SALARIES	8300
5310	Salaries (Midlevel)	8310
5360	Employee Incentives (Midlevel)	8360
5400	MIDLEVEL PROVIDERS — EMPLOYEE RELATED EXPENSES	8400
5410	Payroll Taxes (Midlevel)	8410
5411	Payroll Taxes — FICA/Medicare (Midlevel)	8411
5412	Payroll Taxes — Federal Unemployment Insurance (Midlevel)	8412
5413	Payroll Taxes — State Unemployment Insurance (Midlevel)	8413
5414	Payroll Taxes — Other (Midlevel)	8414
5420	Insurance (Midlevel)	8420
5421	Insurance — Health (Midlevel)	8421
5422	Insurance — Dental (Midlevel)	8422
5423	Insurance — Life (Midlevel)	8423
5424	Insurance — Disability (Midlevel)	8424
5425	Insurance — Workers' Compensation (Midlevel)	8425
5426	Insurance — Other (Midlevel)	8426
5430	Pension and Retirement Benefits (Midlevel)	8430
5431	Deferred Compensation (Midlevel)	8431
5432	Severance Plan (Midlevel)	8432
5435	Professional Development (Midlevel)	8435
5440	Books and Subscriptions (Midlevel)	8440
5445	Dues and Memberships (Midlevel)	8445
5450	Licenses (Midlevel)	8450
5455	Meetings (Midlevel)	8455
5460	Travel (Midlevel)	8460
5465	Medical Reimbursement Plan (Midlevel)	8465
5470	Vehicles (Midlevel)	8470
5475	Parking (Midlevel)	8475
5480	Telephones (Midlevel)	8480
5485	Beepers (Midlevel)	8485
5490	Meals and Entertainment (Midlevel)	8490
5495	Other Benefits (Midlevel)	8495

Reference:

1. (See page 150, paragraph 2.1) Examples of institutional health care providers are hospitals, continuing care retirement communities, skilled nursing facilities, subacute care facilities, multispecialty clinics, and freestanding ambulatory centers.

8

Adapting the Chart of Accounts to Community Health Centers

Eric S. Holzberg, CPA, M.B.A. and Gil Bernhard, CPA

Introduction

This chapter discusses how CRAHCA's *Chart of Accounts for Health Care Organizations* (COA) can be used for a Community Health Center (CHC). The suggested format of the chart of accounts is not an absolute, but rather a guide to CHCs who choose to use this structure as the basis for their own practice's chart of accounts. When developing a chart of accounts, a CHC needs to take into consideration what financial information it will need to be able to extract for various internal monitoring and for external reporting requirements. The various external reporting requirements of CHCs are often unique based on the funding sources and the reporting requirements of those funding sources.

CHCs are not-for-profit ambulatory health care providers that receive funding from various sources in order to provide services in medically underserved areas. As not-for-profit corporations, CHCs are required to follow accounting principles for not-for-profit organizations; therefore, the chapter and the sample chart of accounts' column for not-for-profit organizations should be taken into consideration for CHCs.

CHCs receive funding from the federal, state and local governments through grants and contracts to provide services. They also receive reimbursement from patients and third-party payers such as state Medicaid programs, Medicare, commercial insurance and managed-care organizations (MCOs). CHCs increasingly have gotten more involved in managed care as more and more states are implementing managed-care programs for Medicaid recipients who make up a large portion of a CHC's patient base. As a result of all of these factors, CHCs have substantial reporting requirements that make the designing of the chart of accounts a critical task to the organization. These requirements also make it mandatory for CHCs to keep their accounting records on an accrual basis of accounting.

Many CHCs have developed their chart of accounts without considering all of the internal and external demands on financial information. The combination of this factor and the changing health care environment has led organizations to the conclusion that their chart of accounts does not meet their needs. It is very important for CHCs to make sure they leave room for expansion of new programs and funding sources when developing their chart of accounts. The organization must determine their current requirements, as well as additional requirements that are driven by the organization's plans for the future. By taking these things into consideration and by selecting a flexible information system, the organization should be able to design a chart of accounts that will only require minimal modification and not a complete redesign as the organization grows and requirements change.

Reporting Requirements

Tax Requirements

As not-for-profit corporations, CHCs are required to file "Annual Informational Returns for Tax Exempt Organizations" (Form 990) with the Internal Revenue Service (IRS) for its fiscal year and may be required to file state returns as well. If the organization engages in activities that are not part of its tax-exempt purpose, it is required to file a return for unrelated business income tax (Form 990T). The chart of accounts needs to provide the necessary information in order for the organization to track these activities properly and complete all required tax returns. (See the chapter on not-for-profits for more details.)

Financial Statement Audit Requirements

Virtually all CHCs are required to have their fiscal year end financial statements audited. The federal government and other funding agencies require that these audits meet government audit requirements. The financial statements are required to be in accordance with generally accepted accounting principles (GAAP) and on an accrual basis of accounting. (See the chapter on not-for-profits for more details.)

Funding Agency Requirements

CHCs receive grants and contracts from various sources in order to assist in the support of the services they provide. These funds come from the federal, state and local governments as well as other agencies (i.e., foundations, other not-for-profits, etc.). These funding agencies often have reporting requirements in order to verify that these funds are being spent appropriately. Typically these agencies will request periodic reporting (i.e., quarterly, monthly, etc.) that itemizes how these funds are spent. Usually these reports reflect the expenses for the program for the period, the budgeted amount for the period of funding, how much of the funds were spent cumulatively, and how much of the amount awarded by expense line items are remaining. These are typically referred to as "expense vouchers" and are sometimes not only used to monitor the amount of funding spent, but also to make payments for the services provided by the CHC under the program. These reporting requirements demonstrate the need to capture expenses by funding source in the accounting records, and a segment of the COA can assist in this.

One of the largest grant-funded programs the CHCs receive comes from the U.S. Department of Health and Human Services (DHHS), Bureau of Primary Health Care (BPHC) grants (Section 330). These grants were the initial funding that started a majority of the CHCs across the country. There are a variety of Section 330 grant programs for CHCs to assist them in providing services to the uninsured and special populations on a sliding fee discount basis.

These grants also require reporting back to the BPHC. Similar to the expense vouchers previously noted, the Section 330 grants have a report to verify the amount of the grant funds that were spent. The report, known as the Financial Status Report (FSR), must be filed at the end of the budget period (usually a year). The Section 330 grants are awarded based on a budget that reflects the total expenses of the program, which are funded not only by the Section 330 grant funds, but also by patient services revenue from the patients or third parties plus funding from other nonfederal sources (state and local governments and other agencies). This is referred to as the "scope of the project." There are various types of programs under Section 330, and CHCs can have more than one of these grants. A CHC that has more than one Section 330 grant program is required to report on each one separately. Based on the reporting requirements of the Section 330 grants through the FSR, it is important that the chart of accounts' structure is set up properly to assist in generating the activity for the scope of the project for all Section 330 grants received from the BPHC. The nonfederal grants and contracts may be included in the scope of a Section 330 program but it is not required.

Another report required under the BPHC grants is the Uniform Data System (UDS), which is filed on a calendar-year basis. This report is used to capture data on the services provided with the Section 330 grant funds, and it is used to monitor the grantee. The data captured in this report are both financial and statistical. The financial data comprise costs by cost center; patient services revenue charges, adjustments, collections, bad debts by payer and other revenues. The chart of accounts' structure needs to be set up to provide the financial data needed to complete this report.

Cost Report Requirements

As noted previously, CHCs receive reimbursement for services from patients, as well as third parties (Medicaid, Medicare, private insurance companies, managed care plans and others). The method of reimbursement varies from payer to payer. One method is an all-inclusive, cost-based rate that is determined from a cost report filed by the CHC. This type of reimbursement is required for Medicaid and Medicare through the Federally Qualified Health Center (FQHC) legislation passed by Congress in the late 1980s. The all-inclusive, cost-based rate is determined from the organization's allowable cost of providing services divided by billable visits. The CHC chart of accounts needs to be designed in such a manner as to provide the expenses as required by the cost reports.

Managed Care Requirements

As managed care becomes a larger driving force in the health care environment, it also has an increasing impact on CHCs. Community Health Centers are finding themselves dealing with managed care organizations more and more, especially as states are beginning to implement managed care for Medicaid recipients. With managed care comes additional financial information that CHCs should monitor in order to remain competitive. The CHC chart of accounts should be designed with this in mind.

How to Adapt the COA for CHCs

In designing the format of the chart of accounts, the CHC should consider the suggested categories noted and determine if there are any additional categories that need to be tracked. The general design covers some of the basic items that a CHC may need such as site, cost center and account number. Additional categories that should be taken into consideration are fund, federal grant program and other grants and contracts. There is no set order that these segments are required to be in; the CHC should determine the best order based on their preference and how their accounting software package operates. For example, some accounting software packages require that the account number is the first segment.

The following sections will be detailed discussions on how to adapt the COA account structure and design to CHCs to meet their specific reporting requirements. We will review each of the segments of the sample chart of accounts and discuss what modifications are needed for CHCs, as well as the recommended additional segments and how they should be set up. Each segment represents a level of detailed information that the organization needs to capture as shown in the financial costing format design of the chart of accounts.

Account Number

The chart of accounts Table I in the Appendix provides a comprehensive base for health care organizations and requires a minimal amount of modifications for Community Health Centers. The categories suggested meet the detail required for a majority of the reporting requirements previously identified. There are only a few modifications that need to be made to meet the needs of a CHC.

Exhibit 8.1, Patient Accounts Receivable, provides a sample breakdown of receivables by payer. This allows a CHC to track how much each payer owes and makes it easy to calculate days in accounts receivable by payer. The major payers should be categorized to provide management with relevant information and with the appropriate amount of detail. This information should also be contained in the accounts receivable subsidiary ledger. Summarizing the information by category will allow for more meaningful financial reporting.

EXHIBIT 8.1 Patient Accounts Receivable Detail (Sample)

Account Number	Description
1300	Accounts Receivable — Patients
1310	Accounts Receivable — Medicaid (MCD)
1319	MCD Allowance for Doubtful Accounts
1320	Accounts Receivable — Medicare (MCR)
1329	MCR Allowance for Doubtful Accounts
1330	Accounts Receivable — Self-Pay
1339	Self-Pay Allowance for Doubtful Accounts
1340	Accounts Receivable — Private Insurance
1349	Private Insurance Allowance for Doubtful Accounts
1350	Accounts Receivable — Medicaid Managed Care
1359	Medicaid Managed Care Allowance
1360	Accounts Receivable — Commercial Managed Care
1369	Commercial Managed Care Allowance
1370	Accounts Receivable — Other (Patients)
1379	Accounts Receivable Allowance for Doubtful Accounts

As with patient accounts receivable, the patient services revenue and adjustments should be summarized by the major payer in order to be able to easily calculate the days in accounts receivable by payer. In addition, this information is useful in determining how much patient revenue a CHC is generating. It will assist CHCs in actual as well as budgeted amounts. The patient revenues and adjustments should be information that is contained in the patient accounts receivable subsidiary system, but as previously noted, it is in more detail. Once again, the appropriate categorization of payers makes the information more meaningful and useful to management. Patient services revenue and adjustments by these categories of payers is required to complete Table 9D of the BPHC's UDS.

EXHIBIT 8.2 Patient Services Revenue Detail (Sample)

Account Number	Description
4100	Gross Charges
4110	*Patient Services Revenue — Gross Charges*
4120	*Medicaid*
4121	*Medicaid Retroactive Settlement*
4130	*Medicare*
4131	*Medicare Retroactive Settlement*
4140	*Self-Pay*
4150	*Private Insurance*
4160	*Medicaid Managed Care*
4170	*Commercial Managed Care*
4190	*Other — (Patient)*
4300	Patient Refunds
4400	Fees Collected — Other Revenue
4410	Sales — Medical Related
4420	Patient Records Copying Reimbursement
4430	Fees Collected — Other
4450	Donations Received
4455	*Donated (In-Kind) Goods and Services*
4460	Research/Clinical Studies Income
4470	Grant and Contract Revenue
4480	Miscellaneous Income
4490	Operating Subsidy Income
4500	**ADJUSTMENTS**
4520	*Medicaid Contractual Allowance*
4530	*Medicare Contractual Allowance*
4532	*Medicare — Coinsurance*
4534	*Medicare — Patient Deductibles*
4540	*Self-Pay Sliding Fee Adjustment*
4550	*Private Insurance Contractual Allowance*
4560	*Medicaid Managed Care Contract Allowance*
4570	*Commercial Managed Care Contractual Allowance*
4590	*Other — Patients' Contractual Allowance*

Salary Expenses

Another area where health centers require more detail in the chart of accounts is the salary expense section. The sample chart of accounts details salary expenses for physicians, midlevel providers, ancillary and other staff. (The accounts that are often unique to CHCs are noted in italics.) Note that dental hygienists and oral therapists are included in the midlevel provider category. Pharmacists and pharmacy assistants are included in the ancillary staff category. This level of detail and more is needed by CHCs for cost reports and the UDS.

EXHIBIT 8.3 Salary Detail (Sample)

Account Number	Description
5000	**OPERATING EXPENSES — Salary and Fringe Benefits**
5100	PHYSICIANS — SALARIES
5110	Salaries, Distributions and Incentives (Physician)
5180	*Dentists*
5190	*Psychiatrists*
5300	MIDLEVEL PROVIDERS — SALARIES
5310	Salaries (Midlevel)
5360	Employee Incentives (Midlevel)
5500	ANCILLARY STAFF — SALARIES
5510	Salaries — Radiology
5520	Salaries — Laboratory
5530	Salaries — Optical
5540	Salaries — Physical Therapy
5550	Salaries — Other Ancillary Services
5700	EMPLOYEES — SALARIES
5710	Salaries — General Administrative
5715	Salaries — Business Office
5720	Salaries — Managed Care Administrative
5725	Salaries — Information Services
5730	Salaries — Housekeeping/Maintenance/Security
5735	Salaries — Medical Receptionist
5740	Salaries — Medical Secretaries / Transcribers
5745	Salaries — Medical Records
5750	Salaries — Other Administrative Support
5755	Salaries — Registered Nurses
5760	Salaries — Licensed Practical Nurses
5765	Salaries — Medical Assistants/Nurses Aids
5770	*Salaries — Medical Technicians*
5775	*Salaries — Social Service Professionals*
5780	*Salaries — Other*

Tracking Grants, Contracts, Donations and Different Organizational Units

There are also some additional accounts that may need to be added to the chart of accounts. Grants receivable and refundable advance (liability) accounts most likely will need to be added, as noted in bolded italics in Exhibits 8.4 and 8.5. Since the accounting records for CHCs are maintained on a accrual basis of accounting, there could be amounts due or advances from grantors that need to be reflected.

EXHIBIT 8.4 Additional Accounts (Sample)

Grants and Contracts Receivable	
Account Number	**Description**
1300	*Accounts Receivable — Patients*
1310	*Accounts Receivable — Medicaid (MCD)*
1319	*MCD Allowance for Doubtful Accounts*
1320	*Accounts Receivable — Medicare (MCR)*
1329	*MCR Allowance for Doubtful Accounts*
1330	*Accounts Receivable — Self-Pay*
1339	*Self-Pay Allowance for Doubtful Accounts*
1340	*Accounts Receivable — Private Insurance*
1349	*Private Insurance Allowance for Doubtful Accounts*
1350	*Accounts Receivable — Medicaid Managed Care*
1359	*Medicaid Managed Care Allowance*
1360	*Accounts Receivable — Commercial Managed Care*
1369	*Commercial Managed Care Allowance*
1370	*Accounts Receivable — Other (Patients)*
1379	Accounts Receivable Allowance for Doubtful Accounts
1380	***Grant and Contract Receivables***

EXHIBIT 8.5 Additional Accounts (Sample)

Refundable Advances — Grants and Contracts	
Account Number	**Description**
2360	Estimated Contract Claims Payable
2370	Deferred Revenue — Capitation or Prepaid Plan
2375	Other Deferred Revenue
2380	Deferred Income Taxes — Current Portion
2385	***Refundable Advances — Grants and Contracts***
2390	Other Current Liabilities

CHCs that receive a significant amount of donated (in-kind) goods and services that can be valued and are necessary in the operation of the center (such as specialized skills or items that would normally need to be purchased) should be recorded in the accounting records. In this situation revenue accounts for donated goods and services would be needed to record these items with the debit going to asset or expense accounts as required. An example is Account 4455 noted in bold italics in Exhibit 8.6.

EXHIBIT 8.6 Additional Accounts (Sample)

In-Kind Goods and Services	
Account Number	**Description**
4450	Donations Received
4455	***Donated (In-Kind) Goods and Services***
4460	Research/Clinical Studies Income

Funds

This segment is used to track if grant funds and contributions are unrestricted, temporarily restricted, or permanently restricted as required for not-for-profit organizations by Financial Accounting Standards No. 116 and 117 (see the chapter on not-for-profits). Exhibit 8.7 provides a suggested fund segment to track these funds. Temporarily restricted funds are restricted funds and once the restriction is met should be transferred to unrestricted. Setting up separate temporarily restricted accounts based on the type of restriction is recommended based on the requirement to disclose this in the financial statements. Permanently restricted funds are funds restricted as endowments and may not be used for operations.

EXHIBIT 8.7 Funds (Sample)

Account Number	Description
0	Unrestricted
1	Temporarily Restricted — Strategic Planning
2	Temporarily Restricted — Diabetes Study
9	Permanently Restricted

Federal Grant Programs

As discussed earlier, the Section 330 grants from the BPHC have required reporting whereby it is necessary for CHCs to track the federal program that the grant funds are supporting. This includes all activities (revenues and expenses) within the scope of the project that are included in the grant application (budget). As noted in Exhibit 8.8, a segment for federal grant programs is an easy method to keep track of this activity.

EXHIBIT 8.8 Federal Grant Programs (Sample)

Account Number	Description
0	General
1	Community/Migrant Health Center
2	Homeless Grant
3	Ryan White Title III B
9	Non-Federal

Numbers 1 through 3 identify the BPHC-funded programs and additional numbers can be added to separately track other federal grant programs. The general number 0 is a temporary holding account used to track activity that needs to be allocated to the federal grant programs by month end. It may be necessary to have a segment number to track activity that is not applicable to any of the federal grant programs (i.e., number 9 as shown in Exhibit 8.8). This would represent programs or sites that are not included in the project scope of any of the federal grant programs that are received.

Other Grants And Contracts

This segment is used to track nonfederal grant and contract services funding that the CHC receives. These funds could be a part of the federal grant programs, but also have their own reporting needs as noted previously. By segregating these funds as a separate segment, there is the ability to track them with the federal grant program, if necessary, and still track their activity separately to meet their reporting needs. The activity that needs to be tracked is the revenue from these sources and the related expenses for which these funds are used. Also, this segment can be used to track the receivable or refundable advances on these funds separately, acting as a subsidiary ledger of the main account number.

EXHIBIT 8.9 Other Grants & Contracts (Sample)

Account Number	Description
00	General
01	State Department of Health — WIC
02	City Department of Health — Immunization

Sites

Many CHCs operate out of multiple sites. From a management reporting perspective, it may be necessary to produce financial reports on each of these sites individually in order to monitor how they are doing. To be able to produce these reports the activities of the sites needs to be maintained in the general ledger. By utilizing a segment to track each site's activities, the accounting system must be set up to provide this information.

EXHIBIT 8.10 Sites (Sample)

Account Number	Description
00	Main Site
01	South Site
02	North Site
03	East Site
04	West Site

Departments

Community health centers, like most health care organizations, have various departmental segments that they establish to monitor the activity of the services they provide. These departments in many cases are made up of the service units (specialties) as well as cost centers (support services). The need for this tracking is not only an internal requirement to measure budget to actual activity, but also assists in complying with external reporting requirements. To assist in the preparation of both cost reports and the UDS, it is necessary to be able to determine expenses by function. Departments can be used to provide this information. In addition, as a not-for-profit organization, CHCs are required to disclose in their financial statements expenses by function. Based on how the organization defines the functions, the department segment can also be used to meet these needs.

EXHIBIT 8.11 Departments (Sample)

Account Number	Description
000	Administration
100	Medical
101	Internal Medicine
102	Pediatrics
103	OB/GYN
110	Dental
115	Laboratory
120	Radiology
125	Pharmacy
130	Facility
135	Mental Health
140	Patient Transportation
145	Rehabilitation Therapy
150	Other Health Services
151	Podiatry
152	Optometry
153	Nutrition
160	Community Services
165	Health Education
170	Other Enabling & Outreach Services
175	Fund Raising
180	Data Processing
185	Patient Records

By utilizing the above segments, CHCs should be able to further modify the chart of accounts for their purpose. The example segments that are shown in the exhibits are a basis to use in developing your specific chart of accounts. These segments can be further modified to add items or increase the number of digits needed to meet the practice's exact needs.

9

Adapting the Chart of Accounts to Faculty Practice Plans

Paul V. Calandrella, M.S., J.D. and John R. Fernandez

Introduction

The physician practice chart of accounts (COA) is a critical tool for academic medical centers that can help lead health care finance into the 21st century. Presently, the variation between how physician practices maintain or utilize a chart of accounts has put both academic and nonacademic physicians in a futile position when negotiating or lobbying the government or third-party payers for appropriate and fair compensation for the services they render.

A detailed COA for academic medical practices (AMP) forms the basis for making sound management decisions, including financial and political ones that face the practices daily. In short, the more comparable the detail, the more effective the decision making. The following sections will:

- Provide background and a rationale for standardizing the COA for academic practices
- Review three case studies that demonstrate applications of COA for business and academic planning purposes
- Review some of the complex issues facing academic practices in the near future

In the final analysis, they who have organized leadership will win the war.

Why a Standard COA for Academic Practices?

Simply stated, sound financial management is a necessity given the projections of double-digit reduction in payments by payers.

A chart of accounts serves several purposes in a clinical practice, just as it does in any private, public, profit or not-for-profit organization. It supports financial statement presentation, internal reporting, decision making and implementation of the compensation structure of the organization. This discussion will primarily focus on application of a COA to business decisions and physician compensation structures for a separately incorporated non-profit physician organization operating in affiliation with an academic teaching hospital. However, the application also works well with other corporate structures.

Business Decisions

Traditional accounting controls accompanied by periodic independent audits can reasonably ensure the accuracy of an organization's financial records. The mere accuracy of the information alone, however, makes it neither manageable or meaningful. A well-designed chart of accounts, however, will allow an organization to flexibly manage information in accordance with its decision-making process.

At its most basic level, the chart of accounts should allow for flexible presentation of information in accordance with an organization's structure (i.e., the hierarchy of business units). Individual authority and accountability generally correlate to the business units, culminating with the president, chief executive officer, executive director or similarly titled positions having responsibility for the entire organization's results. It is also common for an organization to view its structure in multiple ways. A physician organization, for example, may wish to view information as it relates to specialty practices or to physical locations regardless of specialty. The ability of the chart of accounts to reflect these variations is equal in importance to its ability to capture and report information at the most discrete level of detail.

The ability to present information in accordance with the organizational structure allows management to determine which units, and thus which individuals, are performing within financial expectations. This is traditional historical variance analysis. Though not completely determinative, it can test the validity of expectations regarding how proposed new ventures or operational changes will manifest themselves in the financial results of a particular business unit. For example, a division that historically has struggled to generate a surplus may be a poor candidate for development of a joint venture or new service line. Management may decide to proceed with the proposal, however, if it provides a mechanism for fixing the problems that drive the unit's historical deficiencies.

Increasing shareholder value is the primary motivator that drives key business decisions in a publicly held corporation. Unlike a corporation, which focuses on shareholder value as its ultimate goal, the missions of an academic teaching facility and its affiliated non-profit physician organizations must encompass the diverse objectives of their many stakeholders. These might include current patients, future patients that may benefit from current research, employees and the community, as well as medical students, residents and others whose career training is carried out within the academic teaching hospital.

In addition to the consideration of various stakeholders, the very nature of affiliations within the academic teaching hospital setting makes the decision process complex. For example, a physician organization, though a separate corporation, may tightly integrate with the corresponding department of the academic teaching hospital (e.g., surgery, medicine, radiology, etc.). Its physicians may operate their practice within the physical confines of the hospital facilities or campus, and they may hold positions or appointments within both the physician organization and the hospital, as well as serve on the faculty of the affiliated medical school. A residency program, while under the auspices of the teaching hospital, may function only via the training provided by the attending physicians employed through the physician organization. Such interdependency and overlap among entities precludes the physician organization from making decisions based strictly upon its own financial interest.

Given its diverse stakeholders and interdependencies with affiliated organizations, a physician organization may have important motivations beyond the financial bottom line. Nonetheless, expenditures should be made consistent with a mission of commitment to patients, the hospital and academic institution's reputation or the profession as a whole.

While an organization in the academic setting must consider the financial realities, those realities will not always drive the final decisions. It is in these circumstances that a detailed and flexible chart of accounts demonstrates its value. A detailed chart of accounts is highly sensitive and reflects even small events that, if compounded, could become unmanageable. While decisions may be necessary for internal reasons, the sensitivity of the chart of accounts reveals the impact of decisions, and therefore the need for the organization to ultimately offset these impacts in other areas to remain solvent as a whole.

Physician Compensation Structures

The manner in which an entity structures physician compensation may directly affect the level of funds available to the organization and its resulting ability to serve its constituents. Physician compensation schemes may range from straight salary without incentives to a purely incentive-based structure tied to a physician's productivity, however that may be defined. At either end of the spectrum, a detailed chart of accounts will further an organization's ability to administer the compensation plan and meet its financial objectives.

A salary-based plan without performance incentives provides little motivation with respect to the volume of reimbursable services provided by physicians. On the other hand, it may remove barriers for physicians who provide indigent patient care, perform research, or undertake other nonrevenue generating activities integral to the organization's mission. In this setting, the individual physicians, their respective departments, and the organization as a whole utilizes the detailed chart of accounts in the same manner previously described with respect to business decisions. The detailed chart of accounts provides for detailed management and accountability for expenses under control of the physicians. A physician's ability to manage expenses while furthering organizational goals is then used as a factor in setting future compensation. The relationship of the chart of accounts to physician compensation becomes even more dynamic with a move toward incentive-based compensation plans.

With an incentive compensation plan, one or more cost centers are associated with each physician for the recording of both income and expenses. Whether for the purposes of the physicians' entire compensation or for strictly performance-based bonuses, proper assignment of revenues and expenses to these physician cost centers requires precise front-end administrative and transaction processing systems, in addition to the detailed chart of accounts. Assuming these front-end systems are in place, entries to these cost centers will occur either through direct charges or allocation of shared charges such as rent or administrative overhead. Because the physicians' compensation depends upon this process, the group will rapidly identify and challenge suspected errors to the chief financial officer or to another individual overseeing administration of physician compensation. While it may be motivated by self-interest, this level of scrutiny effectively creates a financial control and monitoring structure throughout the entire organization. Tracking income and expenses to the physician level also allows senior management to clearly identify which physicians currently fall below expectations so that they may take corrective action.

Once issues regarding physician revenues and expenses are resolved, the information is used to drive the incentive compensation calculation. Exhibit 9.1 illustrates the calculation of a physician surplus or deficit. The inclusion of Physician Salary after calculation of Net Practice Income emphasizes the compensation scheme's incentive feature. Exhibit 9.1 also presents an example of how an individual physician's surplus or deficit is treated. In this case, there could be an impact on the physician's individual compensation, the division's funds or corporate level funds.

EXHIBIT 9.1

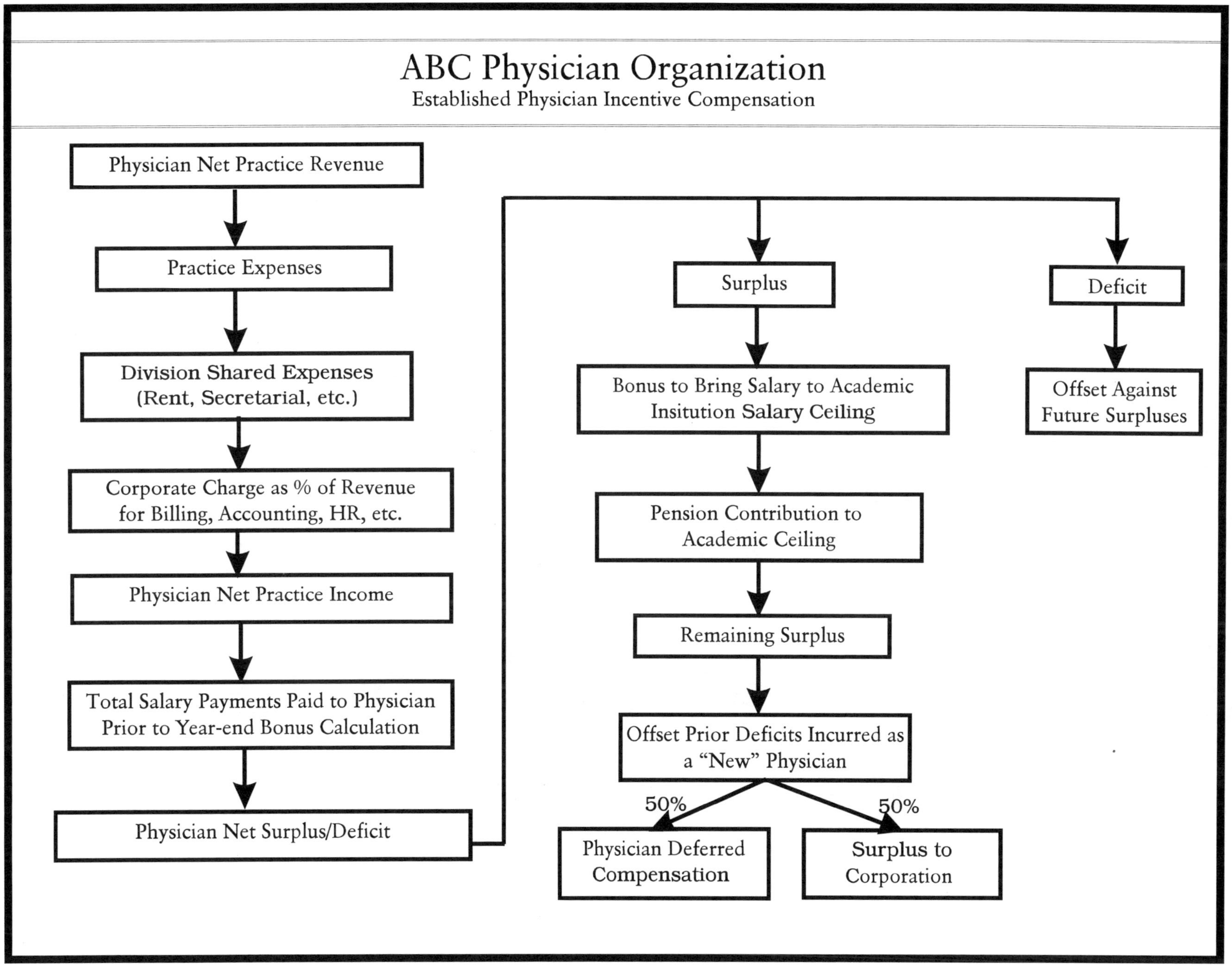
ABC Physician Organization
Established Physician Incentive Compensation
Physician Net Practice Revenue
Practice Expenses
Division Shared Expenses (Rent, Secretarial, etc.)
Corporate Charge as % of Revenue for Billing, Accounting, HR, etc.
Physician Net Practice Income
Total Salary Payments Paid to Physician Prior to Year-end Bonus Calculation
Physician Net Surplus/Deficit
Surplus
Bonus to Bring Salary to Academic Insitution Salary Ceiling
Pension Contribution to Academic Ceiling
Remaining Surplus
Offset Prior Deficits Incurred as a "New" Physician
50%
50%
Physician Deferred Compensation
Surplus to Corporation
Deficit
Offset Against Future Surpluses

In theory, in a pure incentive-based system cost overruns or revenue shortfalls should be offset by a reduction in a physician's compensation. Strict adherence to this approach, however, may be detrimental to an organization over the long run. For example, new members who bring desired talent to the physician organization might need financial leeway to establish their practices. A physician organization could choose to absorb losses associated with new physicians or a new service line during the first few years while guaranteeing a salary for the new physicians during that period. Conversely, if a new physician generates a surplus, the physician organization may retain all or a portion of it during the first few years of employment to offset the risk it absorbs by guaranteeing a salary to the new physician. The absorption of new physician losses and retention of surpluses also may take place at a division level consistent with decentralization of fiscal accountability. Exhibit 9.2 illustrates a compensation structure for new physicians with surplus and loss allocations at both divisional and total corporation levels.

EXHIBIT 9.2

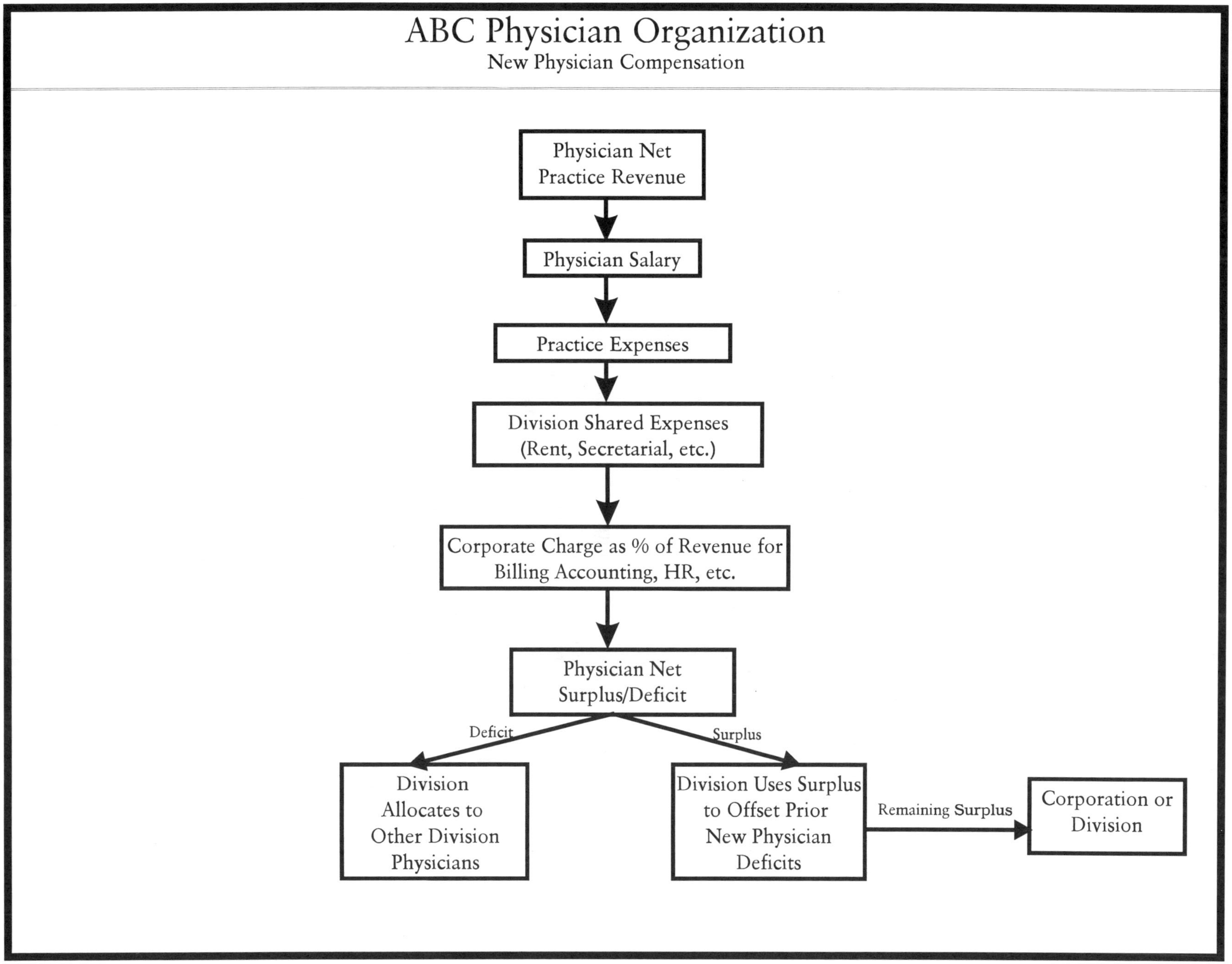
ABC Physician Organization
New Physician Compensation
Physician Net Practice Revenue
Physician Salary
Practice Expenses
Division Shared Expenses (Rent, Secretarial, etc.)
Corporate Charge as % of Revenue for Billing Accounting, HR, etc.
Physician Net Surplus/Deficit
Deficit
Surplus
Division Allocates to Other Division Physicians
Division Uses Surplus to Offset Prior New Physician Deficits
Remaining Surplus
Corporation or Division

Corporate Background

Significant changes have affected health care and health care delivery during the past decade. Sources of income have shifted from Fee-for-Service practices, which operate independently and generate large revenues, to organizations that consolidate practices in order to pool risk. New opportunities may exist for novel applications of health services and support infrastructures. Potential for gains should be identified in the areas of financial services, practice management and office management.

Industry Summary

There exist several types of health organizations whose purpose is to profit from providing financial and/or clinical services to small practices and doctors' offices. The services range from direct ownership of the practice, as in the physician practice management model, to those performing simple office and secretarial services, as in the office management companies. Large, often publicly-traded corporations that purchase physician practices in return for equity have subsequently experienced heavy losses. These physician practice management companies (PPMCs) operate multispecialty clinics, as well as manage independent practice associations (IPAs). Typically, these PPMCs purchase the physician practice whose physicians then become employees of the company. The physicians usually receive a lump-sum (cash or equity in the company) from the PPMC, which then becomes responsible for billing and collecting revenues and performing other management functions.

There are many organizations of this type, including successful and unsuccessful ones. The largest company is Nashville-based Phycor, Inc. It is a PPMC that acquires and operates multispecialty medical clinics and develops and manages IPAs. Currently it operates 60 clinics with about 4,130 physicians in 29 states and manages IPAs with more than 21,900 physicians in 35 markets. Its net revenue increased to $322 million during the first quarter of 1998, compared to $250 million during the first quarter of 1997. However, its expenses similarly increased so much that its net earnings showed a loss, and the PPMC had a negative cash flow of $7.5 million in the first quarter of 1998. Regardless of this, the company has continued to pursue its policy of aggressive takeovers and purchases of physician practices.[1]

Each of these companies utilizes COA information in order to make decisions about valuing or devaluing a practice.

The health care financial service field carries substantial risk and has high barriers to entry. Profits are achieved only when the number of practices served is increased — a system that is unreliable and has a high possibility of collapse. Various models of financial structure require various capital outlays — ranging from several hundred thousand dollars to several hundred million dollars — to finance and initiate working programs. Each of the financial service and clinical models requires substantial capital investment and carries heavy risks. Net profits in these fields have not proven to be easily realized. The health care companies depend upon thin profit margins that grow by expanding the number of contracts and practices they acquire. If growth is difficult or unsustainable, the companies face the threat of insolvency or liquidity.

Industry averages and medians for return on equity and for profit margin are cause for concern. A cross-sectional analysis of eight industry companies with a history of service in the field shows poor earnings and profits. (Licholand Study; not yet published). Products and services range from typical practice management corporations that purchase physician practices to those that offer simple financial services.

Analyses of profits indicate that margins as a percentage of total revenue, including nonoperating income related to net income, are generally slim. The industry average profit margin is 1.0 percent, and the industry median is 1.3 percent. Industry averages indicate that return on equity is 2.2 percent, and the median is 1.8 percent. This is a reflection of a combination of poor net income and relatively high asset-to-liability ratio. Data were collected from annual reports, security disclosures and announcements for data collected in 1997.

Case Studies for Academic Medical Practices (AMP)

There are probably hundreds of versions of the themes presented in the following case studies, which have been developed to illustrate the scope of this section. AMPs are:

- More financially complex than traditional practices
- Often driven by internal or politically-based decisions
- Good examples of why a COA needs to be a management tool, used on a regular basis as opposed to existing as a book on the shelf
- Good examples of why the need for a comprehensive and standardized COA is critical to the success of the AMP
- Good examples of why the future will be more difficult than the past, and why the past will not be a great indicator of future performance.

The following three cases will include:

- A spreadsheet
- A discussion of the spreadsheet
- An overview of how management used the tool
- A summary of what happened as a result of the actions taken

The cases are examples of three of the four quadrants of Diagram A below.

DIAGRAM A

Academic Medical Practice
Chart of Accounts and Management Continuum

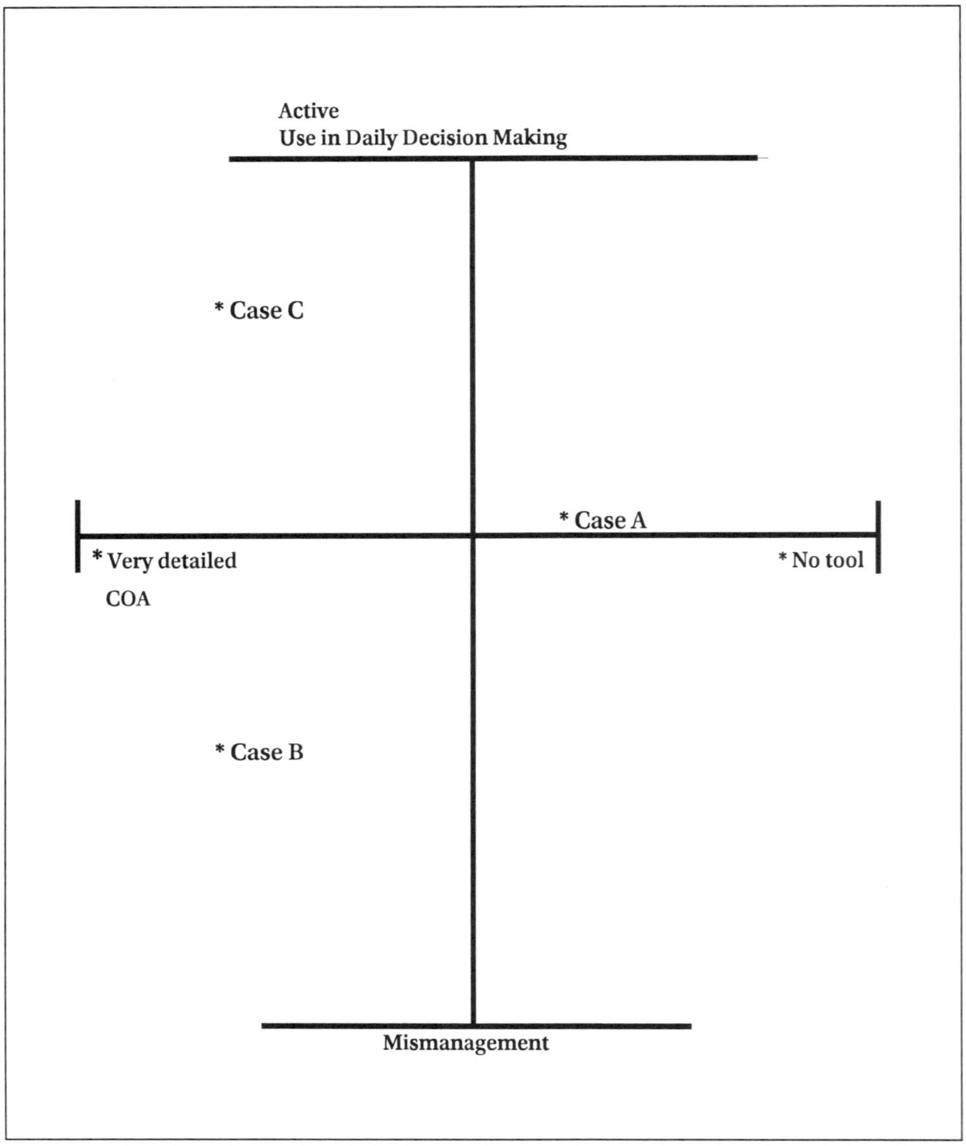

The following is a case study that will examine three stages of a practice's life. It demonstrates how the chart of accounts enhanced the bottom line of the organization by continuing to obtain and then utilize detailed management information. Several of the maneuvers are relevant to a variety of academic practices.

Background: This case study is based on an organization that averages $60 million in annual revenues. The physician complement ranges from 150 to 200 doctors; it is a multispecialty practice. Many of the expenses are fictional and designed to illustrate the points of these case studies. A physician leader and a senior nonphysician executive managed the practice. Salaries were determined by the practice, not by the health system or the medical school. Obviously, each of these assumptions has substantial implications, especially regarding compensation systems, but due to limitations in the scope of this chapter we will not become involved with compensation systems. This practice was part of an "integrated delivery system." Following is a spreadsheet (Exhibit 9.3) showing the continued improved performance of this practice through cases A, B and C.

EXHIBIT 9.3 Chart of Accounts Summary

Account Number	Description	Case A	Case B	Case C
1000	**Assets**			
1100	Cash Unrestricted — Banks	50,000	50,000	50,000
1200	Marketable Securities & Short-Term Investments			
1300	Accounts Receivable	50,000,000	60,000,000	30,000,000
1400	Supply Inventories			
1500	Prepaid Expenses			
1600	**INVESTMENTS — LONG-TERM RECEIVABLES**			
1700	Property, Furniture, Fixtures & Equipment			
1800	Accumulated Depreciation — Property, Furniture, Etc.			
1900	Intangible and Other Assets			
	Subtotal	***50,050,000***	***60,050,000***	***30,050,000***
2000	**Liabilities**			
2100	Current Liabilities — Payables	1,000,000	1,000,000	1,000,000
2200	Current Liabilities — Payroll	2,000,000	2,000,000	2,000,000
2300	Current Liabilities — Other			
2400	Long-Term Liabilities			
	Subtotal	***3,000,000***	***3,000,000***	***3,000,000***
3000	**NET ASSETS (NOT-FOR-PROFIT EQUITY)**	**47,050,000**	**57,050,000**	**27,050,000**
4000	**REVENUES**	**60,000,000**	**60,000,000**	**60,000,000**
4500	Adjustments	-	(4,000,000)	-
	Subtotal	***60,000,000***	***56,000,000***	***60,000,000***
5000	**OPERATING EXPENSES — SALARY & FRINGE BENEFITS**			
5100	Physicians — Salaries	30,000,000	30,000,000	30,000,000
5200	Physicians — Employee Related Expenses	13,500,000	10,500,000	7,500,000
5300	Midlevel Providers — Salaries	700,000	700,000	700,000
5400	Midlevel Providers — Employee Related Expenses	210,000	210,000	210,000
5500	Ancillary Providers — Salaries	500,000	500,000	500,000
5600	Ancillary Providers — Employee Related Expenses	150,000	150,000	150,000
5700	Other Employees — Salaries	700,000	700,000	700,000
5800	Other Employees — Employee Related Expenses	210,000	210,000	210,000
5900	Temporary Employee Salaries — Professional	200,000	200,000	200,000

Exhibit 9-3 continued

Account Number	Description	Case A	Case B	Case C
	Subtotal	***46,170,000***	***43,170,000***	***40,170,000***
6000	**SERVICES AND GENERAL EXPENSE**			
6100	Office and Administrative Expense	150,000	150,000	150,000
6200	Copying (Admin.)	100,000	100,000	100,000
6300	Depreciation	200,000	200,000	200,000
6400	General Supplies	150,000	150,000	150,000
6500	Billing Expense	-	-	-
6600	General Services	50,000	50,000	50,000
6700	Bad Debt Expense	20,000	20,000	20,000
	Subtotal	***670,000***	***670,000***	***670,000***
7000	**CLINICAL EXPENSE**			
7100	Equipment Rentals (Clinical)	100,000	100,000	100,000
7500	Occupancy Expense	400,000	400,000	400,000
7600	Cost of Goods Sold — Medical Related	400,000	400,000	400,000
	Subtotal	***900,000***	***900,000***	***900,000***
8000	**PURCHASED SERVICES/MANAGEMENT FEES**			
8100	Purchased Services — Professional and Medical	7,000,000	8,000,000	-
8200	Purchased Services — Prepaid/Capitation Profess. & Medical	-	-	-
8300	General & Administrative Expense — Purchased Services	4,500,000	8,000,000	12,000,000
8400	Reinsurance	-	-	-
8500	Management Fees — MSO/PPM	4,800,000	4,800,000	4,800,000
	Subtotal	***16,300,000***	***20,800,000***	***16,800,000***
9000	**NONOP REVENUE & EXP., INCOME TAXES & OTHER EXPENSES**			
9100	Nonoperating Revenues	-	(6,000,000)	(8,000,000)
9200	Nonoperating Expenses	-	-	-
9300	Other Income/Expense	-	-	-
	Subtotal	-	***(6,000,000)***	***(8,000,000)***

Exhibit 9-3 continued

Account Number	Description	Case A	Case B	Case C
	Total Operating Expenses	**64,040,000**	**59,540,000**	**50,540,000**
	Net Operating Income	**(4,040,000)**	**460,000**	**9,460,000**
NI = No Information				
	MDs	150	200	150
	Expense/MD	426,933	297,700	336,933
	Revenue/MD	400,000	280,000	400,000

The story goes that ABC Practice had no detailed chart of accounts — just basic expenses, services and limited details to the accounts. The chairman and the president of the practice basically kept a back-of-the-envelope tally as to whom was getting paid what amount and what the various arrangements were for each employee. At that time, the practice had 150 FTE providers with a total salary of $30 million and revenues of $60 million. There were also research activities carried on by this group. Note in the spreadsheet that there were $7 million in purchased services spent on consulting. Net loss for this group was approximately $4 million. This state of affairs (losing $4 million) motivated the practice to look at the existing detail, which caused them to recognize that the salaries were high. However, when the group went to determine action steps, the practice was stuck on whether or not it was feasible to reduce the physicians' salaries and possibly risk the revenue stream. Next they examined the purchased services line, which included approximately $7 million. It was unclear exactly what these monies were for, but it was known to include management fees for billing as well as other activities. Due to limited information in the chart of accounts, they were unable to determine where they might be able to make cuts. They were afraid of taking an across-the-board 10 to 20 percent cut because they lacked the necessary information on exactly what this represented.

The nonphysician manager was fired because the practice lacked all this financial detail. They purchased the MGMA/CRAHCA detailed *Chart of Accounts for Health Care Organizations* and hired a consulting firm to assist them with this transition, while at the same time trying to recruit a new manager.

Now let's move on to Case B or Phase 2 of this practice. In Case B we have the same situation: $60 million in revenues, $30 million in total physician salaries and the same number of physicians. However, this time, after many months of work, there exists extensive financial detail of all expenditures. Again, after much review, it was determined that the fringe benefits structure was a bit high and that some benefits, like car allowances, which were provided to assistant professor-level physicians and above, would be eliminated. This was found in a detail under the fringe benefits accounts. In addition, it was determined that in order to increase productivity, 50 additional physicians needed to be hired for the practice. However, since the practice was in a relatively medium-sized market and already had much of the market share, the revenues did not increase. In addition, detailed information was obtained about the general administrative expenses; much of it had been used for purchasing physician and management services and, therefore, was not something the group felt could be cut immediately. The consultants, along with the new manager, ordered a complete review of the entire chart of accounts from top to bottom. This review cost about $8 million; the practice determined that there were significant revenues to be recovered from this top-to-bottom look.

In the end, this practice barely made a profit, even though it expended significant resources on consulting, on the top-to-bottom approach and in adding new physicians (which yielded no new income). What happened here? Adjustments were made to the revenues generated by several of the high-level academic, salaried physicians who failed to fill out the paperwork and who did not meet their clinical productivity measures. This necessitated a huge correction to the revenue line because of bad billing practices. These revenues were determined to not be collectable in the future.

In summary, this practice had all the details needed, but instead of using the detail in a strategic way it failed because it had weak management that did not analyze the chart of accounts and did not focus its energies in the right areas.

Finally, we come to a group that has essentially the same chart of accounts, with the addition of sound management. It is here that many academic practices can utilize a position in academics as well as multi-institutional arrangements to maximize their position. Several tactics were employed in Case C. For example, although there were 150 physicians (just like in the other two cases) and $30 million in total salaries, the group — through careful analysis — realized that several of its physicians provided hospital-based services and had research grants. Management was able to reduce those physicians' actual fringe benefits rate to 25 percent. They utilized some of their consulting/general administrative dollars to support two grants managers who assisted in obtaining additional non-NIH (National Institutes of Health) funding. These monies were paid directly to the group for clinical research activities and outcomes research, therefore leveraging their intellectual and academic prowess in a way that benefitted the group. The management also decreased the amount of consulting funds by reviewing the cost centers and targeting specific ones where there seemed to be opportunities for improvement.

In addition, it was identified that several of the research and academic activities were being charged to the practice; those expenses were appropriately moved to other organizations. Instead of spending, although there is the same expense line in general administrative expense, these monies were also used to make investments and bridge research projects that generated positive overheads for the department, as opposed to spending money solely on consulting arrangements. Moreover, these funds were directed to the divisions that were both clinically and academically productive, which assisted these groups in becoming more productive. It also helped the bottom line.

In summary, practices with very similar characteristics in terms of number of physicians, total revenues and total physician salaries can vary greatly. It is also important to ensure that sound management is in place so that creative utilization of the chart of accounts benefits the group's managers. Finally, it is necessary to be able to determine the appropriate level of detail so you know exactly where you are spending your money.

Several other examples come to mind, particularly in academic practices. They include funding of physician time for research even though it is being subtracted from clinical practice. This is common for many departments and is a perfectly legitimate way to operate a group practice. It is critical that the salary and other expense components have adequate detail so that when reimbursement to clients or something changes drastically, you know exactly how salary, consulting and other funds are being spent. In this case example, the salary lines were identical in each of the cases but the revenue productivity varied.

It is very clear that without utilizing the strength of a detailed chart of accounts, it is impossible in an academic practice to discern what is being used for academic purposes and what is being used for clinical or revenue-generating purposes. It is clear that a good chart of accounts cannot make up for bad management and that good management can be only moderately successful without a good chart of accounts. It is the combination of the two that is extremely powerful.

This would hold true on checking practices around the country. For example, a practice with large shared expense accounts might have five physicians who unanimously agreed to share equally all the expenses. At the end of the year, these expenses are equally distributed among the practice's physicians. However, without a detailed cost system, the group would be unable to retrace steps and reallocate funds to an individual practitioner if there had been a change in agreement midway through the year. It is this mechanism of shared expense that generally is utilized very skillfully in academic practices. It is a mechanism that may provide division chiefs a means of determining how those monies are spent, whether for research, academics, clinical time, etc.

While there are many cases where this works exceedingly well, it generally breaks down when the group wants to disband and/or when the revenues decrease. It can be difficult to determine who purchased what equipment, services and supplies without a good chart of accounts and financial management personnel. Lacking a good chart of accounts gives the division chief too much latitude on how money is spent and accounted for. Implementation of a detailed chart of accounts provides information that can be utilized by other constituencies to ensure that the power of the purse is being wielded fairly. Large academic practices can clearly benefit from using a detailed chart of accounts, which is as important as sound financial and business managers or physicians.

Future

The future of academic medical centers (AMC) and AMPs usually are tied to numerous external forces that complicate the application of an industry standard for COA. The five major factors are:

1. Integrated delivery systems (IDS) are growing.
2. Specialty care market niche opportunities are expanding.
3. Mergers and affiliations will probably continue and require the use of "their" systems.
4. The legal and regulatory environment continues to make AMPs more complex.
5. The information systems investments for AMPs are expanding, while revenues per patient are decreasing.

With the above challenges being considered, a detailed COA can be an effective management tool depending upon how it is used. Finally, AMC/AMP should be the leaders when developing a standard summary-level COA, but they need to allow for flexibility in the details.

Reference

[1] Liccohai Study

10

Adapting the Chart of Accounts to Hospital-Based Physician Practices

Lisa M. LaCourse

Introduction

This chapter addresses how a hospital that purchases or owns one or more medical group practices could utilize this chart of accounts (COA) for those groups and interface it with the existing hospital COA. Because hospitals and medical groups have very different organizational and cost structures and varying scopes of operations, each has unique reporting needs. It is perhaps not realistic to expect a large hospital system or even an individual hospital to drastically change its general ledger (G/L) format with the addition or incorporation of any medical groups into the corporate entity. Rather, in this chapter, it is assumed that the hospital would maintain an existing COA appropriate for a hospital even when medical practices are part of its overall health care system. The COA in this book will be referenced against the *Chart of Accounts for Hospitals*, created by the Healthcare Financial Management Association (HFMA).[1]

According to an Irving Levin Associates, Inc. survey of publicly announced acquisitions of medical practices that occurred in 1997,[2] there were 306 acquisitions involving 507 groups. Although many of the most recent transactions involve physician practice management companies (PPMCs), an increasing number of hospital mergers and acquisitions over the past four years could indicate a future trend of hospitals buying medical groups as well. Additionally, the survey captures only publicly announced acquisitions and thus misses local hospital purchases of small, independent practices. These types of acquisitions are certainly occurring and warrant attention in this text. Despite the fact that most hospitals project a loss during the first five years in *pro forma* analyses created during the due diligence process of medical group acquisition, long-term strategic plans and other services and geographic diversification needs for the hospital often tip the scale toward buying practices today. Also, as the administrative load on medical groups increases with managed care market penetration across the country, those smaller, independent practices are more frequently seeking buyers for their practices.

Unfortunately, most hospitals do not have the medical practice management expertise in-house, and the accounting, financial, and business concerns of a medical practice lie outside the traditional hospital finance department scope. This chapter will attempt to address these and other more detailed issues for the hospital-owned medical group as they affect both the hospital's and the medical group's accounting practices and structure.

Overall Account Structure

In some cases, hospitals can handle a simpler account structure with respect to details, such as accounting for each capitated-risk contract. In others, hospitals need to maintain a more complex COA overall due to macro-cost reporting issues and stringent, Generally Accepted Accounting Principles (GAAP) and Internal Revenue Service (IRS) requirements. In particular, assets and liabilities are on a much larger and broader scale in a hospital compared to just large medical groups, and revenue centers are more numerous and complex in an acute care hospital.

A hospital that owns medical groups will need to determine how much detail from the medical group must be retained for system-wide financial statements and what reporting requirements for the hospital should be brought into the medical group's COA. Of course, hospitals use an accrual-based accounting system so the medical group should use or convert to this same methodology.

The accounting system that a hospital sets up for its medical groups should be flexible enough to accommodate solo practitioners, as well as multiple groups with various specialty designations. The medical group's chart of accounts should have room so that the number of groups could expand beyond even the current long-range plans. The easiest strategy would be to have each physician in a group or groups, with the group being the common denominator for the medical group's cost centers. A group could have one physician or many. A physician could have multiple physician numbers or codes in the billing system such that the charges or revenue point to the proper group's cost center in the COA.

For example, let's say that a hospital owns four medical group practices. The primary care group has five physicians; the pediatric oncology group has three physicians; the psychiatry group has one physician; and the emergency department has 20 physicians, one of whom covers for the primary care group. This medical group's COA must determine how to separate the assets, liabilities, revenues and expenses for the four groups. For the physician who is part of the two groups, the billing system would assign charges attached to that physician's number to a different cost center depending upon either the location of the service or another distinguishing characteristic in the billing system.

The overall cost structure for the hospital-based medical group could eliminate some of the 20 digits to achieve the level of distinction among practices that the hospital needs. There is a fundamental question about numbering accounts within the medical group's COA with respect to separating revenues and expenses so that each group can generate its own monthly profit and loss (P&L) statements. There are a number of common solutions to this challenge. First, if the medical group maintains the full 20-digit COA structure, the P&L could be run against the different two-digit 'practice' codes in positions 2 and 3. Or each group could simply get a two-digit cost center and keep the account numbers consistent for all practices. Lastly, given the ample room left in the revenue and expense code ranges, unique four-digit revenue and expense accounts (as well as asset and liability accounts for A/R, etc.) could be assigned with a standard fourth digit based on the practice. In this last scenario, the primary care group account numbers would always end in "1," the pediatric oncology group accounts would always end in "2," and so on.

EXHIBIT 10.1

Practice codes

01	*Primary Care*
02	*Pediatric Oncology*
03	*Psychiatry*
04	*Emergency Department*

The practice code would be used as the "entity" designator under the hospital's COA.

Assets

For basic asset accounts, it is wise to have a separate checking account for each medical group's accounts payable (A/P) and daily cash deposits. Medical groups tend to collect many small checks whereas hospitals collect many more large checks. Additionally, more payers, including the government payers like Medicare and Medicaid, are sending payments via electronic funds transfers (EFTs). As part of the normal internal controls' procedures (and so that the medical groups do not have a more difficult time tracking down problem payments or mistakes in posting), the cash assets for daily operations should be kept strictly separate from the hospital's cash. Outside of this concern, a hospital-based medical group practice would, in general, not need as much detail for cash and other assets, such as investments, unless the physicians maintain a certain amount of equity ownership in their practice (i.e., it is a joint venture instead of an outright purchase of all assets and future revenue streams).

If most tangible assets such as real property, furniture, fixtures and equipment are owned by the hospital, then the 1700 - account series of the COA could be greatly simplified if not totally eliminated.

Bad debt has different ramifications for medical groups than it does for hospitals. Hospitals receive reimbursement from the Medicare program for bad debt expenses, whereas medical groups absorb all of those costs. Therefore, these bad debt adjustments to assets could be compiled for the entire hospital system, but the expenses need to be clearly delineated.

Charity care provided by medical groups has a different impact on medical groups than on a hospital. Also, there are important distinctions between a group that is owned by a not-for-profit hospital and a group that is owned by a for-profit organization. This issue is discussed in detail in the chapter on not-for-profit interpretations.

EXHIBIT 10.2 Asset Detail (selected accounts)

Account Number	Description
1000	**ASSETS**
1100	Cash
1110	Cash — Banks
1111	General Checking Accounts
1112	Payroll Checking Accounts
1113	Other Checking Accounts
1120	Cash — On Hand
1121	Change Fund
1122	Petty Cash
1130	Cash — Restricted
1200	Marketable Securities & Short-Term Investments
1210	Valuation Allowance — Short-Term Investments
1300	Accounts Receivable
1301	Accounts Receivable — Fee-for-Service Amounts
1302	Accounts Receivable — Prepaid Contracts
1320	Allowance for Estimated uncollectable Receivables
1321	Allowance for Bad Debts — Patient Accounts
1322	Allowance for Contractual Adjustments
1323	Allowance for Bad Debts — Third-Party Payers
1324	Allowance for Charity Care
1340	Notes Receivable — Short Term
1345	Managed Care Contract — Bonus/Withhold
1350	Other Short-Term Receivables
1351	Interest Receivables
1352	Intercompany Receivables
1353	Due from Employees
1354	Due from Related Parties
1400	Supply Inventories
1401	Drugs and Medications
1402	Medical Supplies
1403	Administrative Supplies
1404	Forms
1405	Housekeeping and Maintenance Supplies

Exhibit 10.2 continued

Account Number	Description
1406	Linen Supplies
1407	Other Supplies
1420	Ancillary Department Supplies
1500	Prepaid Expenses
1501	Prepaid Interest
1502	Prepaid Insurance
1503	Prepaid Rent
1504	Prepaid Taxes
1505	Prepaid Dues
1506	Other Prepaid Expenses
1510	Other Current Assets
1600	INVESTMENTS — LONG-TERM RECEIVABLES
1610	Long-Term Receivables
1630	Long-Term Investments
1635	Valuation Allowance — Long-Term Investments
1640	Investments in Affiliates
1650	Property Held for Future Use
1700	**PROPERTY, FURNITURE, FIXTURES & EQUIPMENT**
1710	REAL PROPERTY
1711	Land
1712	Land Improvements
1713	Buildings
1714	Capital Leases — Buildings
1715	Leasehold Improvements
1716	Construction in Progress
1717	Other Real Property
1750	**FURNITURE, FIXTURES & EQUIPMENT**
1751	Furniture and Fixtures
1752	Capital Leases — Furniture and Fixtures
1753	Equipment
1754	Capital Leases — Equipment
1755	Medical Equipment
1756	Capital Leases — Medical Equipment
1760	Computer
1761	Computer — Hardware
1762	Computer — Software
1763	Computer — Other
1770	Capital Leases — Computer
1771	Capital Leases — Computer — Hardware
1772	Capital Leases — Computer — Software
1773	Capital Leases — Computer — Other
1780	Vehicles
1781	Capital Leases — Vehicles
1790	Ancillary Service Equipment
1791	Laboratory Equipment

Exhibit 10.2 continued

Account Number	Description
1792	Radiology Equipment
1793	Physical Therapy Equipment
1794	Diagnostic Equipment
1795	Capital Leases — Ancillary Service Equipment
1796	Capital Leases — Laboratory Equipment
1797	Capital Leases — Radiology Equipment
1798	Capital Leases — Physical Therapy Equipment
1799	Capital Leases — Diagnostic Equipment

The hospital-based medical group's COA needs to have a high level of detail on the capitated revenue contracts, especially for those primary care practices (PCPs) that are often the initial targets for acquisition by hospitals. These PCPs have a very different revenue stream in many markets than the hospital owner, and the COA will need to accommodate these accounting requirements so that the practices can carefully monitor the profitability or the extent of monthly losses on each capitated contract. This level of detail also will be needed in contra-asset accounts, to handle the individual patient account adjustments and the revenue accounts as well.

EXHIBIT 10.3 Revenues (selected accounts)

Account Number	Description
4000	**REVENUES**
4100	Gross Charges
4110	Gross Charges — Fee-for-Service (FFS)
4120	Gross Charges — Discounted FFS Contracts
4130	Gross Charges — FFS Equivalents for Capitation Plan Patients
4140	Other Gross Charges
4150	Other Revenue
4200	Fees Collected
4210	Fees Collected — FFS
4220	Fees Collected — FFS for Managed Care
4230	Capitated Premium Revenues — Commercial
4240	Capitated Premium Revenues — Medicare
4250	Capitated Premium Revenues — Medicaid
4260	Capitated Premium Revenues — Other
4270	Risk Sharing Revenue
4271	Hospital Risk Sharing — Commercial
4272	Hospital Risk Sharing — Medicare
4273	Hospital Risk Sharing — Medicaid
4274	Hospital Risk Sharing — Pharmacy
4275	Hospital Risk Sharing — Other
4280	Other Managed Care Collected Revenues
4281	Copayments
4282	Coordination of Benefits
4283	Other Prepaid Professional Fees Collected
4290	Reinsurance Recoveries
4300	Patient Refunds
4350	Bad Debt Recovery
4400	Fees Collected — Other Revenue
4410	Sales — Medical Related
4420	Patient Records Copying Reimbursement
4430	Fees Collected — Other
4450	Donations Received (Operating Revenue)
4460	Research/Clinical Studies Income
4470	Grant Revenue
4480	Miscellaneous Income
4490	Operating Subsidy Income
4510	Gross Charges — FFS Discount/Adjustment
4500	**ADJUSTMENTS**
4520	Gross Charges — FFS for Managed Care Discount/Adjustment
4530	Gross Charges — FFS Equivalents for Cap Plan Patients/Adjustment
4540	Other Gross Charges/Adjustments
4550	Other Revenue Discount/Adjustment
4600	Financial Hardship Care Discount/Adjustment
4610	Courtesy Discount/Adjustment
4620	Employee Discount/Adjustment

Exhibit 10.3 continued	
Account Number	**Description**
4630	Charity Care Discount/Adjustment
4700	Third-Party Settlements
4800	Provision for Cash Basis Conversion

Liabilities

In conjunction with asset reallocation to the hospital COA, sometimes as part of the purchase of a practice, a hospital will assume graduate medical education debt from the physicians. This is one of the physicians' predominate liabilities in the first 10 to 15 years of practice, in addition to the practice's past debt financing, so this liability will need to be included in the medical group's COA in detail for each physician under section 2400 — Long-Term Liabilities. Graduate medical education loans are often very complicated. These require constant monitoring and follow-up by the physician even if the hospital assumes the loan. The multiple lenders, which are constantly shifting, must also be kept apprised of the medical group's and the physician's repayment arrangements. Alternatively, these liabilities could be tracked in the COA of the hospital, if they would be more easily assimilated to ensure the timely payment and follow-up on the loans.

Liabilities associated with payroll requirements could be streamlined in the medical group's COA if hospital personnel primarily manage the payroll functions through the hospital's payroll system. This issue is discussed in greater detail later in the chapter. However, there may be additional accounts in the medical group's COA in order to properly and adequately reserve for quarterly or annual bonuses or other payments to physicians, billing companies or medical group staff. These types of compensation and reimbursement arrangements are not common in hospitals. These liability accounts could be included toward the end of section 2100 — Current Liabilities — Payables.

EXHIBIT 10.4 Current liabilities (selected accounts)

Account Number	Description
2000	**LIABILITIES**
2100	**CURRENT LIABILITIES — PAYABLES**
2110	Accounts Payable
2120	Bank Overdrafts Payable
2130	Other Current Liabilities Payable
2131	Intercompany Accounts Payable
2132	Accounts Payable — Employees
2133	Accounts Payable — Related Parties
2134	Accounts Payable — Other
2160	Contract Claims Payable
2200	**CURRENT LIABILITIES — PAYROLL**
2210	Payroll Tax Withholdings Payable
2211	Federal Income Tax Withholdings Payable
2212	State Income Tax Withholdings Payable
2213	FICA/Medicare Tax Withholdings Payable
2214	Local Tax Withholdings Payable
2215	Other Tax Withholdings Payable
2220	Insurance Withholdings Payable
2221	Health Insurance Withholdings Payable
2222	Life Insurance Withholdings Payable
2223	State Disability Insurance Withholdings Payable
2224	Other Insurance Withholdings Payable
2230	Other Payroll Withholdings Payable
2231	401(k) Withholdings Payable
2232	Cafeteria Plan Withholdings Payable
2233	Court Mandated Child Support Withholdings Payable
2234	Other Payroll Withholdings Payable
2250	Accrued Payroll Liabilities
2251	Accrued Payroll
2252	Accrued Vacation, Holiday & Sick Pay (Compensated Absences)
2253	Accrued FICA/Medicare Taxes Payable
2254	Accrued State Unemployment Taxes Payable
2255	Accrued Federal Unemployment Taxes Payable
2256	Accrued Retirement Plan Contribution
2257	Other Accrued Payroll Liabilities
2260	Other Payroll Liabilities
2300	**CURRENT LIABILITIES — OTHER**
2310	Accrued Liabilities — Nonpayroll
2311	Accrued Rent
2312	Accrued Interest
2313	Accrued Insurance
2314	Accrued Income Taxes (Federal/State)
2315	Accrued Property Taxes
2316	Accrued Franchise Taxes

Exhibit 10. 4 Continued

Account Number	Description
2317	Other Accrued Liabilities
2320	Notes and Loans Payable
2321	Current Notes and Loans Payable — Vendors
2322	Current Notes and Loans Payable — Employees
2323	Current Notes and Loans Payable — Stockholders/Partners
2324	Current Other Notes and Loans Payable
2325	Bank Working Capital Line Outstanding
2330	Long-Term Debt — Current Portion
2331	Capital Lease Obligation — Current Portion
2332	Construction Contracts Payable
2333	Other Loans Payable – Current Portion
2340	Advances from Settlements Due to Third-Party Agencies
2350	Patient Deposits
2360	Claims Payable Incurred But Not Reported
2361	Incurred But Not Reported Claims — Commercial
2362	Incurred But Not Reported Claims — Medicare
2363	Incurred But Not Reported Claims — Medicaid
2365	Other Claims Incurred But Not Reported
2370	Deferred Revenue
2371	Deferred Revenue — Fee for Service
2372	Deferred Revenue — Capitated or Prepaid Plan
2375	Other Deferred Revenue
2380	Deferred Income Taxes — Current Portion
2390	Other Current Liabilities

Equity Relationships

This section of the COA will vary in a hospital-based group depending on the extent to which the medical group sells ownership to the hospital entity and what tax status the hospital has. If the physician or a group of physicians retains some equity interests in the practice, then the appropriate partnership or stockholder equity sections should be maintained in the medical group COA. If the medical groups do not have tax-exempt status as a not-for-profit organization but the hospital does, the residual equity gain or loss could be transferred to the fund balance account of the hospital after salaries and applicable bonuses are distributed to the medical group. Another point that could affect the equity accounts and other accounts is how the medical group handles deferred compensation, a familiar payment practice for physicians. There are a number of other permutations of these equity relationships in the COA that would be particular to the entities involved. However these arrangements are handled, it is unlikely that the same level of detail would be needed in the equity section of the COA for the hospital-based medical group compared to a for-profit hospital.

Revenues

Many hospitals buy medical practices and then subsume the ancillary revenues into the corresponding hospital cost centers. Two primary reasons for this are to simplify the accounting and to boost the revenues for those hospital departments. However, those same ancillary revenues traditionally have been a primary source of revenues for medical groups. Removing these revenues and their associated assets in the form of A/R from the medical group accounts is a decision that will affect the bottom line independent of the profitability of these practices. This should be clearly defined and understood up front when determining the corporate structure and business entity relationships. Physicians in some specialties, such as oncology, may not be willing to give up those ancillary revenues to the hospital outpatient departments so readily.

Retail pharmaceuticals and sales of other over-the-counter items such as vitamins and nutritional supplements are other examples of potentially lucrative revenue sources for medical groups. These fall outside of the traditional medical and surgical procedure codes and ancillary services that have been the mainstay of medical practice revenue in the past. Hospital-based groups will want to include separate accounts for the revenue and expenses associated with these items. They also need to include, under the 1300 account series for assets, the value of the inventory of these items.

If a hospital has a central billing function for the medical groups, it may want to consider marketing those services as a management services organization (MSO) or another similar entity. This seems to be a more fiscally sound plan for medical groups that have the backing of the hospital capital and personnel resources compared to an independent practice. Those services could then be contracted out to other physicians and groups. Potential markets for the MSO services would be other physicians in an attached medical office building that the hospital may own or in the community at large. If this becomes a business strategy of the hospital and its associated medical groups, the revenues and their associated expenses generated by those services must have a place in the medical group's COA. One suggestion would be designated accounts under nonoperating revenue and nonoperating expenses in the 9000 series. Or it could be included as nonphysician revenue under Account 4000 and nonpractice billing expenses under Account 6300. An appropriate percentage of central billing office (CBO) staff salaries and benefits could just be charged back to those accounts as well, rather than keeping separate salary and benefits cost centers for the contracted CBO services.

Hospital-based medical groups, and in essence all practices today, must exercise caution about the booking of courtesy discounts or professional write-offs for other physicians, friends, relatives and even hospital employees. The current environment of heightened attention on compliance with federal and other Medicare laws and regulations that prohibit kickbacks for referrals should convince the hospital and the medical group to monitor such a contra-asset account carefully.

Expenses

If the hospital is outsourcing its MSO billing functions as described in the revenues section, it must decide how to record those billing company expenses. Obviously, this will also affect how the hospital would track and record all A/R-associated functions, like collections, to ensure proper reimbursement for those services. In a related matter, if a CBO handles all practice A/R functions, how will these expenses be allocated across the groups if there are multiple groups? This CBO could have one aggregate cost center in the hospital's COA, and the costs could be allocated back to each group as an expense. Or the CBO could remain a cost center in the medical group's COA.

Under the opposite scenario, sometimes the billing functions for the practices are outsourced to a billing company. These billing company fees would be accrued in a separate account under liabilities, and the expenses would be booked separately by practice if the data are available from the contractor, as paid under Account 6100 of the COA.

Under payroll expenses, a hospital-based group would still need to maintain a high level of detail in the COA depending on the types of incentive compensation plans, current and planned, for all employees. This would include both physician and practice staff employees.

The hospital could define 'payments,' company-to-company transfers, or charge-backs by medical groups to the hospital for general administrative costs of hospital employee time to manage the medical groups and the overhead associated with their incorporation into the hospital organization. These costs might include a percentage of salaries and benefits for the information systems department, various affected finance functions, hospital administration, public relations, etc. On the other hand, there may be entire full-time equivalent (FTE) positions that are directly and solely attributable to the medical group. These costs could then be maintained in detail only on the medical group side.

General Ledger Crosswalks

Many issues that are related to hospital-based medical group COA decisions are possible in other related information systems as well. Depending on the hospital payroll system and the calculations necessary to determine medical group salaries for physicians and staff, the hospital should determine the following:

- From which company should it send data to the payroll system?
- Are the physicians and staff employees from the hospital or the medical group?
- How many expense accounts will be needed in each company's COA for salaries?
- What were the other payroll and compensation system issues mentioned earlier in this chapter?

If the hospital's COA can meet the needs defined above with one staff and one physician salary cost center for the medical group subsidiary and leave the level of complexity needed to process payroll in the medical group's COA, the additional cost centers required for the hospital, now and in the future, will be minimized. Additionally, the payroll function will remain fairly automated and will not add a lot of specialized work for the payroll department.

Whoever owns the A/R as an asset (as discussed in the section above) affects how the two COAs interface for the health care system's composite A/R information. Translations into appropriate A/R accounts depend on how the medical group's charge master, or its equivalent in a highly specialized physician billing system, is set up. Important COA decisions also rely on whether the medical groups and the hospital even use the same financial software vendors, much less the same programs.

The hospital and the medical groups should also determine how the materials management, inventory and ordering systems will track supplies and equipment for the practices, particularly if the practices are located off the main hospital campus. If supplies are ordered under the hospital's company number, every supply charge would involve a company-to-company transaction so that the expenses would appear in the medical group COA. An easier solution would be to set up a separate company indicator in the materials management system so that expenses and inventories transfer automatically into the medical group's COA. The same could be said for accounts payable (A/P) functions as well. These A/P transactions affect things like patient or insurance refunds and other check requests for the medical groups.

Conclusion

The specific issues that hospitals face when it owns one or more medical groups can readily be accommodated with minor modifications to the COA contained in this book. Translations between the existing hospital COA and the medical group COA and decisions about which COA will contain the appropriate level of detail are the predominate concerns. With foresight and planning involving administrators, managers and accountants for all involved parties, the joint and independent financial reporting and operations will run smoothly.

References:

1. Ronald Kovener, FHFMA, *Chart of Accounts for Hospitals* (HFMA and McGraw Hill Healthcare Publishing Group, 1998)

2. Denise Morrissey, *The Physician Medical Group Acquisition Report, Third Edition,* 1998 (New Caanan, CT, Irving Levin Associates, Inc., 1998)

11

Adapting the Chart of Accounts to Integrated Delivery Systems

Thomas M. (Mickey) O'Neal, CPA

Introduction

This chapter will address the adaptation of the *Chart of Accounts for Health Care Organizations* (COA) to integrated delivery systems. Keeping in mind that this chart of accounts has been derived from the *Medical Group Practice Chart of Accounts* as most recently published in 1996, the reader should realize that the group practice component of an integrated delivery system will be the focal point.

The key issues to be addressed in adapting the COA to integrated delivery systems include the following:

- Inclusion of multiple components under one financial reporting entity
- The impact of risk-based contracting on the financial reporting entity
- The need for multiple site reporting
- The increased emphasis on tools necessary for cost allocations to be used for sophisticated compensation models
- Heightened emphasis on external reporting requirements

The primary difficulties lie in the fact that no two integrated delivery systems are the same. The chart of accounts structure and its application cannot be absolute and must be considered a flexible system to be adapted to various structures in an orderly and logical manner.

Definition of Integrated Delivery Systems

An integrated delivery system in its most basic form combines two or more components of the health care delivery system into a single entity. Broadly speaking, these components include:

- Physician services
- Hospital services
- Ancillary services

An integrated health care system also includes the following components:

- Financing and risk bearing associated with insurance companies
- Billing and enrollment systems targeted to members
- Marketing to purchasers of health-plan products
- Customer service to members
- Claims adjudication

This chapter will focus on integrated delivery systems as the accounting and financial reporting of an integrated health system. Including all of the reporting responsibilities associated with the health insurance industry is outside the scope of this project.

Partially Integrated Systems *(First-tier Integration)*

Provider integration is usually the first step in the implementation of any form of an integrated system. These affiliations will be termed first tier integration systems as they represent affiliations or associations within one segment of the health care industry. It is important to note that these types of affiliation can and do occur in the hospital and health insurance segments as well.

An ***independent practice association*** (IPA) is a separate entity composed of independent practitioners. The entity is usually formed as a not-for-profit corporation or a limited liability company. The entity's sole purpose is to act as a vehicle for managed care contract negotiation and contracting for its members. The member's practices are not integrated although their contracting methodologies are.

The IPA may contract for physician services with managed-care plans on a fee-for-service or risk-sharing basis. Most successful IPAs enter into capitated contracts and take on many of the administrative functions normally handled by an insurance company including claims adjudication. Accordingly, this type of entity has substantial capitalization requirements and will have a sophisticated infrastructure including a management information system. A physician will usually enter into a participating provider agreement with the physicians and the IPA will normally not employ the doctors, depending upon the state where it is located.

A ***group practice without walls*** usually results from the merger of two or more independent medical practices. The group actually shares a common infrastructure such as upper level management, billings and collections; however, each operating location maintains its own financial independence. The group is able to share more economic risk than an IPA and will usually adopt a compensation system focusing on allocation of common costs and identification of direct expenses associated with separate practice locations. This is usually a transitional vehicle to a more integrated group practice.

The traditional ***group practice*** can either be a single specialty or a multispecialty entity. This entity is characterized by more complete economic integration. The group practice without walls will usually evolve into a group practice with fewer practice sites as leases expire and physicians combine into a more central practice location to take advantage of economies of scale.

A mature group practice may include various types of ancillary services including lab, radiology and other diagnostic services. One of the major advantages of a group practice is to facilitate owner succession. Accordingly a group practice will usually have some form of owner succession plan in the form of a buy-sell or shareholder's agreement.

Partially Integrated Systems *(Second-tier Integration)*

Second-tier integration implies that two or more segments of the health care industry are combining to form a single entity. These affiliations can occur through either contractual relationships or actual ownership arrangements.

A ***physician-hospital organization*** (PHO) is a separate legal entity usually owned and governed jointly by physicians and a hospital or hospital system. The physicians usually will affiliate in an IPA. The IPA then contracts with the PHO. The sole purpose of the PHO is to negotiate managed-care contracts for joint participation between the physicians (IPA) and the hospital. It is important to note that in most states the PHO is a contract negotiation vehicle only and cannot actually enter into managed-care contracts itself. The PHO model is usually seen as a transitional vehicle to a more integrated model of health care delivery.

A ***management services organization*** (MSO) is an entity used to provide practice management and administrative services to medical groups. This entity can be created by a hospital, a medical group or individual investors completely outside of the health care industry. The primary reason for creation of an MSO has been to form an affiliation through a long-term management agreement with a medical practice. Hospitals create them and use them to form alliances with physicians and medical groups. Investor groups and physician practice management companies form them to bring outside capital into the medical group to help build infrastructure necessary to successfully compete in a managed-care environment.

Fully Integrated Systems *(Third-tier Integration)*

A ***medical foundation*** is an example of a fully integrated delivery system. The exact form of the entity depends on state law; however, they are usually formed as not-for-profit corporations as defined by federal and/or state statutes. The foundation model allows a clinic to contract for managed-care services directly with the managed-care company and either contract with or employ the physicians. A fully integrated delivery system will coordinate all aspects of care including:

- Primary-care services
- Specialty-care services
- Outpatient care
- Ancillary services
- Inpatient care
- Skilled nursing facilities
- Long-term care
- Rehabilitation services
- Pharmaceuticals
- Behavioral health

The result is complete vertical integration of health care services including multiple levels of care among multiple types of providers. An integrated delivery system provides for the coordination of care for the patient, to expand the scope of services, the quality of care and to employ economies of scale in an effort to reduce the overall cost of care.

Independent Practice Associations

The Independent Practice Association (IPA) incorporates certain aspects of insurance companies in what is normally a physician owned and controlled company. IPAs can be used for many functions, including group purchasing and discounted fee-for-service contracting. Most mature and successful IPAs eventually enter into risk-contracting arrangements.

In a typical structure, an IPA will contract with a managed-care organization (MCO) to accept a portion of the MCO insurance premium to provide care to its members. The IPA will then contract with a panel of participating providers who agree to provide physician services in exchange for a capitated contract rate or some other form of discounted fee-for-service.

Accordingly, the IPA does accept certain insurance risks associated with providing health care services. The IPA will usually take certain steps to minimize this risk, which include acquiring stop-loss insurance and entering into risk-sharing arrangements to reduce certain costs including inpatient and ancillary services.

The accounting method most appropriate for a risk-sharing entity such as an IPA is the full accrual method of accounting. This primarily results from the necessity of recording a liability for claims incurred but not reported. The IPA receiving capitated contract revenues will invariably be responsible for paying some types of claims for services to be provided on a fee-for-service basis. The liability reflecting the services provided but not paid, and for which no claim has been received, must be recognized for a proper matching of revenues and expenses to occur.

An example of a chart of accounts used by an IPA is reflected in Exhibit 11.1. The following describes some of the accounts that may be found in an IPA chart of accounts and how they might be used:

EXHIBIT 11.1 Independent Practice Association

Account Number	Description	Not-for-Profit	Accrual
	BALANCE SHEET		
1000	**ASSETS**		
1100	Cash Unrestricted — Banks	X	X
1101	General Checking Accounts	X	X
1102	Payroll Checking Accounts	X	X
1321	Hospital Bonus Receivable — Medicare	X	X
1360	Accounts Receivable — Commercial Managed Care	X	X
1361	Hospital Bonus Receivable — Commercial	X	X
1370	A/R Pharmacy Benefits	X	X
1371	Reinsurance Receivable	X	X
1502	Prepaid Insurance	X	X
2000	**LIABILITIES**	X	X
2100	**CURRENT LIABILITIES — PAYABLES**	X	X
2110	Accounts Payable	X	X
2300	**CURRENT LIABILITIES — OTHER**	X	X
2361	Incurred But Not Reported Claims — Commercial	X	X
2362	Incurred But Not Reported Claims — Medicare	X	X
2363	Incurred But Not Reported Claims — Medicaid	X	X
3000	**PARTNERS' EQUITY (PARTNERSHIP)**	X	X
2260	Other Payroll Liabilities		
3010	Contributed Capital (Each Partner)	X	X
3020	Undistributed Earnings	X	X
3030	Partners' Drawing Accounts (Each Partner)	X	X
3040	Current Income/Loss	X	X

Exhibit 11.1 continued

Account Number	Description	Not-for-Profit	Accrual
	REVENUE AND EXPENSE SUMMARY		
4000	**REVENUES**	X	X
4230	Capitated Premiums — Commercial	X	X
4240	Capitated Premiums — Medicare	X	X
4250	Capitated Premiums — Medicaid	X	X
4260	Capitated Premiums — Other	X	X
4271	Hospital Risk Share — Commercial	X	X
4272	Hospital Risk Share — Medicare	X	X
4273	Hospital Risk Share — Medicaid	X	X
4274	Hospital Risk Share — Pharmacy	X	X
4275	Hospital Risk Share — Other	X	X
7000	**CLINICAL EXPENSES — PURCHASED SERVICES — MANAGEMENT FEES**	X	X
7710	Medical Director	X	X
7730	Management Fees — MSO/PPMC	X	X
7831	Management Fees — Commercial	X	X
7832	Management Fees — Medicare	X	X
7833	Management Fees — Medicaid	X	X
7834	Management Fees — Other	X	X
7740	Management Company Incentive	X	X
7800	FFS Purchased Services — Professional and Medical	X	X
7811	FFS Purchased Services — Commercial	X	X
7812	FFS Purchased Services — Medicare	X	X
7813	FFS Purchased Services — Medicaid	X	X
7814	FFS Purchased Services — Other	X	X
7850	Sub-capitation Payments — Primary Care	X	X
7851	Sub-capitation Payments — Primary Care — Commercial	X	X
7852	Sub-capitation Payments — Primary Care — Medicare	X	X
7853	Sub-capitation Payments — Primary Care — Medicaid	X	X
7854	Sub-capitation Payments — Primary Care — Other	X	X
7860	Sub-capitation Payments — Specialty Care	X	X
7861	Sub-capitation Payments — Specialty Care — Commercial	X	X
7862	Sub-capitation Payments — Specialty Care — Medicare	X	X
7863	Sub-capitation Payments — Specialty Care — Medicaid	X	X
7864	Sub-capitation Payments — Specialty Care — Other	X	X
7870	Sub-capitation Payments — Hospitals	X	X
7880	Sub-capitation Payments — Other	X	X

Assets

Accounts receivable includes Accounts 1300 – 1380. The accounts receivable that would normally be recognized on the financial statements of an IPA would include the following:

- **Capitated contract receivables** — this would reflect amounts due under capitated contracts and would be included in Accounts 1340, 1350, 1360 or 1370.
- **Risk pool receivables** — this account would only be used by the IPA with a history of risk pool participation and with the information necessary to evaluate their participation in an inpatient, ancillary service or other type of risk pool. This could be recorded under Account 1321 if it was under a Medicare contract or under Account 1361 if under a commercial contract.
- **Reinsurance recoveries receivables** — this account would be recorded in Account 1371 for the amount of stop-loss claims billed, net of an allowance for uncollectible amounts or anticipated adjustments.

Liabilities

Liabilities, which include accounts payable and accrued expense accounts normally found on the books of an IPA, contain the following:

- **Incurred But Not Reported Claims (IBNR)** should be recorded in Accounts 2361 – 2363 depending on the contract type. This liability represents claims that the IPA is legally responsible to pay for services it has contracted with a managed-care organization for on a capitated basis and pays out to subcontractors on a fee-for-service basis.

  IBNR can be calculated in a number of ways. The most common method is to track the history of claims payment for the specific organization to determine a claims' lag ratio and apply this ratio to current operations. IBNR can also be calculated actuarially based on anticipated utilization of a specific population. Another practical approach is to determine the number of referrals authorized but not billed as of a particular date and apply an average claim amount to these open referrals.
- **Capitated contract payables** could be recorded as accounts payable in Account 2110. These liabilities represent payables of contract amounts due to other providers who are capitated to provide services for the IPA.
- **Accrued management fees** could be recorded in Account 2316 and represent management fees due to a management entity that are unpaid as of the end of a particular accounting period.

Revenues

Revenue sources for an IPA and their related accounts could be presented as follows:

- **Capitated premium revenue** — these represent a portion of the HMO premium assigned to the IPA, usually stated on a per member per month basis, for the specific services the IPA participating providers agree to cover. These should be recorded in Accounts 4230 – 4260 depending upon the nature of the related contract. These contracts are usually negotiated and monitored separately for commercial versus senior or Medicare contracts and accordingly revenue and costs associated with these types of contracts should be segregated by contract type.

- **Risk pool revenue** — these revenue sources represent IPA participation in cost management contracting functions negotiated with an HMO and are usually stated in the form of a risk pool. For instance, a portion of the IPA premium is diverted (withheld) monthly into a separate escrow account. The costs, which are the target of the cost reduction strategies (inpatient, ancillary services or pharmaceuticals, for example), would be charged to the account. The IPA may receive revenue to the extent the withhold exceeded expenses charged against the risk pool. These revenue sources should be recorded in Accounts 4271 – 4274. It should also be noted that risk-pool participation may result in losses to the IPA.

Expenses

Expense accounts, which would normally be utilized by an IPA, include the following:

- **Fee-for-service purchased services,** Accounts 7721 – 7729, would be used to reflect the actual payments to participating providers who have contracted with the IPA for services to be rendered under fee-for-service contracts.

- **Capitation payments,** Accounts 7810 – 7829 should be used to reflect payments to participating providers who are contracted for services under capitated contracts. Most IPAs track these expenses separately between primary care and specialty services, as well as between commercial and Medicare contracts.

- **Management fees** would generally be expensed in Accounts 7841 – 7845 depending on the nature of the contract under management. This arrangement assumes a separate management company is providing most of the general and administrative support services that would otherwise be expenses under the 6000 series of accounts like most other medical practices.

- **Management fee expense payments based on incentive contracts** is reflected by Account 7850.

- **Stop-loss insurance**, Account 6183 is established to reflect payments for premiums associated with reinsurance contracts or those insurance contracts the IPA purchases to insure itself against unusually high claims.

- **Reinsurance recoveries** should be credited to Account 4290. These recoveries reflect the actual amounts received for claims filed against the above mentioned reinsurance policies. The remaining general and administrative expense accounts are similar to those used by most medical groups.

Most IPAs contract with a physician to act as medical director of the IPA. Contract payments to a medical director can be expensed to Account 7710. Likewise, accounts in the 7700 series can be used to reflect payments for case managers for inpatient or other types of concurrent review.

Group Practices

The next type of integrated delivery system that deserves mention is the group practice consisting of multiple providers, specialties and even perhaps multiple locations. The complications arising from adapting the chart of accounts to a large, multispecialty group practice are somewhat similar to that of an IPA as there is essentially a continuum of group practice types. In its simplest form, a group practice consists of two doctors of a similar specialty accepting only fee-for-service contracts and revenues. (Note: MGMA's definition of a group practice sets a three-physician minimum.) In its most complicated form, a group practice can provide virtually all specialties and ancillary services in multiple locations and can participate in risk contracting, even to the extent of taking global risk for hospital or other types of care.

Impact on Compensation Systems

The key issue in large multispecialty, multilocation groups is departmentalized financial reporting. This is a critical issue in being able to properly track revenue and expense items for advanced compensation systems used by most large groups. Practice management software systems used by large groups have the ability to track charges, adjustments and collections by provider; however, expense items need to be allocated among departments in the general ledger for proper inclusion in the financial statements. The *Chart of Accounts for Health Care Organizations* accommodates this through the use of responsibility center fields.

The overall structure of this chart of accounts model provides for a total of nine digits categorized in four fields as detailed below:

Field	Digits	Utilization
Entity	1 (1-9)	Designate separate entities
Basic	4 (0001 – 9999)	Account number
Responsibility Center	2 (01-99)	Department, specialty or location
Provider Number	2 (01-99)	Physician or other provider

The key point to remember about the proposed structure is that it is only a model that will need to be adapted to any particular entity to accommodate the actual structure of that entity. For example, the above structure only allows for 99 providers. Many groups are now made up of many more than 100 physicians, not to mention midlevel providers. The critical issue is to spend adequate time planning when implementing the above structure for any particular group. Also, do not structure the account system around the current group makeup, but rather around the group as its strategic plan projects it to be made up five to ten years in the future.

Most general ledger software programs also provide sufficient flexibility to adopt the above structure or slight adaptations of it. Ten digits are commonly provided for the account coding system while the above only uses nine.

Multispecialty Groups

Assuming you are charged with the task of adapting the above structure to a group practice you will probably only have one entity to deal with; thus eliminating the need for the entity code. Refer to the description chapters to actually choose the accounts to be used. The responsibility center will commonly be used to allocate costs to departments. In a small group the departments may actually be the physician providers. In a large group the responsibility center departments will probably be separate specialties.

In structuring the department coding system one or more administrative departments will normally be used to accumulate costs which need to be allocated to multiple specialties or other departments. A hypothetical responsibility center coding structure could be reflected as follows:

Responsibility Center	Description
01	Administration
02	Billing and collection
03	Marketing
04	Family practice
05	Internal medicine
06	Obstetrics and gynecology
07	General surgery

Using the above responsibility center scheme, expenses of administration, billing and collection and marketing would then be used to accumulate expenses for these departments, which would subsequently be allocated to the specialty departments.

Multilocation Groups

One alternative would be to use the responsibility center codes to designate separate locations and the actual provider number to designate the departments. This would be appropriate in multilocation organizations, especially in the case where the physicians were assigned to specific clinics and did not rotate. In a situation where physicians do rotate among clinics, the entity code could be used to designate the actual clinic location, the responsibility center could be used to designate specialty, and the provider number could be used to designate the individual physicians.

Expense Allocations

Assuming expenses will be accumulated into administrative or other common categories, they will need to be periodically allocated to the specialty departments on some basis. A standardized method of performing this allocation is to identify an account at the end of the general and administrative (G&A) expense series to credit with the amounts allocated to the departments. An example would be to use Account 6999 with a description of "Departmental Allocations" crediting the G&A expenses for responsibility center 01 – 03 in the above example. The expenses would then be charged to departments 04 – 07 using an account such as 6995 styled for administrative expense, billing and collection expense or marketing expense allocation. In this manner each department is able to see how much of the administrative burden is being allocated to its department.

Legal Implications

A final issue in using departments is the impact of the Stark I and II regulations impacting the allocation of ancillary services in a group practice. The regulations are very clear that the revenue and expenses from designated health services such as lab, radiology and diagnostic testing must be pooled and allocated on some basis other than the volume or value of referrals. Therefore, most groups will set up separate responsibility centers for each type of designated health service and are very careful to have an acceptable method of cost allocation for these centers. Alternatively, some groups set up only two responsibility centers for ancillary services: one for Stark-defined services and one for non-Stark-defined services to provide for more flexibility in the allocation of expenses to these important revenue and cost centers.

Management Service Organizations

A management services organization (MSO) typically poses no unique accounting issues for a medical practice. An MSO does, however, usually have an inherent conflict in that most are owned by a hospital or publicly traded physician practice management company, which requires them to reflect operations on the accrual method of accounting. This often creates a conflict, especially when the physician, whose practice is being managed by the MSO, has never had to deal with the concepts of accrual accounting.

Another inherent problem is, that although the MSO usually has the responsibility of billing and collecting, the accounts receivable and the related gross charges, adjustments and collections for physician services belong to the medical group. Accordingly, although accounts receivable may be recorded on the general ledger of the MSO, they are completely removed from the financial statements. This is accomplished through the use of a valuation allowance account (Account 1379) or by reflecting them as deferred revenue (Account 2375) at an amount equal to the balance of accounts receivable on the books.

The primary revenue source for an MSO is from management fee income. The management fee may be set at an amount usually equivalent to a billing service if the MSO is only performing billing and collection functions, or it may be as high as the typical overhead percentage if performing all administrative functions for the medical practice. A typical scenario is to reflect all charges, adjustments and collections from physician services on the books of the MSO. These items are then backed out at 100 percent on a separate line item in the general ledger and financial statements only to be replaced with the actual amount of the MSO management fee for the period. An example of this presentation is as follows:

	Month	Year
Gross charges	$100,000	$1,200,000
Adjustments	30,000	400,000
Net charges	70,000	800,000
Collection	68,000	750,000
Refunds	2,000	24,000
Net revenue applicable to managed physician	(66,000)	(750,000)
Management fee revenue	33,000	363,000
General and administrative expense (in detail)	34,000	370,000
Net income (usually net loss)	$(1,000)	$(7,000)

Accordingly, the only revenue item on most MSO books could be reflected in Account 4485 (miscellaneous income) and styled as Management Fee Income. Likewise, the only general and administrative expense (6000 series) on the books of a managed physician might be Account 5240—Management Fees MSO/PPMC. One of the distinct changes in this edition of the *Chart of Accounts for Health Care Organizations* is the categorization of general and administrative expenses into the 6000 series and the categorization of clinical expenses into the 7000 series. This will result over time in allowing for more comparability between the financial statements of physicians managed by an MSO or other type of management entity and those that are not.

Physician-Hospital Organization

The typical physician-hospital organization has a very simple chart of accounts and financial reporting system. The fact that these organizations usually do not enter directly into contracts themselves but mainly just negotiate contracts on behalf of a physician-owned IPA and a hospital has been mentioned earlier. Accordingly, the entity may only have cash and some furniture and fixtures as its only assets. Likewise, revenue sources would be limited to fees derived off of negotiated contracts or annual dues received from members. Expenses would normally be limited to salaries and related payroll costs. All of these items have been dealt with in other parts of this chapter.

Fully Integrated Delivery Systems

The accounting method preferable for the small group practice is still the cash method of accounting. Accrual accounting would generally be used by fully integrated delivery systems accepting global risk contracts. In such instances, the entity would adopt many of the accounts and accounting policies described above for an IPA. Accrual accounting adopted by a group practice accepting global risk contracts would include utilization of the following accounts:

Description	Accounts
Capitated Contract Receivables	1340, 1350, 1360, 1370
Risk-Pool Receivables	1321, 1361
Reinsurance Recoveries Receivable	1371
IBNR Claims	2361, 2362, 2363
Capitated Contract Payables	2110
Capitated Contract Revenue (premium revenue)	4230, 4240, 4250, 4260
Risk-Pool Revenue	4271, 4272, 4273, 4274
Capitation Payments (medical expense)	7810 – 7829
Fee-For-Service Purchased Services	7721 – 7729

Adopting the accrual method of accounting for a delivery system, including a medical group providing traditional fee-for-service medical services concurrently with full-risk contracting poses some unique accounting problems having to do with revenue recognition and accounting for income taxes.

Revenue Recognition

Fee-for-service revenue for a medical practice is extremely difficult to measure. A large medical group may see patients whose reimbursement for medical services is provided in literally hundreds of different ways. The amount of revenue, for example, to be received by a general surgeon performing an appendectomy on a patient can vary based on the type of patient and what insurance contract that patient is covered by. Reimbursement can change based on the diagnosis used to bill the service, the time frame under which the service was billed, whether or not any complications arose during surgery requiring the use of a modifier, and whether or not the patient was under the concurrent care of another physician. These are but a few of the reasons why a billed charge may be paid at one rate versus another or not paid at all.

These complications make it virtually impossible to precisely estimate the realizable value of accounts receivable. Accordingly, to recognize revenue as accurately as possible, a medical group utilizing the full accrual method of accounting will be relying heavily on accounts such as the allowance for doubtful accounts receivable. These are 'contra' accounts used to reduce the value of the accounts receivable to an estimate of the net realizable value and include the following:

Description	Accounts	Contractual Adj. Acct.
Medicaid Allowance for Doubtful Accounts	1319	4520
Medicare Allowance for Doubtful Accounts	1329	4530
Self-Pay Allowance for Doubtful Accounts	1339	4540
Private Insurance Allowance for Doubtful Accounts	1349	4550
Medicaid Managed-Care Allowance for Doubtful Accounts	1359	4560
Commercial Allowance for Doubtful Accounts	1369	4570
AR Other (patients) Allowance for Doubtful Accounts	1379	4590

The allowance accounts listed above are credit balance accounts used to reduce their related accounts receivable asset accounts to the estimated amount to actually be received. The calculation of the allowance would be based on a historical analysis of collections by payer type; for example, the gross collection ratio may be used comparing total collections to gross charges. The contractual adjustment account listed above is the offsetting account in the income statement used to record the debit entry to reduce the associated revenue to its estimated collectable amount.

Income Tax Accounting

Most medical groups utilize the cash method of accounting for federal income tax reporting. Accordingly, federal income tax expense is not recognized until a tax liability is actually paid. Because most medical groups are organized as professional associations and have traditionally had little need to accumulate capital, most earnings have been paid out to physician shareholders resulting in little or no income tax at the corporate or group practice level. Managed care is changing all of that.

An IPA exclusively performing risk contracting where all revenue is received in the form of capitated contract revenues may want to adopt the accrual method for federal income tax reporting purposes. The IRS has allowed IPAs in certain situations to deduct the reserve for claims incurred but not reported. Likewise, it stands to reason, that an integrated delivery system entering into full-risk contracts is also performing the types of activities formerly limited exclusively to insurance companies. These entities may consider adopting the accrual method of reporting for federal income tax reporting purposes. This, of course, assumes a delivery system organized as a for-profit venture as opposed to a not-for-profit corporation.

Large groups and delivery systems have also come to the realization that dealing with managed care requires staff, equipment and information systems that are expensive. Retained earnings, once a term never used in a medical group setting, is now receiving some amount of consideration as groups see tremendous needs for capital and few sources of legally attracting that capital without losing complete control of their destiny.

Accordingly, more and more situations arise in an integrated delivery system where income tax expense is actually recognized. Additionally, there are now increasing trends for revenue and expense to be reported at different times for financial reporting purposes versus for federal income tax reporting purposes, resulting in the recognition of deferred income tax assets as well as liabilities. A complete discussion of accounting for income taxes is beyond the scope of this chapter, except to point out the accounts to be used for these purposes. These accounts and a brief description of their usage are presented on the next page:

Description	Account	Usage
Income Tax Receivable — current	1390	Record current income tax receivable
Deferred Tax Asset — current	1515	Record current deferred tax charge
Deferred Tax Asset — noncurrent	1970	Record noncurrent deferred tax charge
Accrued Income Tax Payable — current	2314	Record current tax liability payable
Deferred Tax Liability — current	2380	Record current deferred tax liability
Deferred Tax Liability — noncurrent	2475	Record noncurrent deferred tax liability
Current Federal Income Tax Expense	9231	Record current FIT expense
Deferred Federal Income Tax Expense	9233	Record deferred FIT expense

Medical Foundations

A medical foundation is typically an integrated delivery system organized as a not-for-profit corporation. Accordingly, all of the above accounting issues and accounts used for full accrual and risk contracting come into play for a medical foundation. Because they are exempt for federal income tax reporting purposes, the above noted accounts for income tax expense would not come into play. They also follow most principles detailed in the related chapter "Adapting the Chart of Accounts to Not-for-Profit Health Care Organizations."

Conclusion

The above analysis has attempted to define integrated delivery systems as actually encountered in the health care industry today and to describe adapting this chart of accounts to those organizations. Naturally more complete integrated delivery systems would include components of inpatient care, home-health care, ambulatory surgery centers, long-term care and behavioral health, to name a few. Each of these types of health care delivery activities have developed industry standards for financial reporting. The purpose of this chapter has not been to outline or redefine those standards but to address how they could be integrated into a comprehensive reporting entity. Each of those activities represent separate lines of business, and the generally accepted accounting principles has adopted well established principles for reporting in these situations.

12

Adapting the Chart of Accounts to the MGMA Surveys

Lisa Pieper, M.B.A., M.S.H.A.

MGMA Surveys

The MGMA Survey Operations Department conducts several annual surveys of the MGMA member practices. These surveys query the membership on critical topics, such as operating costs, physician compensation and staffing ratios. The published survey report and accompanying "Respondent Ranking Report" provide medical practice administrators and executives with critical information tools necessary to better manage their practices.

The *Cost Survey*, a comprehensive financial survey of medical practices, is MGMA's oldest survey — conducted since 1948. This survey reports charges, revenue, support staffing ratios, general operating and provider costs and accounts receivable data. To control for differences in practice size, data are reported on a per-physician, per-provider or percent-of-revenue basis. Data are reported for 19 different types of single specialty practices, for multispecialty practices, and for categories of multispecialty practices such as geographic section or group size. Practices use the survey data to benchmark their own organizations and identify areas for improvement. This process can help practices become more efficient while reducing costs.

The *Physician Compensation and Production Survey* reports individual physician and midlevel provider compensation data. In addition, several measures of productivity data are reported. These measures include professional gross charges, ambulatory encounters and hospital encounters, surgical/anesthesia cases and RBRVS work relative value units. The data are used to calculate ratios of compensation to gross charges and compensation per RVU. The survey reports data by provider specialty and other individual characteristics such as years in specialty and gender. Practice characteristics are also factored in, such as type of practice (single or multispecialty), geographic section, size of practice and level of managed care.

Another compensation survey conducted by MGMA is the *Management Compensation Survey*. In addition to compensation information, the report includes bonus and retirement benefit amounts for middle- and upper-level managers and physician executives. Information is available for approximately 40 position titles. Users of the report can assess compensation levels nationally or by geographic section, the type of practice (single or multispecialty), the amount of total net medical revenue, the size of the practice and the number of clinic locations.

MGMA also conducts three parallel surveys in the academic sector similar to the ones described above. The *Faculty Practice Activities Survey*, conducted jointly with the Association of American Medical Colleges, reports clinical science department revenue and expenses, staffing and payer mix. The *Academic Practice Faculty Compensation and Production Survey* provides compensation and productivity levels for faculty physicians. Finally, clinical science and practice plan managerial compensation and benefit information is reported in the *Academic Practice Management Compensation Survey*.

Information Needs

The MGMA surveys focus mainly on financial and operational indices. Respondents to the survey pull data from a variety of sources to complete the questionnaires. The income statement, balance sheet, chart of accounts and appointment schedule are standard sources of information found in medical practices. Patient billing systems, clinical information systems, payroll and other special reports also provide survey information. Special surveys, inventories and assessments are needed to collect data on the number of FTE physicians and employees or satellites and square footage for the facility.

One way to measure production is to track gross charges off a patient billing system. Other measures of provider productivity can be obtained through ad hoc production reports. The number of visits, encounters, patients, procedures or RBRVS relative value units are other important measures of productivity.

Benefits of Using the COA to Complete Surveys

One valuable tool used to simplify data collection of the *Cost Survey* and other MGMA surveys is a standardized chart of accounts. The chart of accounts can be used to report the information requirements in the *Cost Survey* including revenue, charges, and general support staff and provider cost. In exhibit 12.1, the information requirements are listed for the *Cost Survey* along with the corresponding chart of accounts code.

The chart of accounts presents several advantages to the survey process:

1. **Ease in data retrieval:** Categorizing financial information by use of a chart of accounts simplifies the data retrieval process, whether it is for a survey or a management report. Data already collected in an organized manner can be easily extracted from an accounting or information management system.

2. **Reduction of reporting error:** The proper organization of financial data reduces reporting error as data can be retrieved without performing complicated calculations or manual reclassifications. There is more

confidence in the data because of understanding what should or should not be included in a specific category.

3. **Achieve data comparability:** An important aspect of survey participation is the alignment of internal measures with the survey definitions. When this alignment does not occur, data are reported inconsistently and the validity of the survey declines. A chart of accounts ensures that data are reported the same way across all respondents.

4. **Information to be utilized for comparison is tracked and tracked appropriately:** The chart of accounts provides the structure that allows users to track the information needed in many financial or operational surveys. Many times, respondents do not complete a question or entire sections of a survey because their system does not track the information or the information is tracked in a different manner. The chart of accounts allows data to be tracked the same way.

Benchmarking

health care organizations need to closely monitor their performance to successfully manage increasing competition and the changing landscape of health care. The chart of accounts allows managers an intimate knowledge and understanding of an organization's financial and operational picture. This knowledge coupled with comparisons, assessments and action plans provide the framework for the benchmarking process. This process turns data into useful information. Benchmarking helps practices develop effective measures of their success. It also increases flexibility, which allows an organization to act quickly in a changing environment while maintaining profitability.

The surveys play a two-fold role in the benchmarking process. First, by using the chart of accounts to complete the surveys, managers gain a thorough knowledge of the organization's performance and can provide detailed financial information. Secondly, the survey report provides the comparison component of the benchmarking process on several different levels.

1. **Data comparison:** The surveys provide users several different comparison options. Comparisons can be performed nationally against all practices. Or, a practice may choose similar practices, such as those of the same type (single specialty or multispecialty), specialty, size or region. "Better performing" practices are identified in the *Cost Survey* based on the attainment of particular goals. These goals are related to operating cost and the level of net revenue after operating expenses.

2. **Data standardization:** To account for differences in size, most financial data are standardized to provide a more useful measure. For example, reporting raw revenue is not very helpful when differences between high and low levels are due to size and not performance. Reporting revenue per FTE physician provides a much more meaningful measure.

   The *Cost Survey* provides several standardization options. Data are reported on a per-physician, per-provider, per-RVU, per-patient and per-square foot basis as well as by the percent of total net medical revenue. This allows benchmarking on a unit basis and organization size is factored out.

3. **Assessment:** An important aspect of performing benchmark comparisons is analyzing the differences between an organization's data and the benchmark data. This can be done several ways. Actual differences can be tallied for each benchmark measure. Although this identifies where the variances are, calculating the percent of the difference provides a better understanding of the *scope* of the difference. Charts and graphs are useful to illustrate and explain the findings to others.

4. **Internal and external benchmarks:** Once an organization is tracking financial information via a chart of accounts system, the possibilities are endless for benchmarking. Benchmarking data comes from a variety of sources — current and prior period budgets and internal and external data.

Reviewing data outside the practice takes on new meaning when it can be related to a practice's own performance. Comparing financial indicators over time allows organizations to assess whether action plans have been effective in meeting goals and objectives.

Benchmarking is not limited to external analysis. Managers can learn a lot about their organizations by tracking certain indicators either at a point in time or over time. The same benefits of external benchmarking apply to internal benchmarking, i.e., identification of variances, action plan effectiveness, etc.

EXHIBIT 12.1 Data Requirements for Cost Survey

Question Number	Measure	Previous COA*	New COA
MEDICAL CHARGES AND REVENUE			
22	Gross FFS charges	3100, 3200	4110, 4120
23	Adjustments to FFS charges	4100, 4200, 4500-4700	4510, 4520, 4600-4700
24	Bad debts due to FFS activity	7720-7740	6710, 6720
25	Net FFS revenue	3500, 3600, 3900, 4900	4210, 4220, 4292, 4300
26	Usual and customary charges for patients covered by capitation contracts	3300	4130
27	Gross capitation revenue	3710-3730, 3740-3790, 4300	4230-4283, 4530, 4291
28	Purchased services for capitation patients	7200	7800
29	Net capitation revenue	Calculated	Calculated
30	Other medical revenue	3400, 3800	4140, 4150, 4420-4480, 4540, 4550
31	Revenue from the sale of medical goods and services	3400, 3800, 4400	4140, 4410, 4540
32	Gross revenue from other medical activities	Calculated	Calculated
33	Cost of sales and/or cost of other medical activities	6300	7600
34	Net other medical revenue	Calculated	Calculated
35	Total gross charges	Calculated	Calculated
36	Total medical revenue	Calculated	Calculated
SUPPORT STAFF OPERATING COST			
37	General administrative	5160, 5610, 5620, 5660, 5670, 7360	5710, 8170, 8370
38	Business office	5630, 5640, 7360	5715
39	Managed care administrative		5720
40	Information services	5650	5725
41	Housekeeping, maintenance, security	5700	5730
42	Medical receptionists	5530	5735
43	Medical secretaries, transcribers	5540	5740
44	Medical records	5550	5745
45	Other administrative support	5680, 5690, 7360	5750
46	Registered nurses	5510	5755
47	Licensed practical nurses	5520	5760
48	Medical assistants, nurse's aides	5520	5765
49	Clinical laboratory	5410	5520
50	Radiology and imaging	5420	5510
51	Other medical support services	5430-5490, 5560-5590, 5800	5530-5550
52	Total employed support staff compensation	Calculated	Calculated
53	Total employed support staff benefit cost	5911-5920, 5930-5990	5610-5695, 5810-5895
54	Total contracted support staff		5903, 5904, 5913, 5914, 7710
55	Total support staff cost	Calculated	Calculated
GENERAL OPERATING COST			
56	Information services	6660, 6760, 7370, 7610	6120, 6220, 6304, 6420, 6430, 6520, 6530, 7120
57	Medical and surgical supply	6110-6130, 6170-6190	7010, 7020, 7030, 7040, 7060

Exhibit 12.1 continued

Question Number	Measure	Previous COA*	New COA
58	Building and occupancy	6160, 6410-6430, 6460-6500, 6900, 7810	6150, 7070, 7510-7544, 7560, 7570, 7590, 7595
59	Furniture and equipment	6610, 6650, 6670-6690, 6710, 6750, 6770-6790, 6830, 6890	6110, 6115, 6301-6303, 6305-6307, 6510, 6515, 6580, 7100, 7110, 7161
60	Administrative supplies and services	6140, 6150, 6180, 6190, 7350, 7390, 7630-7650	6130, 6140, 6160, 6190-6210, 6370, 6380, 6400, 6540-6570, 6600, 6650, 6730, 7130, 7140, 7720
61	Professional liability insurance premiums	7510	6185-6189
62	Other insurance premiums	6450, 6820, 7520, 7530	6180-6184, 7580
63	Outside professional fees	7310-7340, 7380	6310-6360
64	Promotion and marketing	7620, 7660, 7710	6170, 7050
65	Clinical laboratory	6210, 6220, 6620, 6720, 6840, 7130	7022, 7163
66	Radiology and imaging	6230, 6630, 6730, 6850, 7140	7021, 7162
67	Other ancillary services	6260-6290, 6640, 6740, 6880	7023
68	Management fees paid to a PPMC,MSO, hospital or parent organization		7730-7740
69	Miscellaneous operating cost	7420-7490, 7670, 7690, 7760-7790	6230-6270, 6390, 6410, 6440, 7150, 7550
70	Total general operating cost	Calculated	Calculated
TOTAL OPERATING COST AND TOTAL MEDICAL REVENUE AFTER OPERATING COST			
71	Total operating cost	Calculated	Calculated
72	Total medical revenue after operating cost	Calculated	Calculated
PROVIDER STAFFING AND COST			
73	Midlevel provider compensation	5300	8310-8360, 8380
74	Midlevel provider benefit cost		8410-8495
75	Total midlevel provider	Calculated	Calculated
76	Provider consultant cost	7110, 7120, 7150-7190	5901, 5902, 5911, 5912
77	Primary care physicians	N/A	N/A
78	Nonsurgical specialty physicians	N/A	N/A
79	Surgical specialty physicians	N/A	N/A
80	Total physicians compensation	5110-5150	8110-8160, 8180
81	Total physician compensation		8210-8295
82	Total physician	Calculated	Calculated
83	Total provider	Calculated	Calculated
NONMEDICAL REVENUE AND COST			
84	Nonmedical revenue	8100, 8400	9110-9160, 9300
85	Financial support for operating costs		4490, 9170
86	Nonmedical cost	8200, 8300, 8500	9200-9243, 9300
87	Net nonmedical income	Calculated	Calculated
88	Net practice income or loss	Calculated	Calculated

Exhibit 12.1 continued

Question Number	Measure	Previous COA*	New COA
BALANCE SHEET DATA			
89	Current assets	1100-1300	1110-1550
90	Noncurrent and all other assets	1400-1900	1600-1961
91	Total assets	Calculated	Calculated
92	Current liabilities	2100-2300	2100-2390
93	Noncurrent and all other liabilities	2400	2400-2480
94	Total liabilities	Calculated	Calculated
95	Total net worth	2500-2700	3000-3090

* Previous COA refers to the 1996 edition titled *Medical Group Practice Chart of Accounts*

13

Adapting the Chart of Accounts to PSPA

Kathryn P. Glass, M.B.A., M.S.H.A.

Introduction

Physician Services Practice Analysis (PSPA) software is a practice management tool developed by MGMA/CRAHCA that uses the Health Care Financing Administration's (HCFA's) Resource-Based Relative Value Scale (RBRVS) to measure provider productivity and calculate a practice's cost per procedure based on utilization. The productivity is analyzed through three monthly files downloaded from the practice's billing system:

- detailed procedure file
- provider unique patient count file
- specialty encounter file

Building on this utilization data, PSPA's Cost Accounting module calculates unit costs using year-to-date expense information input from the Profit and Loss accounting statements. What does any of this have to do with a cost-based chart of accounts? More than one may think.

In this era of managed care, a medical practice needs to know the cost of providing each procedure in order to successfully negotiate contracts that would allow the practice to remain financially viable. PSPA calculates the cost per procedure and compares it to third-party payer reimbursement to analyze profitability. This type of analysis was not so critical under the traditional fee-for-service (FFS) payment systems because increasing the fees or increasing the number of patients seen on a daily or weekly basis could negate any loss in revenue. However, with revenues increasingly generated from managed-care contracts, this analysis has become critical because health care organizations are at-risk for potential heavy financial losses if costs and patient care are not carefully monitored. The traditional "more is better" philosophy has been replaced by the "maybe less is better" philosophy since lower patient volume under managed-care contracts results in more revenue being retained in the practice. (Thus, the reason that most medical practices with capitated contracts stress preventive care is to catch any potential problems before they become expensive problems.) Knowing the costs of providing those services covered under the contracts gives the medical practice a huge advantage at the negotiating table. How can an educated decision be made *without* this knowledge?

Three RVU Components; Three RVU Costs

PSPA calculates the cost per relative value unit (RVU) for the physician work, practice expense (overhead), and professional liability (malpractice) components of a given procedure code using year-to-date expenses broken out into general categories for provider compensation, overhead and malpractice. Why not just use total expenses instead of breaking it out? The RBRVS comprises the "Physician's Current Procedural Terminology," fourth edition (CPT-4) codes (copyrighted by the American Medical Association) and the RVUs assigned to each code. These RVUs are divided into physician work, practice expense and professional liability components. As part of the Medicare Physician's Fee Schedule, HCFA has also determined, by locality across the United States, Geographic Practice Cost Indices (GPCIs) that are also divided into physician work, practice expense and professional liability components. (GPCIs are used to adjust for the differences in practice operating costs across the country.) Since the RBRVS, the Medicare Physician's Fee Schedule, and the GPCIs all use these three components, it is only logical (and not a coincidence) that the expense categories used to determine the cost per RVU (and ultimately the cost per procedure) are also divided into the same three components.

Cost Category Structure

Using this cost-based *Chart of Accounts for Health Care Organizations,* it is much easier to pull together the accounts that correspond to overhead, physician and midlevel compensation and professional liability insurance. Why? The structure of the *Chart of Accounts for Health Care Organizations* is based on this question: "Who is responsible for these expenses?" (**Note:** Balance sheet accounts [assets, liabilities and owners' equity] are excluded from the cost input categories in PSPA. PSPA calculates the cost per procedure; thus, only income statement expense account categories are used. It compares the *cost* per procedure to the collected charges per procedure based on the billing system downloads.) This structure makes it easy to decide what goes into provider compensation versus practice expense because the physician and midlevel expense categories are broken out. The other expense accounts (including those for ancillary providers) fall into either overhead or professional liability (malpractice).

If certain accounts are simply not used within a practice, it is easy to eliminate them when rolling up the sub-accounts into the major account categories. Just because an account is listed in the *Chart of Accounts for Health Care Organizations* does not mean it has to be included. Each practice will tweak this particular chart of accounts to its specific needs.

Physician vs. Provider

If HCFA used "physician work" as the component definition for both the RVU and the GPCI, why does PSPA call it "provider compensation"? With the advent of managed care, practices have expanded their use of physician extenders (i.e., midlevel providers). Midlevel providers do many of the same procedures a physician does and can bill for those services using their own unique provider identification (ID) code. So what's the difference? The cost to the practice is less with midlevels since their compensation package is less than what physicians receive. If a practice compensates providers based on productivity, the more procedures performed by midlevels instead of physicians results in a cost savings to the practice. Commercial insurance companies reimburse the same regardless of whether it was a midlevel or physician who provided the service. (Medicare reimburses midlevel providers who bill with their own Provider Identification Number (PIN) at 85 percent of the Physician's Fee Schedule.) Since both midlevels and physicians are doing the "physician work" and getting reimbursed for it, the categories are combined to form "provider work" and/or "provider compensation."

A caveat to this is that not all midlevel providers bill under their own provider ID code for the services they provide. Some midlevels use the physician's ID code instead. Why does this matter? PSPA tracks productivity through CPT-4 codes and patient visits as billed each month using individual provider ID codes. If a midlevel provider uses the physician's ID code rather than his or her own ID, then the physician would be credited with those CPT-4 codes on the PSPA procedure billing download file and with those patient visits on the provider patient count file. The rule of thumb is that if a midlevel bills for services using his or her own provider ID code and receives productivity credit and reimbursement for those services in return, then those midlevels should be included within the provider compensation category (and added to the PSPA System module under the Provider Data section). Any midlevel who bills for his or her services under a physician's ID, and therefore is not credited for productivity by procedure code, should be included in the general practice expense (overhead) category.

Provider Compensation Expenses

As previously discussed, the provider compensation expense category should include both physicians and midlevels if the midlevel providers are to be included in the PSPA data analysis. If midlevels do not bill for services using their own individual provider ID code, then the data analysis would include only physicians and the provider compensation would include only physician expenses. If midlevels were not included in the provider compensation category, their salaries and related expenses would be included with the practice expense (overhead) category.

Components of Provider Compensation Expense

There is currently no hard-and-fast rule about exactly what is and is not included in this category when calculating the cost per work RVU. It is really based on what the individual organization considers to comprise "provider compensation." Obviously, this does not help in cost benchmarking clarifications! Until nationwide standardization occurs, there are a few common schools of thought, two of which will be discussed in this chapter. The first includes salaries and all fringe benefits for both physicians and midlevel providers; thus providing a more accurate picture of true provider expenses within the organization. The second includes strictly standard compensation packages for both physicians and midlevel providers; thus allowing for more accurate benchmarking when comparing outside the organization on a regional or national basis. Neither of these options is any more "correct" than the other one. It all depends on what you are attempting to achieve: accurate cost accounting for strictly internal use or accurate comparative information for external use.

School of Thought #1

Exhibit 13.1 displays both salaries and fringe benefits. Why would fringe benefits be included as part of the provider compensation field? Remember that the *Chart of Accounts for Health Care Organizations* structure is based on the question: "Who is responsible for these expenses?" The total compensation package is rarely just salary and a bonus plan. Fringe benefits, which include expenses such as insurance, travel and professional development are often part of that package, too. The reasoning is that if it were not for the physicians and midlevels, the practice would not incur the expenses associated with their benefits. In legalese terms ask yourself: "But for these physicians and midlevel providers, would these expenses occur?" That will define what can be considered direct provider expenses. If you abide by School of Thought #1, the fringe benefits are considered directly related to the physicians and midlevels; therefore, all direct provider expenses should be included as part of their compensation expense.

EXHIBIT 13.1

Account Number	Description
5900	Temporary Employee Salaries
5901	Physician Salaries
5902	Midlevel Provider Salaries
5910	Temporary Employee Benefits
5911	Physician Benefits
5912	Midlevel Provider Salaries
8000	**PROVIDER — RELATED EXPENSES**
8100	PHYSICIAN — SALARIES
8110	Salaries, Distributions and Incentives (Physician)
8200	PHYSICIAN — EMPLOYEE-RELATED EXPENSES
8210	Payroll Taxes (Physician)
8220	Insurance (Physician)
8230	Pension and Retirement Benefits (Physician)
8235	Professional Development (Physician)
8240	Books and Subscriptions (Physician)
8245	Dues and Memberships (Physician)
8250	Licenses (Physician)
8255	Meetings (Physician)
8260	Travel (Physician)
8265	Medical Reimbursement Plan (Physician)
8270	Vehicles (Physician)
8275	Parking (Physician)
8280	Telephones (Physician)
8285	Beepers (Physician)
8290	Meals and entertainment (Physician)
8295	Other Benefits (Physician)
8300	MIDLEVEL PROVIDERS — SALARIES
8310	Salaries, Distributions and Incentives (Midlevel)
8400	MIDLEVEL PROVIDERS — EMPLOYEE-RELATED EXPENSES
8410	Payroll Taxes (Midlevel)
8420	Insurance (Midlevel)
8430	Pension and Retirement Benefits (Midlevel)
8435	Professional Development (Midlevel)
8440	Books and Subscriptions (Midlevel)
8445	Dues and Memberships (Midlevel)
8450	Licenses (Midlevel)
8455	Meetings (Midlevel)
8460	Travel (Midlevel)
8465	Medical Reimbursement Plan (Midlevel)
8470	Vehicles (Midlevel)
8475	Parking (Midlevel)
9480	Telephones (Midlevel)
8485	Beepers (Midlevel)

Exhibit 13.1 continued

Account Number	Description
8490	Meals and Entertainment (Midlevel)
8495	Other Benefits (Midlevel)

Overhead Expenses

Exhibit 13.2 outlines the expense accounts included in the practice expense (overhead) section in PSPA's Cost Accounting module. Although it is not mandatory to use all of these account categories, the overhead expenses should include the roll-ups into the major accounts. What does overhead include? In general, both Ancillary Providers' Salaries and Related Expenses (Accounts 5500 – 5690) and Other Employees' Salaries and Related Expenses (Accounts 5700 – 5790) are included as overhead. Basically, everything under the Services and General Expense Accounts 6000 – 8400 is included *except* for Accounts 6186 (Physician Malpractice Insurance) and 6187 (Midlevel Provider Malpractice Insurance). The 9200 – 9300 Expense Accounts under the Non-Operating Expenses, Income Taxes and Other Expenses category are also included.

Perhaps it would be easier to designate the exclusions rather than all the inclusions! Physicians' salaries and fringe benefits are *not* considered part of overhead. Midlevel providers *who bill for their services under their own individual provider ID code* are *not* considered part of overhead. If the midlevel providers do not bill out for their services *using their own unique provider ID code,* then their salaries and fringe benefits *should* be included in overhead expenses. Physician malpractice insurance is not considered an overhead expense. If the midlevels' expenses are included with provider compensation, then the midlevels' malpractice expense should be included in the Professional Liability Insurance expense category with the physicians' malpractice insurance. If the midlevels' expenses are included in the overhead category, so should the midlevels' malpractice insurance be included in overhead.

EXHIBIT 13.2

Account Number	Description
5000	OPERATING EXPENSES — Salary and Fringe Benefits
5500	ANCILLARY STAFF — SALARIES Include all sub-accounts under 5500
5600	ANCILLARY STAFF — EMPLOYEE-RELATED EXPENSES Include all sub-accounts under 5600
5700	EMPLOYEES — SALARIES Include all sub-accounts under 5700
5800	EMPLOYEES — EMPLOYEE-RELATED EXPENSES Include all sub-accounts under 5800
5900	Temporary Employee Salaries and Benefits Do *not* include sub-accounts 5901, 5902, 5911 and 5912 (temporary employee salaries and benefits for physicians and midlevels)
6000	SERVICES AND GENERAL EXPENSE Include all sub-accounts under 6000 - 7600 except as noted
6100	Office and Administrative Expense Include all sub-accounts under 6100 *except* 6186 and 6187 for physician and midlevel malpractice insurance
6500	Billing Expense
6700	Bad Debt Expense
7000	Clinical Expense
7500	Occupancy Expense
7600	Cost of Goods Sold — Medical Related
7700	PURCHASED SERVICES/MANAGEMENT FEES Include all sub-accounts under 7700 - 7800 as applicable
9200	Nonoperating Expenses Include all sub-accounts under 9200 - 9300 as applicable

Malpractice Expenses

What about malpractice? In the *Chart of Accounts for Health Care Organizations* those expenses are listed as Services and General Expense categories of 6185 – 6187. Account 6185 (Malpractice Insurance) is the roll-up category for the sub-accounts of 6186 (Physician Malpractice) and 6187 (Midlevel Provider Malpractice). The malpractice expense includes both physician and midlevels if the midlevel providers are included in the PSPA data analysis. To be included in the data analysis, a midlevel must bill for his or her medical services under each one's own individual provider identification code. Exhibit 13.3 details the accounts included in the malpractice expense component.

Note that there are two additional malpractice sub-accounts (6188 for ancillary providers and 6189 for global coverage), which should be included with the general overhead expenses. Why? Since the provider compensation field excludes ancillary providers' compensation, the malpractice expense field should also exclude ancillary to follow the pattern of matching expense categories to the provider.

EXHIBIT 13.3

Account Number	Description
6185	Malpractice Insurance
6186	Physicians
6187	Midlevel Providers

School of Thought #2

The second School of Thought is based on the belief that bonuses should not be included in the work component because bonus is only related to profit and is not a true salary. Likewise, incentives should not be included because they are often built around specific contracts, which are not permanent. Exhibit 13.4 includes the provider compensation accounts that would be included if using this particular methodology.

In this methodology, the salary accounts of 8120 (Salaries — Physician Owner/ Stockholder), 8150 (Salaries — Physician Employees), 8170 (Salaries — Physician Administrators), 8320 (Salaries — Midlevel Providers Owner/Stockholder), 8350 (Salaries — Midlevel Provider Employees) and 8370 (Salaries — Midlevel Provider Administrators) are included as provider compensation (work component); any incentive and distribution accounts are excluded. If used, temporary employee salary accounts (5901 for physicians and 5902 for midlevel providers) would also be included as part of the work component.

Also included are the payroll tax accounts for physicians (8210 – 8214), standard insurance accounts for physicians (8220 – 8226), the defined pension benefit account for Physicians (8230), the payroll tax accounts for midlevel providers (8410 – 8414), standard insurance accounts for midlevels (8420 – 8426), and the defined pension benefit account for midlevels (8430). These are all standard compensation package accounts that would be used by all employers, thus the logic behind their inclusion and the exclusion of other accounts.

The additional benefit accounts are included as part of general physician expense for Accounts 8240 – 8270 and general (overhead) expense for midlevel provider expense Accounts 8440 – 8490 rather than provider compensation in this methodology. Why not include them in the provider compensation component? One reason is that not all employers offer these benefits. The second reason is that these benefits are 'add-ons' to a generic compensation package. If you want to be standardized to compare with other practices across the nation, use the basics without the fringe as in this School of Thought # 2.

Remember that midlevel providers who bill for their services under their own individual provider ID code are *included* in the Provider Compensation category. If the midlevel providers do *not* bill out for their services *using their own unique provider ID code*, then their salaries and related expenses should be included in overhead expenses, not Provider Compensation.

EXHIBIT 13.4

Account Number	Descriptions
8120	Salaries — Owner/Stockholder (Physician)
8150	Employee Salaries (Physician)
8170	Administrative Salaries (Physician)
8210	Payroll Taxes (Physician)
8211	Payroll Taxes — FICA/Medicare (Physician)
8212	Payroll Taxes — Federal Unemployment Insurance (Physician)
8213	Payroll Taxes — State Unemployment Insurance (Physician)
8214	Payroll Taxes — Other (Physician)
8220	Insurance (Physician)
8221	Insurance — Health (Physician)
8222	Insurance — Dental (Physician)
8223	Insurance — Life (Physician)
8224	Insurance — Disability (Physician)
8225	Insurance — Workers' Compensation (Physician)
8226	Insurance — Other (Physician)
8230	Pension and Retirement Benefits (Physician)
8320	Salaries — Owner/Stockholder (Midlevel)
8350	Employee Salaries (Midlevel)
8370	Administrative Salaries (Midlevel)
8410	Payroll Taxes (Midlevel)
8411	Payroll Taxes — FICA/Medicare (Midlevel)
8412	Payroll Taxes — Federal Unemployment Insurance (Midlevel)
8413	Payroll Taxes — State Unemployment Insurance (Midlevel)
8414	Payroll Taxes — Other (Midlevel)
8420	Insurance (Midlevel)
8421	Insurance — Health (Midlevel)
8422	Insurance — Dental (Midlevel)
8423	Insurance — Life (Midlevel)
8424	Insurance — Disability (Midlevel)
8425	Insurance — Worker's Compensation (Midlevel)
8426	Insurance — Other (Midlevel)
8430	Pension and Retirement Benefits

Exhibit 13.4 continued

Account Number	Descriptions
5900	Temporary Employee Salaries
5901	Physician Salaries
5902	Midlevel Provider Salaries

Overhead Expenses

The overhead expenses for School of Thought #2 include all the expenses in School of Thought #1 plus the accounts that were eliminated from the provider compensation in this particular model. Exhibit 13.5 shows the categories of overhead expenses for School of Thought #2. Although it is not mandatory to use all of these account categories, the overhead expenses should include the roll-ups into the major accounts. Rather than summarize all the account *inclusions* (which are many), here is a summary of the account *exclusions* (which are relatively few): 8120, 8150, 8170, 8210 – 8214, 8221 – 8226, 8230, 8320, 8350, 8370, 8410 – 8414, 8421 – 8426, 8430, 5901, 5902, 6186 and 6187. Those 30 or so accounts are either physician or midlevel provider compensation or provider malpractice insurance accounts.

EXHIBIT 13.5

Account Number	Descriptions
5000	OPERATING EXPENSES — Salary and Fringe Benefits
5500	ANCILLARY STAFF — SALARIES Include all sub-accounts under 5500
5600	ANCILLARY STAFF — EMPLOYEE-RELATED EXPENSES Include all sub-accounts under 5600
5700	EMPLOYEES — SALARIES Include all sub-accounts under 5700
5800	EMPLOYEES — EMPLOYEE-RELATED EXPENSES Include all sub-accounts under 5800
5900	Temporary Employee Salaries Include all sub-accounts under 5900 except 5901, 5902 (temporary employee salaries for physicians and midlevels)
6000	SERVICES AND GENERAL EXPENSE Include all sub-accounts under 6000 - 7000 except as noted
6100	Office and Administrative Expense Include all sub-accounts except 6186 and 6187 (malpractice insurance for physicians and midlevel providers)
6500	Billing Expense
6600	General Services
6700	Bad Debt Expense
7000	Clinical Expense
7500	Occupancy Expense
7600	Cost of Goods Sold — Medical Related
7000	PURCHASED SERVICES/MANAGEMENT FEES Include all sub-accounts under 7700 - 7800
9200	Nonoperating Expenses Include all sub-accounts under 9200 - 9300

Malpractice Expense

This is a very simple category including just one or two accounts: 6186 (for physicians) and 6187 (for midlevel providers if their compensation is included in the provider compensation field). Exhibit 13.6 displays these accounts.

As with School of Thought #1, note that there are two additional malpractice sub-accounts (6188 for Ancillary Providers and 6189 for Global Coverage), which should be included with the general overhead expenses. Why? Since the provider compensation field *excludes* ancillary providers' compensation, the malpractice expense field should also exclude ancillary malpractice to follow the pattern of matching expense categories to the provider.

EXHIBIT 13.6

Account Number	Descriptions
6185	Malpractice Insurance
6186	Physicians
6187	Midlevel Providers

PSPA's Cost Input screen

Where are these expenses entered in PSPA? In PSPA version 6.6x, the entries are made in the Cost Input Screen found under Cost Accounting: Maintenance: Group. Illustration 13.1 is a sample screen shot that illustrates the three categories. PSPA's Cost Accounting module uses year-to-date figures only; thus, all expenses should be year-to-date rather than a specific month or quarter. If your practice operates on a cash or modified-cash accounting basis, you should also make adjustments for year-end expenses when calculating expenses. If you do not make any adjustments, you may find a huge spike in costs at year-end. That, in turn, will skew the average cost per procedure compared to the other 11 months of the year.

Note in Illustration 13.2 that the Cost/RVU Components on the bottom row do not add up to the Cost/RVU (blended), which is $38.63. Why? Mathematically speaking, it is because of the weighting of the numerators and denominators used in calculating the ratios. Should they add up? No. It is appropriate to sum the total expenses and divide by the total RVUs to arrive at a generic Cost/RVU. It is not appropriate, algebraically speaking, to expect the sum of the Cost/RVU Components to equal the whole. Different weights are applied to each component, so it would be like comparing apples to oranges. Ask your resident math expert if you still have doubts.

ILLUSTRATIONS 13.1 and 13.2

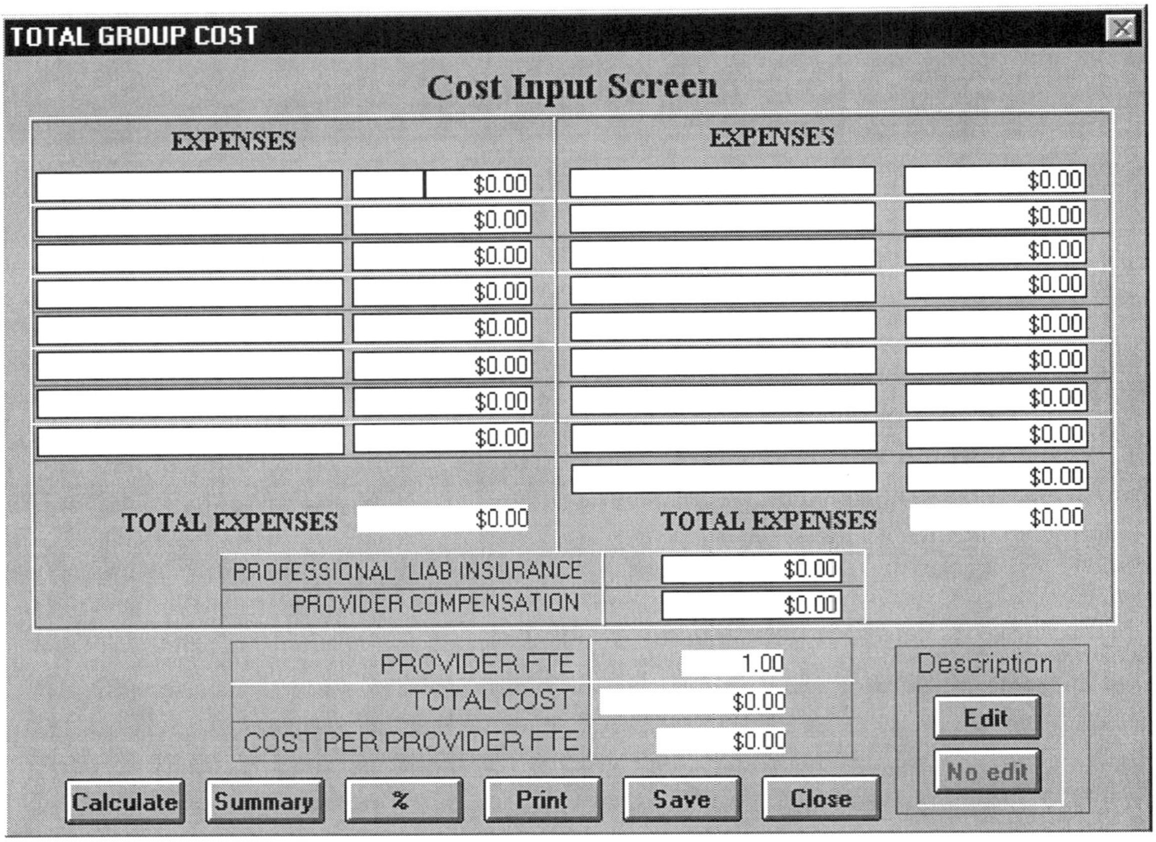

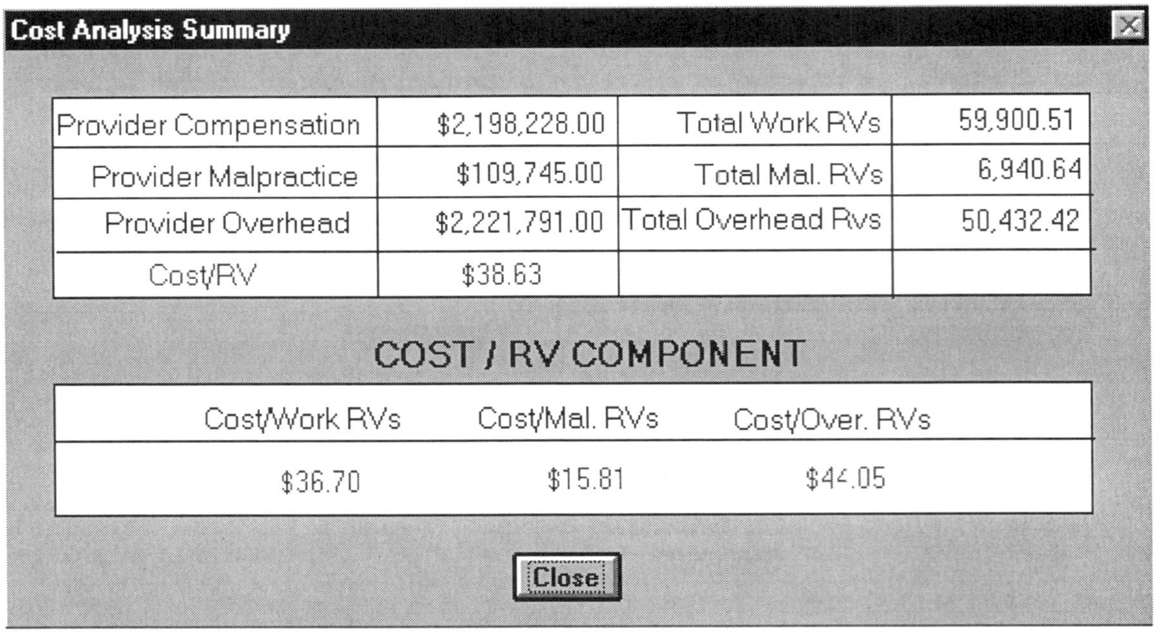

There are 17 fields on the top half of the Cost Input Screen under "Expense" for the major overhead categories, but not all of the 17 fields need to be used. (The 17 fields are only there to give the user multiple expense categories if desired. The reason the fields are split into two columns is simply to fit it on one screen.) The "Professional Liability Insurance" field is where the year-to-date sum of the malpractice Accounts 6186 and 6187 are entered. "Provider Compensation" includes the year-to-date sum of those accounts previously discussed.

Illustration 13.2 shows the summary screen that displays the three totals for the expense categories plus the total of each of the three RVU categories. The total expenses divided by the total RVUs results in the cost per blended RVU (Cost/RVU). This figure is the "bottom line" payment per RVU that should be used when negotiating managed-care contracts. It is the break even point when analyzing contracts based on RVUs and payments per RVU.

The bottom half of the screen displays the cost per component RVU. The Cost/Work RVU is calculated by dividing the total provider compensation by the total work RVUs. Likewise, the Cost/Malpractice RVU is derived by dividing the total malpractice expense by the total malpractice RVUs. Can you guess how the cost per overhead (practice expense) RVU is calculated?

Summary

Although there is not a hard-and-fast-rule on what comprises provider compensation versus practice expense, there are two prevailing schools of thought. One theory is to use all direct expenses associated with physicians and midlevel providers when calculating the total provider compensation. This may be a good theory to use when estimating the cost per RVU for internal users. The other theory emphasizes a much stricter rule when determining provider compensation: include only physician and midlevel provider salaries, payroll taxes, standard insurance categories and define retirement benefits. This makes it easy to perform benchmarking with outside organizations because that compensation package is fairly standard throughout the United States. Whichever theory an organization uses should be guided by the purpose behind the lumping of categories. Consistency is key.

Glossary

Accounts Payable: Amounts on open account owed by the organization to outside persons or entities for goods and services received by the organization. These accounts are usually control accounts for individual accounts payable balances that may be contained in a subsidiary ledger.

Accounts Receivable: The open account amounts (debts) owed to the organization by other entities (including customers, patients and third-party payers) as a result of the services provided to its customers and patients. Amounts assigned to "Accounts receivable" are due to "Gross fee-for-service charges." Assignment of a charge into "Accounts receivable" is initiated at the time an invoice is submitted for payment. For example, if an obstetrics practice establishes an open account for accumulation of charges when a patient is accepted into a prenatal program, and the charges will not be posted until after delivery, then "Accounts receivable" will not reflect these charges until an invoice is created. Deletion of charges from "Accounts receivable" is done when the account is paid, turned over to a collection agency or written off as bad debt. "Accounts payable (refunds) to patients and payers" are subtracted from "Accounts receivable" before reporting "Accounts receivable."

Accounts Receivable Write-Offs: Differences between adjusted gross charges and the amount actually collected as settlements for particular accounts. These write-offs may be the result of negotiating a payment less than adjusted gross charges with an individual patient or third-party agency (contractual adjustment).

Accrual: An accounting method where revenues are recorded as earned when services are performed rather than when cash is received. Cost is recorded in the period during which it is incurred, that is, when the asset or service is used, regardless of when cash is paid. Costs for goods and services that will be used to produce revenues in the future are reported as assets and recorded as costs in future periods. The accrual method balance sheet includes not only the assets and liabilities from the cash basis balance sheet, but also includes the receivables from patients, prepayments, and deferrals of costs, accruals of costs and revenues and payables owed to suppliers.

Accrued Liabilities: Current liabilities accrued at the end of an accounting period to reflect the proper amount of expenses for the organization under the accrual basis of accounting. Generally, no invoices or other billings are received within the accounting period, and the liability for these items is estimated or obtained from other sources.

Accrued Payroll Liabilities: Actual or estimated liabilities for payroll obligations. These accounts are credited (increased) when the payroll expense is incurred and are debited (decreased) when payment is made to the appropriate employee, agency or authority.

Adjustment: Adjustments represent the value of services performed for which payment is not expected to be received.

Advances from Settlements Due to Third-Party Agencies: Amounts owed to third-party agencies for current financing and other advances that are due and payable within one year. An example of a settlement due to a third-party agency would include amounts owed Medicare or Medicaid resulting from overpayments due to inaccurate claims.

Allowance for Change in Net Unrealized Gains/Losses on Investments: For-profit medical organizations should record changes in fair market value of investments that are classified as "available for sale" in this account.

Allowance for Charity Care: An account that tracks the patient services in which payment was neither sought nor collected by request of an authority (such as a physician or executive manager) within the organization or hospital.

Allowance for Estimated Uncollectible Receivables: Estimated amount of uncollectible receivables. An historical analysis of bad debt write-offs as well as contractual adjustments is usually required to determine periodic credits to this account.

Amortization: As a general rule, amortization is used to record the consumption or utilization over time of intangible property. Accumulated amortization is a contra-account to the related *intangible* asset. Amortization is recorded periodically, that is monthly, as an expense of the profit/loss or income statement. The offsetting entry is to increase (credit) accumulated amortization.

Assets: Resources owned by the business. Assets may be tangible (physical in character) such as land, buildings and equipment, or a direct right to tangible property such as amounts due from patients and third-party agencies, or they can be intangible such as goodwill, patents, licenses and leaseholds.

Bad Debt Expense: This account is used for uncollectible accounts receivable and notes receivable. An historical analysis of bad debt write-offs is usually required to determine periodic credits to this account. Other methods may be used, but a consistent and justifiable method of estimating the periodic charge to provision for bad debts (and the corresponding credit to either the Allowance for Estimated Uncollectible Receivables account or the Allowance for Bad Debts — Patients Account) should be applied systematically.

Bad Debt Recovery: Recovered revenues from collections that were originally written off as bad debt.

Balance Sheet: Also known as the Statement of Financial Position because it lists the organization's assets, liabilities and owners' equity (capital) at a particular point in time. It is a snapshot of the financial situation on a given date.

Bank Overdrafts Payable: Overdrafts on banks having no other free balances in amounts sufficient to offset.

Bonus: Managed-care contracts may have provisions for a bonus that would be paid after the accounts are reconciled at year-end. Bonuses are commonly linked to the achievement of predetermined goals typically based on either total plan performance or on the reduction of medical expenses.

Business Corporation: A legal entity whose shareholders need *not* be licensed to practice the profession practiced by the corporation.

Capital Contributed in Excess of Par: Capital contributed by owners in excess of the par or stated value of the capital stock.

Capital Lease Obligation — Long-Term Portion: Present value of future lease payments, excluding interest and finance charges, that will be made beyond one year on leases that have been capitalized.

Capital Leases: A capital lease meets any of the following criteria:

- Lease transfers ownership to lessee during or at the end of the lease term.
- Lease contains a bargain purchase option.
- Lease term (including any bargain renewal options) is 75 percent or more of estimated economic life of property.
- Present value of the minimum lease payments (excluding tax credits and executory costs, for example, maintenance, taxes and insurance) equals 90 percent or more of fair market value of leased property, minus investment tax credit.

Capitalization: Expensing of the costs of furniture, fixtures and equipment over time. A common criterion for capitalization is a unit cost of $500 or more. Other criteria for capitalization include:

- A unit cost sufficiently large to justify the cost of control incident to an equipment or property ledger.
- Depreciable life of two years or more but less than the life of buildings to which the equipment or fixtures may be affixed.
- Used in organizational operations.
- Sufficient individuality and size to make control feasible by means of identification tags or numbers.

Capitated Premium Revenues — Commercial: Net revenue actually collected from capitation payments, risk-sharing revenues and other revenues paid to the organization by an HMO for assigned enrollees under a patient-care contract.

Capitation: A set amount of money received or paid out according to a managed-care contract. Also known as a "cap rate," capitation is based on the number of enrollees in a health plan (membership) rather than on actual services delivered. It is usually expressed in units of per-member per-month (PMPM). A health plan may adjust the capitation rate based on such factors as age and sex of the enrollee. A capitation contract is one in which the practice agrees to provide medical services to a defined population for a fixed price per beneficiary per month, regardless of the actual services provided. Capitated contracts, which always contain an element of risk, include commercial HMO, Medicare and Medicaid capitation contracts.

Cash — Restricted: Cash restricted for other than general operating purposes. Even though the cash may be restricted for use with noncurrent budget items, it may still be expended within one year.

Cash — Unrestricted: This account is for cash that is typically used for general operating purposes. Unrestricted cash on-hand covers both a change fund and/or a petty cash fund. Unrestricted cash on deposit in banks is immediately available for current operations.

Cash-Basis Accounting: An accounting method where revenues are recorded when cash is received and costs are recorded when cash is paid out. Receivables, payables, accruals and deferrals arising from operations are ignored. On a pure cash basis, long-lived (fixed) assets are expensed when acquired, leaving cash and investments as the only assets, and borrowings and payroll withholdings as the only liabilities.

Cash Surrender Value of Life Insurance Policies: Amounts that recognize the accumulated buildup in value inside a life insurance policy that could be used for loan purposes and/or that would be available upon the termination of a policy.

Charity Care: Patients who come to the practice for care where no payment is expected or collected.

Claims Payable Incurred But Not Reported: Liability account used to record an estimation of the amounts owed to providers outside the organization for medical services to prepaid patients of the organization for which invoices have not been received. These are normally estimated using historical lag factors. When invoiced, the claims should be transferred to Contract Claims Payable.

Collection Agency Write-Offs: Any accounts turned over to a collection agency. The corresponding accounts receivable should be credited.

Common Stock: A type of stock whereby equity claims are held by the "residual owners" of the organization, who are the last to receive any distribution of earning or assets. It represents the stated or par value of stock issued to owners.

Community Health Center: An ambulatory clinic serving an area with limited health services or with special health needs. The funding authority for these centers occurs under the Public Health Services Act. CHCs coordinate federal, state, and local resources in a single organization capable of delivering both health care and related social services to a defined population. While such centers may not directly provide all types of health care, they arrange for all medical services needed by their patients.

Contract Claims Payable: This account is related to Claims Payable Incurred But Not Reported (IBNR). Once determined or invoiced, the contract claims from that account should be transferred to this account. Contract Claims Payable records amounts owed by the organization to providers outside the organization for medical services to patients assigned to the organization.

Contributions: Amounts paid out by the organization to recognized non-profit entities or to charitable causes.

Coordination of Benefits: Policy guidance within the National Association of Insurance Commissioners (NAIC) to prevent double payment for services when an enrollee has coverage from two or more sources. It is used to ensure that the insured's benefits from all sources do not exceed 100 percent of allowable.

Copayments: Revenues generated from payment-sharing arrangements between the insurance carriers or federal entity and the patient, which often includes the concept of a specific amount of money per visit.

Corporation: A for-profit organization recognized by law as a business entity separate and distinct from its shareholders. A medical practice organized as a corporation can either be a 'C' corporation or a 'S' corporation as designated by the Internal Revenue Code. The primary difference between these two types of entities is the way they are taxed and how distributions are made. A 'S' corporation is a flow-through entity, meaning all the income whether or not distributed is taxed at the individual shareholder level. A 'C' corporation can retain earnings and be taxed at both a corporate and individual level if there are dividend distributions. *See also Business Corporation, Professional Corporation.*

Covered Lives: The number of individual lives enrolled in a prepaid/capitated insurance plan serviced by the medical practice. A covered life is considered a member and is also known as an enrollee. A member is not considered a patient unless services are received during a particular month. (i.e., A covered life, enrollee, or member is one whose health care facility or provider receives monthly payments from the enrollee's insurance carrier. They become patients when services are rendered by their health care provider.)

CPT-4 Code: *Physician's Current Procedural Terminology, Fourth Edition,* copyrighted by the American Medical Association.

Current Assets: Cash and other assets that are expected to be converted to cash, sold or consumed in the normal course of operations within one year.

Current Liabilities: Liabilities that mature and require payment from current assets or through the creation of other liabilities within one year.

Deferred Revenue: Revenue received in one period applicable to services to be rendered in some future period.

Deficit: The excess of expenses and other outflows over revenues and other inflows.

Depreciation: As a general rule, depreciation is used to record the consumption or utilization over time of tangible property. Accumulated depreciation is a contra-account to the related fixed asset. Depreciation is recorded periodically, that is monthly, as an expense on the profit/loss or income statement earnings in the statement of operations. The offsetting entry is to increase (credit) accumulated depreciation.

Donated Capital: Increase in owners' equity due to assets contributed to the corporation.

Donations: Any endowment or gift received by the organization.

Encounter: An encounter includes only procedures from the evaluation and management chapter (CPT codes 99201 - 99499) or the medicine chapter (CPT codes 90800 - 99199) of the *Physician's Current Procedural Terminology, Fourth Edition,* copyrighted by the American Medical Association.

Faculty Practice Plan (FPP): A faculty practice plan is a formal framework that structures the clinical practice activities of a medical school faculty. The plan performs a range of services including billing, collections, contract negotiations and the distribution of income. Plans may form a separate legal organization or may be affiliated with the medical school through a clinical science department or teaching hospital. Faculty associated with the plan must provide patient care as part of a teaching or research program.

Federally Qualified Health Center (FQHC): A facility located in a medically underserved area that provides Medicare beneficiaries preventive primary medical care under the general direction of a physician.

Goodwill: Excess of costs over the fair market value of identifiable assets in the purchase of an entire organization.

Grant Revenue: Includes federal, state, or local government or private foundation grants to provide indigent patient care or for case management of the frail and elderly.

Gross Charges — FFS Equivalents for Capitation Plan Patients: Gross charges under capitation contracts for assigned enrollees under a patient-care contract are recorded in this account. This account is used to record accrual-basis revenues under risk-sharing arrangements such as bonuses and risk-pool allocations; however, the Fees Collected account series should be used to reflect revenues actually collected on these accounts.

Gross Charges: Established usual and customary rates are the full price for services before charge restrictions imposed by Medicare or contractual adjustments required by third-party payers, such as commercial insurance carriers or other adjustments. Services include all medical/surgical services provided by physicians and midlevel providers as well as professional and technical components of ancillary services such as radiology and laboratory.

Group Practice Without Walls (GPWW): A business entity formed by independent physicians or medical practices in order to create centralized management and decision-making structure and to share administrative, billing and purchasing costs. The result is an organization with multiple sites. The physicians and medical practices retain their independence by maintaining their private offices and practice styles.

Health Maintenance Organization (HMO): An insurance company indemnifies an insured party against a specified loss in return for premiums paid, as stipulated by a contract. A Health Maintenance Organization (HMO), for-profit or not-for-profit, accepts responsibility for providing and delivering a predetermined set of comprehensive health maintenance and treatment services to a voluntarily enrolled population for a negotiated and fixed periodic premium.

Income Statement: It is a measure of the results of operations representing the difference between revenue and expense for the reported period. The income statement is used to summarize results of business operations for a period of time, not longer than one year, to determine if the organization is operating efficiently.

Incurred But Not Reported (IBNR): This liability represents claims that the organization is legally responsible to pay for services it has contracted with a managed care organization for on a capitated basis and pays to subcontractors on a fee-for-service basis. It is an amount of money that the organization accrues for future medical expenses. These are medical expenses that the authorization system has not captured and for which claims have not yet been processed. IBNR can be calculated in a number of ways. The most common method is to track the history of claims payment for the specific organization to determine a claims' lag ratio and apply this ratio to current operations. IBNR can also be calculated actuarially based on anticipated utilization of a specific population. Another practical approach is to determine the number of referrals authorized but not billed as of a particular date and apply an average claim amount to these open referrals.

Independent Practice Association/Organization (IPA/IPO): An organization or network of licensed providers. This organization is a separate legal entity, usually on a for-profit basis. Typically, the primary purpose of the IPA/IPO is to secure and maintain contractual relationships between providers and health plans.

Intangible Assets: Property rights without physical substance that will benefit future operations of the organization. Intangible assets are purchased from external sources, provide future benefit and are relatively long-lived. Other assets include long-term prepayments, deferred charges, goodwill and assets not included in other categories.

Intercompany Accounts Payable: Amounts owed *by* the organization to other entities consolidated for financial reporting purposes.

Intercompany Receivables: Amounts owed *to* the organization by other entities consolidated for financial reporting purposes.

Interest Expense: Interest incurred on borrowings.

Interest Income: Interest earned on marketable securities, certificates of deposit, savings accounts and/or other short-term investments.

Interest Receivables: Interest that has been earned but not yet received.

Investments — Long-Term Receivables: Long-term investments in securities, property (not used for operations) and receivables due beyond one year. Assets recorded in these accounts will not be used to finance operations.

Keyman Insurance: Contracts that insure the lives of certain owners or management of the organization against certain business risks.

Lag Study: A report that displays the age of the processed claims and how much money is paid out each month. The report compares these figures to the amount of money that was accrued for those expenses each month and calculates the lag ratio. Lag ratios are used to determine whether the organization's reserves are adequate to meet all expenses.

Liabilities: Liabilities are debts or obligations owed by the organization to creditors. These debts arise as a result of the purchase of goods and services from others on credit and through cash borrowings to finance business operations. Liabilities are also obligations of responsibility to transfer other assets or to provide services to another entity.

Limited Liability Company: A legal entity that is a hybrid between a corporation and a partnership providing limited liability to owners like a corporation, while passing profits and losses through to owners like a partnership.

Long-Term Assets: Assets that are not expected to be converted to cash, sold or otherwise consumed in the normal course of operations within one year.

Long-Term Liabilities: Liabilities that will mature and require payment at some future time beyond one year.

Malpractice Insurance: Premiums or self-insurance cost for coverage of professional liability claims.

Managed Care Organization (MCO): A generic term applied to a managed-care plan.

Management Company Incentive: Management companies are increasingly becoming encouraged to be better performers by entering into contracts in which they get paid a bonus based on performance. This account can be used to reflect the incentive portion of that management fee.

Management Fees: Amounts paid in accordance with managed service organization, physician practice management company, hospital or other parent organization agreements for covered services including management, administrative and/or related support services.

Medical Foundation: A not-for-profit corporation that is exempt from paying federal income taxes under Section 501(c) of the Internal Revenue Service (IRS) code. Typically, the medical foundation is legally integrated with another organization that also has a tax-exempt status. The foundation may employ physicians or may contract with independent physicians for the delivery of health care services.

Medical Group: A medical practice consisting of at least three or more physicians who are engaged in the practice of medicine and share management and support staff personnel, facilities, equipment and medical records.

Medical Practice: An organization consisting of at least one physician and/or midlevel provider who delivers health care services. A medical practice need not be a single legal entity.

Medical Services Organization: An organization that provides services and/or nonphysician support staff to practices but does not provide health care services. Typically, the MSO is owned by a hospital, health system or by a group of investors. The MSO may purchase facilities, equipment and furniture from practices and then lease it back.

Midlevel Providers: Specially trained and licensed nonphysician providers (also known as physician extenders), employed or contracted, who can provide medical care and bill for services without continuous supervision by a physician.

Modified Cash-Basis Accounting: An accounting method that is primarily a cash-basis system as previously defined, but allows the cost of long-lived (fixed) assets to be expensed through depreciation. The modified cash system recognizes inventories of goods intended for resale as assets. Under a modified cash system, purchases of buildings and equipment, leasehold improvements, and payments of insurance premiums applicable to more than one accounting period are normally recorded as assets. Costs for these assets are allocated to accounting periods in a systematic manner over the length of time the practice benefits from the assets.

Net Assets: Excess of the not-for-profit entity's assets over its liabilities. The balances in these accounts are the cumulative results of original investments, grants, gifts, donations, and revenues and expenditures.

Noncurrent Expenses Paid in Advance: Costs incurred (payments) for goods or services that will benefit future operations (beyond a year).

Nonoperating Revenues: Revenues not directly related to patient care or the provision of medical services.

Notes Payable — Long-Term: Notes payable that mature more than one year from financial statement date. The current portion of any long-term liability should be included in Long-Term Debt — Current Portion, except those obligations to be refinanced or paid from a sinking fund.

Notes Receivable — Short-Term: Amounts owed to the organization by other entities where the obligation is represented by a note with a maturity of one year or less.

Not-For-Profit Entity: A legal entity that has obtained special exemption under Section 501(c) of the Internal Revenue Service code that qualifies the organization to be exempt from federal income taxes. To qualify as a tax-exempt organization, an entity, practice or faculty practice plan has to provide advance evidence of a planned charitable, educational or research purpose.

Occupancy Expense: Expenses related to the occupancy and use of land and buildings. In the event that another legal entity owns the land or buildings, any rental fees, commissions or charges paid to the other entity are charged to this account. For the purpose of peer comparison (for example, comparative data or cost survey), a fair market rental value may be charged to this account even if no rent is otherwise charged to the organization by the owning entity.

Operating Expenses: Expired costs incurred in the process of providing medical services to the organization's patients. Excludes all costs pertaining to nonoperating activities such as general investments, endowments, etc.

Operating Subsidy Income: Operational support (operating subsidies) received by medical practices from a parent organization such as a hospital, health system, PPMC, MSO or other large integrated system.

Organization Costs: Costs incurred in the original incorporation and start-up of a business operation. These costs are generally amortized over a period of five years.

Owners' Equity: A residual interest or claim of the owners to the assets after creditor claims are settled. (Legally, creditors are first in line to receive reimbursement.) Owners' equity derives from two sources:

1) contributed capital, which is the investment of cash or other assets by the owner or owners; and/or

2) retained earnings, the accumulative results of income, less losses and withdrawals over the years.

Partnership: A legal entity where two or more individuals have agreed that they will share profits and losses and assets and liabilities, although not necessarily on an equal basis. The partnership agreement is typically formalized in writing.

Patient: A unique patient is one who is counted only once per month regardless of the number of times that patient sees a specific physician or midlevel provider. This patient count is per physician or midlevel provider. If the patient sees more than one physician or midlevel provider during a certain month, each physician or midlevel provider would receive a patient count of one. If the patient does not receive any services during a particular month, the patient is not counted in that month's total patients.

Patient Refunds: Refunds of amounts collected from patients that should not have been collected or that need to be returned for some other reason. The corresponding credit is cash or accounts payable. This account should be used only if the specific revenue in which the payment was originally recorded is not used.

Payroll Tax Withholdings Payable: Actual liabilities for Payroll Tax Withholdings. These accounts are credited (increased) for amounts withheld from employees and are debited (decreased) when payment is made to the appropriate agency, authority or plan.

Permanently Restricted Net Assets: Net assets with donor restrictions that do not expire with the passage of time and cannot be removed by any actions taken by the medical organization other than for its restricted use. Endowment funds are an example.

Physician Hospital Organization (PHO): A legal entity created by the joining together of a physician contracting network and a hospital to create a managed care contracting network consisting of both physicians and hospital(s).

Physician Practice Management Company (PPMC): An independent business that provides a menu of management, administrative and/or related support services to one or more practices for a fee as specified by contract.

Preferred Provider Organization (PPO): Independent health care providers that contract with a managed-care plan to provide services at a discount. A PPO may or may not be risk-bearing entities.

Preferred Stock: A type of stock whose holders are given certain priority over common stockholders in the payment of dividends and liquidation/termination of the entity. Usually the dividend rate is fixed at the time of stock issue.

Prepaid Expenses: Payments for goods or services that will benefit future operations.

Procedure Code: Typically the CPT-4 code performed by a provider, but it could also be a home-grown or other recognized code from the McGraw-Hill scale, for instance. In PSPA CPT download files, these codes are associated with the provider that performed them.

Professional Corporation: A legal entity whose shareholders must typically all be licensed to practice in the same profession as that practiced by the organization. State law determines whether all shareholders must be licensed.

Provision for Cash Basis Conversion: An account used to convert revenues recorded on the accrual basis to collections recorded on the cash basis. This adjustment is optional and is provided for the organization that may wish to compute revenues on both the cash and accrual basis.

RBRVS: Resource-Based Relative Value Scale developed by the Health Care Financing Administration (HCFA) for use by Medicare. Relative values are assigned to each CPT-4 code based on the amount of resources used to provide a given service.

Realized Gains and Losses — Investments: Gains or losses recognized on closed and sold securities during the period.

Reinsurance Recoveries: Amounts received as a result of a stop-loss policy issued by an insurance carrier that specializes in underwriting the risks associated with the insurance industry.

Reinsurance: Stop-loss insurance (reinsurance) coverage of catastrophic claims, emergency care outside the contract parameters and insolvency.

Relative Value Unit (RVU): A nonmonetary standard unit of measure that indicates the value of services provided by physicians, midlevel providers and other health care professionals.

Research/Clinical Studies Income: Research stipends for activities such as pharmaceutical studies and educational subsidies used to train residents. Also includes revenue received from research activities during the fiscal year. Sponsored funding comes from external sources (i.e., grants and contracts) and is awarded for specific research activities.

Retained Earnings — Appropriated: Restrictions placed on portions of earnings retained in the corporation. These restrictions may temporarily limit the amount of dividends available for distribution to owners. This account should be used to record creation of unfunded reserves required by state HMO laws or regulations.

Retained Earnings — Unappropriated: Net income (or loss) over the life of the corporation minus all distributions to owners and appropriations of retained earnings carried in the Retained Earnings — Appropriated Account.

Revenue and Expense Summary: A summary account for use in the closing of revenue and expense accounts when financial statements are prepared.

Revenues: Inflows of cash and other items of value received or to be received for services rendered. There are different measures of these inflows of cash for fee-for-service (FFS) revenues, depending upon whether the organization identifies gross charges, adjustments and allowances; whether the organization uses the cash, modified cash or accrual basis of accounting; and whether a prepaid plan pays discounted FFS or capitation.

Risk Sharing Revenues: Any mechanism that gives incentive to providers to render cost-effective, high-quality health care.

Sinking Fund: An actual depository account established to pay off a specific liability.

Stockholders' Equity: Net assets of the corporation; that is, the excess of the corporate entity's assets over its liabilities. The balances in these accounts are the cumulative result of the owners' investments and the equity originating from net earnings retained by the corporation.

Surplus: The excess of revenues and other inflows over expenses and other outflows.

Temporarily Restricted Net Assets: Donor-restricted net assets that can be used by the medical organization for their specified purpose once the donor's restriction is met. Generally, these restrictions are met either by the passage of time or by actions taken by the entity, such as the use of funds for the purpose intended.

Third-Party Settlements: Under a retrospective rate-setting system, third parties usually determine an interim payment rate and, during the rate period, pay the medical organization for services rendered using the rate. After the rate period has ended, the medical organization may be entitled to receive additional payments or may be required to refund amounts received in excess of amounts earned under the system.

Treasury Stock: Capital stock repurchased by the corporation that has not been retired. Treasury stock is usually carried on the balance sheet at acquisition cost.

Undistributed Earnings: Difference between revenues and expenses allocated to the partners as earned capital. This account tracks the prior year's net earnings/losses.

Unrealized Gains and Losses — Investments: The accounting recognition of the difference between the fair market value of carried investments and the adjusted cost (current "book" value) of those investments for the period.

Unrestricted Net Assets: Unrestricted equity of the not-for-profit entity. Equity resulting from incurring revenues for providing or agreeing to provide health care services, receiving unrestricted contributions and/or grants, or receiving dividend or interest from investing in income-producing assets minus expenses incurred in providing or agreeing to provide health care services or other community benefits and performing administrative functions.

Valuation Allowance: Adjustments to investments to reflect the unrealized appreciation or depreciation in the fair market value of the investment at the end of the period. At the end of the period, changes in the fair market value of equity and debt securities of a not-for-profit medical organization should be recorded here.

Withhold: A percentage of the primary care capitation rate that is withheld every month and used to cover the cost overruns (excess medical expenses) in referral or organizational services. Typically used in capitation contracts or other risk-sharing arrangements, this account is reconciled at year-end. If the entire amount of the withhold was not required to cover cost overruns, the remainder may be distributed or kept in the account to fund the risk pool as determined by contract terms.

APPENDIX
Tables I - VI

Chart of Accounts for Health Care Organizations

TABLE I

General - Detailed Format

Account Number	Description	Accrual	Modified Cash	Cash
	BALANCE SHEET			
1000	**ASSETS**			
1100	Cash	X	X	X
1110	Cash - Banks	X	X	X
1111	General Checking Accounts	X	X	X
1112	Payroll Checking Accounts	X	X	X
1113	Other Checking Accounts	X	X	X
1120	Cash - On hand	X	X	X
1121	Change Fund	X	X	X
1122	Petty Cash	X	X	X
1130	Cash - Restricted	X	X	X
1200	Marketable Securities & Short-Term Investments	X	X	X
1210	Valuation Allowance - Short-Term Investments	X	X	X
1300	Accounts Receivable	X		
1301	Accounts Receivable - Fee-for-Service Amounts	X		
1302	Accounts Receivable - Prepaid Contracts	X		
1320	Allowance for Estimated Uncollectible Receivables	X		
1321	Allowance for Bad Debts - Patient Accounts	X		
1322	Allowance for Contractual Adjustments	X		
1323	Allowance for Bad Debts - Third-Party Payers	X		
1324	Allowance for Charity Care	X		
1340	Notes Receivable - Short Term	X	X	X
1345	Managed Care Contract - Bonus/Withhold	X		
1350	Other Short-Term Receivables	X	X	X
1351	Interest Receivables	X		
1352	Intercompany Receivables	X	X	X
1353	Due from Employees	X	X	X

Chart of Accounts for Health Care Organizations

TABLE I

General - Detailed Format

Account Number	Description	Accrual	Modified Cash	Cash
1354	Due from Related Parties	X	X	X
1400	Supply Inventories	X	X	
1401	Drugs and Medications	X	X	
1402	Medical Supplies	X	X	
1403	Administrative Supplies	X	X	
1404	Forms	X	X	
1405	Housekeeping and Maintenance Supplies	X	X	
1406	Linen Supplies	X	X	
1407	Other Supplies	X	X	
1420	Ancillary Department Supplies	X	X	
1500	Prepaid Expenses	X	X	
1501	Prepaid Interest	X	X	
1502	Prepaid Insurance	X	X	
1503	Prepaid Rent	X	X	
1504	Prepaid Taxes	X	X	
1505	Prepaid Dues	X	X	
1506	Other Prepaid Expenses	X	X	
1550	Other Current Assets	X	X	
1600	INVESTMENTS - LONG-TERM RECEIVABLES	X	X	X
1610	Long-Term Receivables	X	X	X
1630	Long-Term Investments	X	X	X
1635	Valuation Allowance - Long-Term Investments	X	X	X
1640	Investments in Affiliates	X	X	X
1650	Property Held for Future Use	X	X	
1700	PROPERTY, FURNITURE, FIXTURES & EQUIPMENT			

Chart of Accounts for Health Care Organizations

TABLE I

General - Detailed Format

Account Number	Description	Accrual	Modified Cash	Cash
1710	REAL PROPERTY	X	X	
1711	Land	X	X	
1712	Land Improvements	X	X	
1713	Buildings	X	X	
1714	Capital Leases - Buildings	X		
1715	Leasehold Improvements	X	X	
1716	Construction in Progress	X	X	
1717	Other Real Property	X	X	
1750	FURNITURE, FIXTURES & EQUIPMENT	X	X	
1751	Furniture and Fixtures	X	X	
1752	Capital Leases - Furniture and Fixtures	X		
1753	Equipment	X	X	
1754	Capital Leases - Equipment	X		
1755	Medical Equipment	X	X	
1756	Capital Leases - Medical Equipment	X		
1760	Computer	X	X	
1761	Computer - Hardware	X	X	
1762	Computer - Software	X	X	
1763	Computer - Other	X	X	
1770	Capital Leases - Computer	X		
1771	Capital Leases - Computer - Hardware	X		
1772	Capital Leases - Computer - Software	X		
1773	Capital Leases - Computer - Other	X		
1780	Vehicles	X	X	
1781	Vehicles	X	X	
1782	Capital Leases - Vehicles	X		
1790	Ancillary Service Equipment	X	X	
1791	Laboratory Equipment	X	X	

Chart of Accounts for Health Care Organizations

General - Detailed Format

Account Number	Description	Accrual	Modified Cash	Cash
1792	Radiology Equipment	X	X	
1793	Physical Therapy Equipment	X	X	
1794	Diagnostic Equipment	X	X	
1795	Capital Leases - Ancillary Service Equipment	X		
1796	Capital Leases - Laboratory Equipment	X		
1797	Capital Leases - Radiology Equipment	X		
1798	Capital Leases - Physical Therapy Equipment	X		
1799	Capital Leases - Diagnostic Equipment	X		
1800	ACCUMULATED DEPRECIATION - PROPERTY, FURNITURE, ETC.			
1810	ACCUMULATED DEPRECIATION - REAL PROPERTY	X	X	
1812	Accum Depreciation - Land Improvements	X	X	
1813	Accum Depreciation - Buildings	X	X	
1814	Accum Depreciation - Capital Leases - Buildings	X		
1815	Accum Depreciation - Leasehold Improvements	X	X	
1817	Accum Depreciation - Other Real Property	X	X	
1850	ACCUM DEPRECIATION - FURNITURE, FIXTURES & EQUIPMENT	X	X	
1851	Accum Depreciation - Furniture and Fixtures	X	X	
1852	Accum Depreciation - Capital Leases - Furniture and Fixtures	X		
1853	Accum Depreciation - Equipment	X	X	
1854	Accum Depreciation - Capital Leases - Equipment	X		
1855	Accum Depreciation - Medical Equipment	X	X	
1856	Accum Depreciation - Capital Leases - Medical Equipment	X		
1860	Accum Depreciation - Computer	X	X	
1861	Accum Depreciation - Computer - Hardware	X	X	
1862	Accum Depreciation - Computer - Software	X	X	
1863	Accum Depreciation - Computer - Other	X	X	
1870	Accum Depreciation - Capital Leases - Computer	X		

Chart of Accounts for Health Care Organizations

General - Detailed Format

Account Number	Description	Accrual	Modified Cash	Cash
1871	Accum Depreciation - Capital Leases - Computer Hardware	X		
1872	Accum Depreciation - Capital Leases - Computer Software	X		
1873	Accum Depreciation - Capital Leases - Computer - Other	X		
1880	Accum Depreciation - Vehicles	X	X	
1881	Accum Depreciation - Vehicles	X	X	
1882	Accum Depreciation - Capital Leases - Vehicles	X		
1890	Other Accum Depreciation - Ancillary Service Equipment	X	X	
1891	Accum Depreciation - Laboratory Equipment	X	X	
1892	Accum Depreciation - Radiology Equipment	X	X	
1893	Accum Depreciation - Physical Therapy Equipment	X	X	
1894	Accum Depreciation - Diagnostic Equipment	X	X	
1895	Accum Depreciation - Capital Leases - Ancillary Service Equipment	X		
1896	Accum Depreciation - Capital Leases - Laboratory Equipment	X		
1897	Accum Depreciation - Capital Leases - Radiology Equipment	X		
1898	Accum Depreciation - Capital Leases - Physical Therapy Equipment	X		
1899	Accum Depreciation - Capital Leases - Diagnostic Equipment	X		
1900	INTANGIBLE AND OTHER ASSETS			
1910	Organization Costs	X	X	
1915	Accumulated Amortization - Organization Costs	X	X	
1920	Goodwill	X	X	
1925	Accumulated Amortization - Goodwill	X	X	
1930	Other Intangible Assets	X	X	
1940	Deposits	X	X	
1950	Noncurrent Expenses Paid in Advance	X	X	
1951	Noncurrent Interest Paid in Advance	X	X	
1952	Noncurrent Insurance Paid in Advance	X	X	
1953	Noncurrent Rent Paid in Advance	X	X	

Chart of Accounts for Health Care Organizations **TABLE I**

General - Detailed Format

Account Number	Description	Accrual	Modified Cash	Cash
1954	Noncurrent Taxes Paid in Advance	X	X	
1955	Noncurrent Dues Paid in Advance	X	X	
1956	Other Noncurrent Expenses Paid in Advance	X	X	
1960	Other Assets	X	X	
1961	Cash Surrender Value of Life Insurance Policies	X	X	
2000	**LIABILITIES**	X		
2100	CURRENT LIABILITIES - PAYABLES	X		
2110	Accounts Payable	X		
2120	Bank Overdrafts Payable	X		
2130	Other Current Liabilities Payable	X		
2131	Intercompany Accounts Payable	X		
2132	Accounts Payable - Employees	X		
2133	Accounts Payable - Related Parties	X		
2134	Accounts Payable - Other	X		
2160	Contract Claims Payable	X		
2200	CURRENT LIABILITIES - PAYROLL	X		
2210	Payroll Tax Withholdings Payable	X	X	X
2211	Federal Income Tax Withholdings Payable	X	X	X
2212	State Income Tax Withholdings Payable	X	X	X
2213	FICA/Medicare Tax Withholdings Payable	X	X	X
2214	Local Tax Withholdings Payable	X	X	X
2215	Other Tax Withholdings Payable	X	X	X
2220	Insurance Withholdings Payable	X	X	X
2221	Health Insurance Withholdings Payable	X	X	X
2222	Life Insurance Withholdings Payable	X	X	X

Chart of Accounts for Health Care Organizations

TABLE I

General - Detailed Format

Account Number	Description	Accrual	Modified Cash	Cash
2223	State Disability Insurance Withholdings Payable	X	X	X
2224	Other Insurance Withholdings Payable	X	X	X
2230	Other Payroll Withholdings Payable	X	X	X
2231	401(k) Withholdings Payable	X	X	X
2232	Cafeteria Plan Withholdings Payable	X	X	X
2233	Court Mandated Child Support Withholdings Payable	X	X	X
2234	Other Payroll Withholdings Payable	X	X	X
2250	Accrued Payroll Liabilities	X		
2251	Accrued Payroll	X		
2252	Accrued Vacation, Holiday, & Sick Pay (Compensated Absences)	X		
2253	Accrued FICA/Medicare Taxes Payable	X		
2254	Accrued State Unemployment Taxes Payable	X		
2255	Accrued Federal Unemployment Taxes Payable	X		
2256	Accrued Retirement Plan Contribution	X	X	
2257	Other Accrued Payroll Liabilities	X		
2260	Other Payroll Liabilities	X		
2300	CURRENT LIABILITIES - OTHER	X		
2310	Accrued Liabilities - Nonpayroll	X		
2311	Accrued Rent	X		
2312	Accrued Interest	X		
2313	Accrued Insurance	X		
2314	Accrued Income Taxes (Federal/State)	X		
2315	Accrued Property Taxes	X		
2316	Accrued Franchise Taxes	X		
2317	Other Accrued Liabilities	X		
2320	Notes and Loans Payable	X	X	X
2321	Current Notes and Loans Payable - Vendors	X	X	X

Chart of Accounts for Health Care Organizations

TABLE I

General - Detailed Format

Account Number	Description	Accrual	Modified Cash	Cash
2322	Current Notes and Loans Payable - Employees	X	X	X
2323	Current Notes and Loans Payable - Stockholders/Partners	X	X	X
2324	Current Other Notes and Loans Payable	X	X	X
2325	Bank Working Capital Line Outstanding	X	X	X
2330	Long-Term Debt - Current Portion	X	X	X
2331	Capital Lease Obligation - Current Portion	X		
2332	Construction Contracts Payable	X	X	X
2333	Other Loans Payable - Current Portion	X	X	X
2340	Advances from Settlements Due to Third-Party Agencies	X	X	X
2350	Patient Deposits	X	X	
2360	Claims Payable Incurred But Not Reported	X		
2361	Incurred But Not Reported Claims - Commercial	X		
2362	Incurred But Not Reported Claims - Medicare	X		
2363	Incurred But Not Reported Claims - Medicaid	X		
2365	Other Claims Incurred But Not Reported	X		
2370	Deferred Revenue	X		
2371	Deferred Revenue - Fee for Service	X		
2372	Deferred Revenue - Capitated or Prepaid Plan	X		
2375	Other Deferred Revenue	X		
2380	Deferred Income Taxes - Current Portion	X		
2390	Other Current Liabilities	X		
2400	LONG-TERM LIABILITIES	X	X	X
2410	Long-Term Notes Payable	X	X	X
2420	Construction Loans	X	X	X
2430	Capital Lease Obligation - Long-Term Portion	X		
2440	Other Loans Payable - Long-Term Portion	X	X	X
2450	Deferred Third-Party Revenue	X		

Chart of Accounts for Health Care Organizations

TABLE I

General - Detailed Format

Account Number	Description	Accrual	Modified Cash	Cash
2451	Deferred Third-Party Revenue - Medicare	X		
2452	Deferred Third-Party Revenue - Medicaid	X		
2453	Deferred Third-Party Revenue - Other	X		
2460	Deferred Compensation	X		
2465	Severance Plan	X		
2470	Deferred Income Taxes - Long-Term Portion	X		
2480	Other Long-Term Liabilities	X		
	Owners' Equity Accounts			
3000	**PARTNERS' EQUITY (PARTNERSHIP)**	X	X	X
3010	Contributed Capital (Each Partner)	X	X	X
3020	Undistributed Earnings	X	X	X
3030	Partners' Drawing Accounts (Each Partner)	X	X	X
3040	Current Income/Loss	X	X	X
3000	**STOCKHOLDERS' EQUITY (CORPORATION)**	X	X	X
3010	Preferred Stock	X	X	X
3020	Common Stock	X	X	X
3030	Capital Contributed in Excess of Par	X	X	X
3040	Donated Capital	X	X	X
3050	Allowance for Change in Net Unrealized Gains/Losses on Investments	X	X	
3060	Dividends and Distributions	X	X	X
3070	Retained Earnings - Unappropriated	X	X	X
3075	Retained Earnings - Appropriated	X	X	X
3080	Current Income/Loss	X	X	X
3090	Treasury Stock	X	X	X

Chart of Accounts for Health Care Organizations **TABLE I**

General - Detailed Format

Account Number	Description	Accrual	Modified Cash	Cash
3000	**NET ASSETS (NOT-FOR-PROFIT EQUITY)**	X	X	X
3010	Unrestricted Net Assets	X	X	X
3030	Temporarily Restricted Net Assets	X	X	X
3040	Permanently Restricted Net Assets	X	X	X
3050	Current Surplus/Deficit	X	X	X
3000	**LIMITED LIABILITY COMPANY/PARTNERSHIP**	X	X	X
3010	Members' Capital/Limited Partners' Interest	X	X	X
3020	Members' Distributions/Limited Partners' Distributions	X	X	X
3030	Current Income/Loss	X	X	X
	INCOME STATEMENT ACCOUNTS			
4000	**REVENUES**	X	X	X
4100	GROSS CHARGES	X		
4110	Gross Charges - Fee-for-Service (FFS)	X		
4120	Gross Charges - Discounted FFS Contracts	X		
4130	Gross Charges - FFS Equivalents for Capitation Plan Patients	X		
4140	Other Gross Charges	X		
4150	Other Revenue	X		
4200	Fees Collected		X	X
4210	Fees Collected - FFS		X	X
4220	Fees Collected - FFS for Managed Care		X	X
4230	Capitated Premium Revenues - Commercial		X	X
4240	Capitated Premium Revenues - Medicare		X	X
4250	Capitated Premium Revenues - Medicaid		X	X
4260	Capitated Premium Revenues - Other		X	X
4270	Risk Sharing Revenue		X	X

Chart of Accounts for Health Care Organizations

TABLE I

General - Detailed Format

Account Number	Description	Accrual	Modified Cash	Cash
4271	Hospital Risk Sharing - Commercial		X	X
4272	Hospital Risk Sharing - Medicare		X	X
4273	Hospital Risk Sharing - Medicaid		X	X
4274	Hospital Risk Sharing - Pharmacy		X	X
4275	Hospital Risk Sharing - Other		X	X
4280	Other Managed Care Collected Revenues	X	X	X
4281	Copayments	X	X	X
4282	Coordination of Benefits	X	X	X
4283	Other Prepaid Professional Fees Collected	X	X	X
4290	Recoveries	X	X	X
4291	Reinsurance Recoveries	X	X	X
4292	Bad Debt Recovery	X		
4300	Patient Refunds	X	X	X
4400	Fees Collected - Other Revenue	X	X	X
4410	Sales - Medical Related	X	X	X
4420	Patient Records Copying Reimbursement	X	X	X
4430	Fees Collected - Other	X	X	X
4450	Donations Received (Operating Revenue)	X	X	X
4460	Research/Clinical Studies Income	X	X	X
4470	Grant Revenue	X	X	X
4480	Miscellaneous Income	X	X	X
4490	Operating Subsidy Income	X	X	X
4500	ADJUSTMENTS	X		
4510	Gross Charges - FFS Discount/Adjustment	X		
4520	Gross Charges - Discounted FFS Contracts Adjustment	X		
4530	Gross Charges - FFS Equivalents for Cap Plan Patients/Adjustment	X		

Chart of Accounts for Health Care Organizations

TABLE I

General - Detailed Format

Account Number	Description	Accrual	Modified Cash	Cash
4540	Other Gross Charges/Adjustments	X		
4550	Other Revenue Discount/Adjustment	X		
4600	Financial Hardship Care Discount/Adjustment	X		
4610	Courtesy Discount/Adjustment	X		
4620	Employee Discount/Adjustment	X		
4630	Charity Care Discount/Adjustment	X		
4700	Third-Party Settlements	X	X	X
4800	Provision for Cash Basis Conversion		X	X
5000	**OPERATING EXPENSES - Salary and Fringe Benefits**	X	X	X
5100	PHYSICIAN - SALARIES *			
5200	PHYSICIAN - EMPLOYEE-RELATED EXPENSES *			
5300	MIDLEVEL PROVIDERS - SALARIES *			
5400	MIDLEVEL PROVIDERS - EMPLOYEE-RELATED EXPENSES *			
5500	ANCILLARY STAFF - SALARIES	X	X	X
5510	Salaries - Radiology	X	X	X
5520	Salaries - Laboratory	X	X	X
5530	Salaries - Optical	X	X	X
5540	Salaries - Physical Therapy	X	X	X
5550	Salaries - Other Ancillary Services	X	X	X
5600	ANCILLARY STAFF - EMPLOYEE-RELATED EXPENSES	X	X	X
5610	Payroll Taxes (Ancillary)	X	X	X
5611	Payroll Taxes - FICA/Medicare (Ancillary)	X	X	X

Chart of Accounts for Health Care Organizations

TABLE I

General - Detailed Format

Account Number	Description	Accrual	Modified Cash	Cash
5612	Payroll Taxes - Federal Unemployment Insurance (Ancillary)	X	X	X
5613	Payroll Taxes - State Unemployment Insurance (Ancillary)	X	X	X
5614	Payroll Taxes - Other (Ancillary)	X	X	X
5620	Insurance (Ancillary)	X	X	X
5621	Insurance - Health (Ancillary)	X	X	X
5622	Insurance - Dental (Ancillary)	X	X	X
5623	Insurance - Life (Ancillary)	X	X	X
5624	Insurance - Disability (Ancillary)	X	X	X
5625	Insurance - Workers' Compensation (Ancillary)	X	X	X
5626	Insurance - Other (Ancillary)	X	X	X
5630	Pension and Retirement Benefits (Ancillary)	X	X	X
5631	Pension (Ancillary)	X	X	X
5632	Deferred Compensation (Ancillary)	X	X	X
5633	Severance Plan (Ancillary)	X	X	X
5635	Professional Development (Ancillary)	X	X	X
5640	Books and Subscriptions (Ancillary)	X	X	X
5645	Dues and Memberships (Ancillary)	X	X	X
5650	Licenses (Ancillary)	X	X	X
5655	Meetings (Ancillary)	X	X	X
5660	Travel (Ancillary)	X	X	X
5665	Medical Reimbursement Plan (Ancillary)	X	X	X
5670	Vehicle (Ancillary)	X	X	X
5675	Parking (Ancillary)	X	X	X
5680	Telephones (Ancillary)	X	X	X
5685	Beepers (Ancillary)	X	X	X
5690	Meals and Entertainment (Ancillary)	X	X	X
5695	Other Benefits (Ancillary)	X	X	X

Chart of Accounts for Health Care Organizations

TABLE I

General - Detailed Format

Account Number	Description	Accrual	Modified Cash	Cash
5700	EMPLOYEES - SALARIES	X	X	X
5710	Salaries - General Administrative	X	X	X
5715	Salaries - Business Office	X	X	X
5720	Salaries - Managed Care Administrative	X	X	X
5725	Salaries - Information Services	X	X	X
5730	Salaries - Housekeeping/ Maintenance / Security	X	X	X
5735	Salaries - Medical Receptionist	X	X	X
5740	Salaries - Medical Secretaries / Transcribers	X	X	X
5745	Salaries - Medical Records	X	X	X
5750	Salaries - Other Administrative Support	X	X	X
5755	Salaries - Registered Nurses	X	X	X
5760	Salaries - Licensed Practical Nurses	X	X	X
5765	Salaries - Medical Assistants / Nurses' Aids	X	X	X
5800	EMPLOYEES - EMPLOYEE-RELATED EXPENSES	X	X	X
5810	Payroll Taxes (Other)	X	X	X
5811	Payroll Taxes - FICA/Medicare (Other)	X	X	X
5812	Payroll Taxes - Federal Unemployment Insurance (Other)	X	X	X
5813	Payroll Taxes - State Unemployment Insurance (Other)	X	X	X
5814	Payroll Taxes - Other (Other)	X	X	X
5820	Insurance (Other)	X	X	X
5821	Insurance - Health (Other)	X	X	X
5822	Insurance - Dental (Other)	X	X	X
5823	Insurance - Life (Other)	X	X	X
5824	Insurance - Disability (Other)	X	X	X
5825	Insurance - Workers' Compensation (Other)	X	X	X
5826	Insurance - Other (Other)	X	X	X
5830	Pension and Retirement Benefits (Other)	X	X	X

Chart of Accounts for Health Care Organizations

TABLE I

General - Detailed Format

Account Number	Description	Accrual	Modified Cash	Cash
5831	Pension (Other)	X	X	X
5832	Deferred Compensation (Other)	X	X	X
5833	Severance Plan (Other)	X	X	X
5835	Professional Development (Other)	X	X	X
5840	Books and Subscriptions (Other)	X	X	X
5845	Dues and Memberships (Other)	X	X	X
5850	Licenses (Other)	X	X	X
5855	Meetings (Other)	X	X	X
5860	Travel (Other)	X	X	X
5865	Medical Reimbursement Plan (Other)	X	X	X
5870	Vehicle (Other)	X	X	X
5875	Parking (Other)	X	X	X
5880	Telephones (Other)	X	X	X
5885	Beepers (Other)	X	X	X
5890	Meals and Entertainment (Other)	X	X	X
5895	Other Benefits (Other)	X	X	X
5900	Temporary Employee Salaries	X	X	X
5901	Physician Salaries	X	X	X
5902	Midlevel Provider Salaries	X	X	X
5903	Ancillary Staff Salaries	X	X	X
5904	Administrative and Other Staff	X	X	X
5910	Temporary Employee Benefits	X	X	X
5911	Physician Benefits	X	X	X
5912	Midlevel Provider Benefits	X	X	X
5913	Ancillary Staff Benefits	X	X	X
5914	Administrative and Other Staff	X	X	X

Chart of Accounts for Health Care Organizations — **TABLE I**

General - Detailed Format

Account Number	Description	Accrual	Modified Cash	Cash
6000	**SERVICES AND GENERAL EXPENSE**	X	X	X
6100	Office and Administrative Expense	X	X	X
6110	Equipment Rentals (Admin)	X	X	X
6115	Equipment Maintenance (Admin)	X	X	X
6120	Telephone (Admin)	X	X	X
6130	Postage (Admin)	X	X	X
6140	Courier and Overnight Delivery (Admin)	X	X	X
6150	Security	X	X	X
6160	Library/Books and Subscriptions	X	X	X
6170	Advertising and Marketing	X	X	X
6180	General Business and Other Insurance	X	X	X
6181	Officers' and Directors' Liability	X	X	X
6182	Other Liability	X	X	X
6183	Reinsurance for Capitation Contracts	X	X	X
6184	Keyman and Overhead Insurance	X	X	X
6185	Malpractice Insurance	X	X	X
6186	Physicians	X	X	X
6187	Midlevel Providers	X	X	X
6188	Ancillary and Clinical Staff	X	X	X
6189	Global Coverage	X	X	X
6190	Printing (Admin)	X	X	X
6200	Copying (Admin)	X	X	X
6210	Medical Forms	X	X	X
6220	Answering Service	X	X	X
6230	Meals and Entertainment	X	X	X
6240	Cafeteria	X	X	X
6250	Employee Relations	X	X	X
6260	Physician Recruitment	X	X	X

Chart of Accounts for Health Care Organizations

TABLE I

General - Detailed Format

Account Number	Description	Accrual	Modified Cash	Cash
6270	Nonphysician Recruitment	X	X	X
6300	Depreciation/Amortization	X	X	
6301	Furniture and Fixtures	X	X	
6302	Capital Leases	X		
6303	Equipment	X	X	
6304	Computers	X	X	
6305	Vehicles	X	X	
6306	Amortization	X	X	
6307	Other Depreciation	X	X	
6310	Accounting Services	X	X	X
6320	Legal Services	X	X	X
6330	Actuarial Services	X	X	X
6340	Pension Administration Expense	X	X	X
6350	Consulting Services	X	X	X
6360	Other Professional Services	X	X	X
6370	Medical Transcription	X	X	X
6380	Payroll Services	X	X	X
6390	Business Transportation	X	X	X
6400	General Supplies	X	X	X
6410	Taxes - Excise and Other Business Taxes	X	X	X
6420	Computer Supplies	X	X	X
6430	Computer Software	X	X	X
6440	Other Office and Administrative Expense	X	X	X
6500	Billing Expense	X	X	X
6510	Equipment Rentals (Billing)	X	X	X
6515	Equipment Maintenance (Billing)	X	X	X
6520	Electronic Data Processing	X	X	X

Chart of Accounts for Health Care Organizations

TABLE I

General - Detailed Format

Account Number	Description	Accrual	Modified Cash	Cash
6530	Telephone (Billing)	X	X	X
6540	Postage (Billing)	X	X	X
6550	Courier and Overnight Delivery (Billing)	X	X	X
6560	Printing (Billing)	X	X	X
6570	Copying (Billing)	X	X	X
6580	Depreciation	X	X	X
6600	General Services	X	X	X
6650	Other Billing Expense	X	X	X
6700	Bad Debt Expense	X		
6710	Accounts Receivable Write-Offs	X		
6720	Collection Agency Write-Offs	X		
6730	Collection Expenses	X	X	X
7000	**Clinical Expense**	X	X	X
7010	Drugs and Medications	X	X	X
7020	Medical Supplies	X	X	X
7021	Radiology	X	X	X
7022	Laboratory	X	X	X
7023	Other Ancillary Supplies	X	X	X
7030	Linen Supplies	X	X	X
7040	Uniforms and Laundry	X	X	X
7050	Patient Education	X	X	X
7060	Photography	X	X	X
7070	Biohazardous Waste Removal	X	X	X
7100	Equipment Rentals (Clinical)	X	X	X
7110	Equipment Maintenance (Clinical)	X	X	X
7120	Telephone (Clinical)	X	X	X
7130	Postage (Clinical)	X	X	X

Chart of Accounts for Health Care Organizations

TABLE I

General - Detailed Format

Account Number	Description	Accrual	Modified Cash	Cash
7140	Medical Record Supplies	X	X	X
7150	Other Clinical Expense	X	X	X
7160	Depreciation (Clinical)	X	X	X
7161	General Clinical	X	X	X
7162	Radiology	X	X	X
7163	Laboratory	X	X	X
7500	Occupancy Expense	X	X	X
7510	Rent/Lease	X	X	X
7520	Condominium Assessments/Monthly Maintenance Fees	X	X	X
7530	General Maintenance	X	X	X
7540	Utilities	X	X	X
7541	Utilities - Water	X	X	X
7542	Utilities - Electricity	X	X	X
7543	Utilities - Waste Disposal	X	X	X
7544	Other Utilities	X	X	X
7550	Property Taxes	X	X	X
7560	Housekeeping/Maintenance Services	X	X	X
7570	Other Occupancy Expense	X	X	X
7580	Insurance (Occupancy)	X	X	X
7590	Deprcciation (Occupancy)	X	X	
7595	Amortization - Leasehold Improvements (Occupancy)	X	X	
7600	Cost of Goods Sold - Medical Related	X		
7700	PURCHASED SERVICES/MANAGEMENT FEES	X	X	X
7710	Medical Directorships	X	X	X

Chart of Accounts for Health Care Organizations

TABLE I

General - Detailed Format

Account Number	Description	Accrual	Modified Cash	Cash
7720	General and Administrative Expense - Purchased Services	X	X	X
7730	Management Fees - MSO/PPMC	X	X	X
7731	Management Fees - Commercial	X	X	X
7732	Management Fees - Medicare	X	X	X
7733	Management Fees - Medicaid	X	X	X
7734	Management Fees - Other	X	X	X
7740	Management Company Incentive	X	X	X
7800	Purchased Services for HMO/PPO Patients - Professional and Medical	X	X	X
7810	FFS Purchased Services for HMO/PPO Patients	X	X	X
7811	FFS Purchased Services for HMO/PPO Patients - Physicians	X	X	X
7812	FFS Purchased Services for HMO/PPO Patients - Nonphysicians	X	X	X
7813	FFS Purchased Services for HMO/PPO Patients - Laboratory	X	X	X
7814	FFS Purchased Services for HMO/PPO Patients - Radiology	X	X	X
7815	FFS Purchased Services for HMO/PPO Patients - Hospital Inpatient	X	X	X
7816	FFS Purchased Services for HMO/PPO Patients - Hospital Emergency Room	X	X	X
7817	FFS Purchased Services for HMO/PPO Patients - Ambulance	X	X	X
7818	FFS Purchased Services for HMO/PPO Patients - Out-of-Area Emergency Care	X	X	X
7819	FFS Purchased Services for HMO/PPO Patients - Other Professional and Medic	X	X	X
7850	Sub-capitation Payments - Primary Care	X	X	X
7851	Sub-capitation Payments - Primary Care - Commercial	X	X	X
7852	Sub-capitation Payments - Primary Care - Medicare	X	X	X
7853	Sub-capitation Payments - Primary Care - Medicaid	X	X	X
7854	Sub-capitation Payments - Primary Care - Other	X	X	X
7860	Sub-capitation Payments - Specialty Care	X	X	X
7861	Sub-capitation Payments - Specialty Care - Commercial	X	X	X
7862	Sub-capitation Payments - Specialty Care - Medicare	X	X	X
7863	Sub-capitation Payments - Specialty Care - Medicaid	X	X	X
7864	Sub-capitation Payments - Specialty Care - Other	X	X	X

Chart of Accounts for Health Care Organizations

General - Detailed Format

Account Number	Description	Accrual	Modified Cash	Cash
7870	Sub-capitation Payments - Hospitals	X	X	X
7880	Sub-capitation Payments - Other	X	X	X
8000	**PROVIDER-RELATED EXPENSES**			
8100	PHYSICIANS - SALARIES	X	X	X
8110	Salaries, Distributions and Incentives (Physician)	X	X	X
8120	Salaries - Owner/Stockholder (Physician)	X	X	X
8130	Distributions and Incentives (Physician)	X	X	X
8140	Global/Capitation Distributions (Physician)	X	X	X
8150	Employee Salaries (Physician)	X	X	X
8160	Employee Incentives (Physician)	X	X	X
8170	Administrative Salaries (Physician)	X	X	X
8180	Other Compensation (Physician)	X	X	X
8200	PHYSICIAN - EMPLOYEE-RELATED EXPENSES	X	X	X
8210	Payroll Taxes (Physician)	X	X	X
8211	Payroll Taxes - FICA/Medicare (Physician)	X	X	X
8212	Payroll Taxes - Federal Unemployment Insurance (Physician)	X	X	X
8213	Payroll Taxes - State Unemployment Insurance (Physician)	X	X	X
8214	Payroll Taxes - Other (Physician)	X	X	X
8220	Insurance (Physician)	X	X	X
8221	Insurance - Health (Physician)	X	X	X
8222	Insurance - Dental (Physician)	X	X	X
8223	Insurance - Life (Physician)	X	X	X
8224	Insurance - Disability (Physician)	X	X	X
8225	Insurance - Workers' Compensation (Physician)	X	X	X
8226	Insurance - Other (Physician)	X	X	X

General - Detailed Format

Account Number	Description	Accrual	Modified Cash	Cash
8227	Insurance - Officers' Life (Physician)	X	X	X
8230	Pension and Retirement Benefits (Physician)	X	X	X
8231	Pension (Physician)	X	X	X
8232	Deferred Compensation (Physician)	X	X	X
8233	Severance Plan (Physician)	X	X	X
8235	Professional Development (Physician)	X	X	X
8240	Books and Subscriptions (Physician)	X	X	X
8245	Dues and Memberships (Physician)	X	X	X
8250	Licenses (Physician)	X	X	X
8255	Meetings (Physician)	X	X	X
8260	Travel (Physician)	X	X	X
8265	Medical Reimbursement Plan (Physician)	X	X	X
8270	Vehicle (Physician)	X	X	X
8271	Leased Motor Vehicles (Physician)	X	X	X
8275	Parking (Physician)	X	X	X
8280	Telephone (Physician)	X	X	X
8285	Beepers (Physician)	X	X	X
8290	Meals and Entertainment (Physician)	X	X	X
8295	Other Benefits (Physician)	X	X	X
8300	MIDLEVEL PROVIDERS - SALARIES	X	X	X
8310	Salaries, Distributions and Incentives (Midlevel)	X	X	X
8320	Salaries - Owner/Stockholder (Midlevel)	X	X	X
8330	Distributions and Incentives (Midlevel)	X	X	X
8340	Global/Capitation Distributions (Midlevel)	X	X	X
8350	Employee Salaries (Midlevel)	X	X	X
8360	Employee Incentives (Midlevel)	X	X	X
8370	Administrative Salaries (Midlevel)	X	X	X

Chart of Accounts for Health Care Organizations **TABLE I**

General - Detailed Format

Account Number	Description	Accrual	Modified Cash	Cash
8380	Other Compensation (Midlevel)	X	X	X
8400	MIDLEVEL PROVIDERS - EMPLOYEE-RELATED EXPENSES	X	X	X
8410	Payroll Taxes (Midlevel)	X	X	X
8411	Payroll Taxes - FICA/Medicare (Midlevel)	X	X	X
8412	Payroll Taxes - Federal Unemployment Insurance (Midlevel)	X	X	X
8413	Payroll Taxes - State Unemployment Insurance (Midlevel)	X	X	X
8414	Payroll Taxes - Other (Midlevel)	X	X	X
8420	Insurance (Midlevel)	X	X	X
8421	Insurance - Health (Midlevel)	X	X	X
8422	Insurance - Dental (Midlevel)	X	X	X
8423	Insurance - Life (Midlevel)	X	X	X
8424	Insurance - Disability (Midlevel)	X	X	X
8425	Insurance - Workers' Compensation (Midlevel)	X	X	X
8426	Insurance - Other (Midlevel)	X	X	X
8430	Pension and Retirement Benefits (Midlevel)	X	X	X
8431	Pension (Midlevel)	X	X	X
8432	Deferred Compensation (Midlevel)	X	X	X
8433	Severance Plan (Midlevel)	X	X	X
8435	Professional Development (Midlevel)	X	X	X
8440	Books and Subscriptions (Midlevel)	X	X	X
8445	Dues and Memberships (Midlevel)	X	X	X
8450	Licenses (Midlevel)	X	X	X
8455	Meetings (Midlevel)	X	X	X
8460	Travel (Midlevel)	X	X	X
8465	Medical Reimbursement Plan (Midlevel)	X	X	X
8470	Vehicle (Midlevel)	X	X	X
8475	Parking (Midlevel)	X	X	X

Chart of Accounts for Health Care Organizations

TABLE II

General - Detailed Format

Account Number	Description	Profit	Not-for-Profit
	BALANCE SHEET		
1000	**ASSETS**		
1100	Cash	X	X
1110	Cash - Banks	X	X
1111	General Checking Accounts	X	X
1112	Payroll Checking Accounts	X	X
1113	Other Checking Accounts	X	X
1120	Cash - On hand	X	X
1121	Change Fund	X	X
1122	Petty Cash	X	X
1130	Cash - Restricted	X	X
1200	Marketable Securities & Short-Term Investments	X	X
1210	Valuation Allowance - Short-Term Investments	X	X
1300	Accounts Receivable	X	X
1301	Accounts Receivable - Fee-for-Service Amounts	X	X
1302	Accounts Receivable - Prepaid Contracts	X	X
1320	Allowance for Estimated Uncollectible Receivables	X	X
1321	Allowance for Bad Debts - Patient Accounts	X	X
1322	Allowance for Contractual Adjustments	X	X
1323	Allowance for Bad Debts - Third-Party Payers	X	X
1324	Allowance for Charity Care	X	X
1340	Notes Receivable - Short Term	X	X
1345	Managed Care Contract - Bonus/Withhold	X	X
1350	Other Short-Term Receivables	X	X
1351	Interest Receivables	X	X
1352	Intercompany Receivables	X	X
1353	Due from Employees	X	X
1354	Due from Related Parties	X	X

Chart of Accounts for Health Care Organizations **TABLE II**

General - Detailed Format

Account Number	Description	Profit	Not-for-Profit
1400	Supply Inventories	X	X
1401	Drugs and Medications	X	X
1402	Medical Supplies	X	X
1403	Administrative Supplies	X	X
1404	Forms	X	X
1405	Housekeeping and Maintenance Supplies	X	X
1406	Linen Supplies	X	X
1407	Other Supplies	X	X
1420	Ancillary Department Supplies	X	X
1500	Prepaid Expenses	X	X
1501	Prepaid Interest	X	X
1502	Prepaid Insurance	X	X
1503	Prepaid Rent	X	X
1504	Prepaid Taxes	X	X
1505	Prepaid Dues	X	X
1506	Other Prepaid Expenses	X	X
1550	Other Current Assets	X	X
1600	INVESTMENTS - LONG-TERM RECEIVABLES	X	X
1610	Long-Term Receivables	X	X
1630	Long-Term Investments	X	X
1635	Valuation Allowance - Long-Term Investments	X	X
1640	Investments in Affiliates	X	X
1650	Property Held for Future Use	X	X
1700	PROPERTY, FURNITURE, FIXTURES & EQUIPMENT		
1710	REAL PROPERTY	X	X
1711	Land	X	X

Chart of Accounts for Health Care Organizations

TABLE II

General - Detailed Format

Account Number	Description	Profit	Not-for-Profit
1712	Land Improvements	X	X
1713	Buildings	X	X
1714	Capital Leases - Buildings	X	X
1715	Leasehold Improvements	X	X
1716	Construction in Progress	X	X
1717	Other Real Property	X	X
1750	FURNITURE, FIXTURES & EQUIPMENT	X	X
1751	Furniture and Fixtures	X	X
1752	Capital Leases - Furniture and Fixtures	X	X
1753	Equipment	X	X
1754	Capital Leases - Equipment	X	X
1755	Medical Equipment	X	X
1756	Capital Leases - Medical Equipment	X	X
1760	Computer	X	X
1761	Computer - Hardware	X	X
1762	Computer - Software	X	X
1763	Computer - Other	X	X
1770	Capital Leases - Computer	X	X
1771	Capital Leases - Computer - Hardware	X	X
1772	Capital Leases - Computer - Software	X	X
1773	Capital Leases - Computer - Other	X	X
1780	Vehicles	X	X
1781	Vehicles	X	X
1782	Capital Leases - Vehicles	X	X
1790	Ancillary Service Equipment	X	X
1791	Laboratory Equipment	X	X
1792	Radiology Equipment	X	X
1793	Physical Therapy Equipment	X	X

Account Number	Description	Profit	Not-for-Profit
1794	Diagnostic Equipment	X	X
1795	Capital Leases - Ancillary Service Equipment	X	X
1796	Capital Leases - Laboratory Equipment	X	X
1797	Capital Leases - Radiology Equipment	X	X
1798	Capital Leases - Physical Therapy Equipment	X	X
1799	Capital Leases - Diagnostic Equipment	X	X
1800	ACCUMULATED DEPRECIATION - PROPERTY, FURNITURE, ETC.		
1810	ACCUMULATED DEPRECIATION - REAL PROPERTY	X	X
1812	Accum Depreciation - Land Improvements	X	X
1813	Accum Depreciation - Buildings	X	X
1814	Accum Depreciation - Capital Leases - Buildings	X	X
1815	Accum Depreciation - Leasehold Improvements	X	X
1817	Accum Depreciation - Other Real Property	X	X
1850	ACCUM DEPRECIATION - FURNITURE, FIXTURES & EQUIPMENT	X	X
1851	Accum Depreciation - Furniture and Fixtures	X	X
1852	Accum Depreciation - Capital Leases - Furniture and Fixtures	X	X
1853	Accum Depreciation - Equipment	X	X
1854	Accum Depreciation - Capital Leases - Equipment	X	X
1855	Accum Depreciation - Medical Equipment	X	X
1856	Accum Depreciation - Capital Leases - Medical Equipment	X	X
1860	Accum Depreciation - Computer	X	X
1861	Accum Depreciation - Computer - Hardware	X	X
1862	Accum Depreciation - Computer - Software	X	X
1863	Accum Depreciation - Computer - Other	X	X
1870	Accum Depreciation - Capital Leases - Computer	X	X
1871	Accum Depreciation - Capital Leases - Computer Hardware	X	X
1872	Accum Depreciation - Capital Leases - Computer Software	X	X

Chart of Accounts for Health Care Organizations

TABLE II

General - Detailed Format

Account Number	Description	Profit	Not-for-Profit
1873	Accum Depreciation - Capital Leases - Computer - Other	X	X
1880	Accum Depreciation - Vehicles	X	X
1881	Accum Depreciation - Vehicles	X	X
1882	Accum Depreciation - Capital Leases - Vehicles	X	X
1890	Other Accum Depreciation - Ancillary Service Equipment	X	X
1891	Accum Depreciation - Laboratory Equipment	X	X
1892	Accum Depreciation - Radiology Equipment	X	X
1893	Accum Depreciation - Physical Therapy Equipment	X	X
1894	Accum Depreciation - Diagnostic Equipment	X	X
1895	Accum Depreciation - Capital Leases - Ancillary Service Equipment	X	X
1896	Accum Depreciation - Capital Leases - Laboratory Equipment	X	X
1897	Accum Depreciation - Capital Leases - Radiology Equipment	X	X
1898	Accum Depreciation - Capital Leases - Physical Therapy Equipment	X	X
1899	Accum Depreciation - Capital Leases - Diagnostic Equipment	X	X
1900	INTANGIBLE AND OTHER ASSETS		
1910	Organization Costs	X	X
1915	Accumulated Amortization - Organization Costs	X	X
1920	Goodwill	X	X
1925	Accumulated Amortization - Goodwill	X	X
1930	Other Intangible Assets	X	X
1940	Deposits	X	X
1950	Noncurrent Expenses Paid in Advance	X	X
1951	Noncurrent Interest Paid in Advance	X	X
1952	Noncurrent Insurance Paid in Advance	X	X
1953	Noncurrent Rent Paid in Advance	X	X
1954	Noncurrent Taxes Paid in Advance	X	X
1955	Noncurrent Dues Paid in Advance	X	X

Chart of Accounts for Health Care Organizations

TABLE II

General - Detailed Format

Account Number	Description	Profit	Not-for-Profit
1956	Other Noncurrent Expenses Paid in Advance	X	X
1960	Other Assets	X	X
1961	Cash Surrender Value of Life Insurance Policies	X	X
2000	**LIABILITIES**	X	X
2100	CURRENT LIABILITIES - PAYABLES	X	X
2110	Accounts Payable	X	X
2120	Bank Overdrafts Payable	X	X
2130	Other Current Liabilities Payable	X	X
2131	Intercompany Accounts Payable	X	X
2132	Accounts Payable - Employees	X	X
2133	Accounts Payable - Related Parties	X	X
2134	Accounts Payable - Other	X	X
2160	Contract Claims Payable	X	X
2200	CURRENT LIABILITIES - PAYROLL	X	X
2210	Payroll Tax Withholdings Payable	X	X
2211	Federal Income Tax Withholdings Payable	X	X
2212	State Income Tax Withholdings Payable	X	X
2213	FICA/Medicare Tax Withholdings Payable	X	X
2214	Local Tax Withholdings Payable	X	X
2215	Other Tax Withholdings Payable	X	X
2220	Insurance Withholdings Payable	X	X
2221	Health Insurance Withholdings Payable	X	X
2222	Life Insurance Withholdings Payable	X	X
2223	State Disability Insurance Withholdings Payable	X	X
2224	Other Insurance Withholdings Payable	X	X
2230	Other Payroll Withholdings Payable	X	X

Chart of Accounts for Health Care Organizations

TABLE II

General - Detailed Format

Account Number	Description	Profit	Not-for-Profit
2231	401(k) Withholdings Payable	X	X
2232	Cafeteria Plan Withholdings Payable	X	X
2233	Court Mandated Child Support Withholdings Payable	X	X
2234	Other Payroll Withholdings Payable	X	X
2250	Accrued Payroll Liabilities	X	X
2251	Accrued Payroll	X	X
2252	Accrued Vacation, Holiday, & Sick Pay (Compensated Absences)	X	X
2253	Accrued FICA/Medicare Taxes Payable	X	X
2254	Accrued State Unemployment Taxes Payable	X	X
2255	Accrued Federal Unemployment Taxes Payable	X	X
2256	Accrued Retirement Plan Contribution	X	X
2257	Other Accrued Payroll Liabilities	X	X
2260	Other Payroll Liabilities	X	X
2300	CURRENT LIABILITIES - OTHER	X	X
2310	Accrued Liabilities - Nonpayroll	X	X
2311	Accrued Rent	X	X
2312	Accrued Interest	X	X
2313	Accrued Insurance	X	X
2314	Accrued Income Taxes (Federal/State)	X	X
2315	Accrued Property Taxes	X	X
2316	Accrued Franchise Taxes	X	X
2317	Other Accrued Liabilities	X	X
2320	Notes and Loans Payable	X	X
2321	Current Notes and Loans Payable - Vendors	X	X
2322	Current Notes and Loans Payable - Employees	X	X
2323	Current Notes and Loans Payable - Stockholders/Partners	X	X
2324	Current Other Notes and Loans Payable	X	X

Chart of Accounts for Health Care Organizations

TABLE II

General - Detailed Format

Account Number	Description	Profit	Not-for-Profit
2325	Bank Working Capital Line Outstanding	X	X
2330	Long-Term Debt - Current Portion	X	X
2331	Capital Lease Obligation - Current Portion	X	X
2332	Construction Contracts Payable	X	X
2333	Other Loans Payable - Current Portion	X	X
2340	Advances from Settlements Due to Third-Party Agencies	X	X
2350	Patient Deposits	X	X
2360	Claims Payable Incurred But Not Reported	X	X
2361	Incurred But Not Reported Claims - Commercial	X	X
2362	Incurred But Not Reported Claims - Medicare	X	X
2363	Incurred But Not Reported Claims - Medicaid	X	X
2365	Other Claims Incurred But Not Reported	X	X
2370	Deferred Revenue	X	X
2371	Deferred Revenue - Fee for Service	X	X
2372	Deferred Revenue - Capitated or Prepaid Plan	X	X
2375	Other Deferred Revenue	X	X
2380	Deferred Income Taxes - Current Portion	X	
2390	Other Current Liabilities	X	X
2400	LONG-TERM LIABILITIES	X	X
2410	Long-Term Notes Payable	X	X
2420	Construction Loans	X	X
2430	Capital Lease Obligation - Long-Term Portion	X	X
2440	Other Loans Payable - Long-Term Portion	X	X
2450	Deferred Third-Party Revenue	X	X
2451	Deferred Third-Party Revenue - Medicare	X	X
2452	Deferred Third-Party Revenue - Medicaid	X	X
2453	Deferred Third-Party Revenue - Other	X	X

Chart of Accounts for Health Care Organizations

TABLE II

General - Detailed Format

Account Number	Description	Profit	Not-for-Profit
2460	Deferred Compensation	X	X
2465	Severance Plan	X	X
2470	Deferred Income Taxes - Long-Term Portion	X	
2480	Other Long-Term Liabilities	X	X
3000	**Owners' Equity Accounts**		
3000	**PARTNERS' EQUITY (PARTNERSHIP)**	X	
3010	Contributed Capital (Each Partner)	X	
3020	Undistributed Earnings	X	
3030	Partners' Drawing Accounts (Each Partner)	X	
3040	Current Income/Loss	X	
3000	**STOCKHOLDERS' EQUITY (CORPORATION)**	X	
3010	Preferred Stock	X	
3020	Common Stock	X	
3030	Capital Contributed in Excess of Par	X	
3040	Donated Capital	X	
3050	Allowance for Change in Net Unrealized Gains/Losses on Investments	X	
3060	Dividends and Distributions	X	
3070	Retained Earnings - Unappropriated	X	
3075	Retained Earnings - Appropriated	X	
3080	Current Income/Loss	X	
3090	Treasury Stock	X	
3000	**NET ASSETS (NOT-FOR-PROFIT EQUITY)**		X
3010	Unrestricted Net Assets		X
3030	Temporarily Restricted Net Assets		X

Chart of Accounts for Health Care Organizations — **TABLE II**

General - Detailed Format

Account Number	Description	Profit	Not-for-Profit
3040	Permanently Restricted Net Assets		X
3050	Current Surplus/Deficit		X
3000	**LIMITED LIABILITY COMPANY/PARTNERSHIP**	X	
3010	Members' Capital/Limited Partners' Interest	X	
3020	Members' Distributions/Limited Partners' Distributions	X	
3030	Current Income/Loss	X	
	INCOME STATEMENT ACCOUNTS		
4000	**REVENUES**	X	X
4100	GROSS CHARGES	X	X
4110	Gross Charges - Fee-for-Service (FFS)	X	X
4120	Gross Charges - Discounted FFS Contracts	X	X
4130	Gross Charges - FFS Equivalents for Capitation Plan Patients	X	X
4140	Other Gross Charges	X	X
4150	Other Revenue	X	X
4200	Fees Collected	X	X
4210	Fees Collected - FFS	X	X
4220	Fees Collected - FFS for Managed Care	X	X
4230	Capitated Premium Revenues - Commercial	X	X
4240	Capitated Premium Revenues - Medicare	X	X
4250	Capitated Premium Revenues - Medicaid	X	X
4260	Capitated Premium Revenues - Other	X	X
4270	Risk Sharing Revenue	X	X
4271	Hospital Risk Sharing - Commercial	X	X
4272	Hospital Risk Sharing - Medicare	X	X
4273	Hospital Risk Sharing - Medicaid	X	X

Chart of Accounts for Health Care Organizations

TABLE II

General - Detailed Format

Account Number	Description	Profit	Not-for-Profit
4274	Hospital Risk Sharing - Pharmacy	X	X
4275	Hospital Risk Sharing - Other	X	X
4280	Other Managed Care Collected Revenues	X	X
4281	Copayments	X	X
4282	Coordination of Benefits	X	X
4283	Other Prepaid Professional Fees Collected	X	X
4290	Recoveries	X	X
4291	Reinsurance Recoveries	X	X
4292	Bad Debt Recovery	X	X
4300	Patient Refunds	X	X
4400	Fees Collected - Other Revenue	X	X
4410	Sales - Medical Related	X	X
4420	Patient Records Copying Reimbursement	X	X
4430	Fees Collected - Other	X	X
4450	Donations Received (Operating Revenue)	X	X
4460	Research/Clinical Studies Income	X	X
4470	Grant Revenue	X	X
4480	Miscellaneous Income	X	X
4490	Operating Subsidy Income	X	X
4500	ADJUSTMENTS	X	X
4510	Gross Charges - FFS Discount/Adjustment	X	X
4520	Gross Charges - Discounted FFS Contracts Adjustment	X	X
4530	Gross Charges - FFS Equivalents for Cap Plan Patients/Adjustment	X	X
4540	Other Gross Charges/Adjustments	X	X
4550	Other Revenue Discount/Adjustment	X	X
4600	Financial Hardship Care Discount/Adjustment	X	X
4610	Courtesy Discount/Adjustment	X	X

Chart of Accounts for Health Care Organizations TABLE II

General - Detailed Format

Account Number	Description	Profit	Not-for-Profit
4620	Employee Discount/Adjustment	X	X
4630	Charity Care Discount/Adjustment	X	X
4700	Third-Party Settlements	X	X
4800	Provision for Cash Basis Conversion	X	X
5000	**OPERATING EXPENSES - Salary and Fringe Benefits**	X	X
5100	PHYSICIAN - SALARIES *		
5200	PHYSICIAN - EMPLOYEE-RELATED EXPENSES *	*** (See Accounts**	
5300	MIDLEVEL PROVIDERS - SALARIES *	**8100-8400)**	
5400	MIDLEVEL PROVIDERS - EMPLOYEE-RELATED EXPENSES *		
5500	ANCILLARY STAFF - SALARIES	X	X
5510	Salaries - Radiology	X	X
5520	Salaries - Laboratory	X	X
5530	Salaries - Optical	X	X
5540	Salaries - Physical Therapy	X	X
5550	Salaries - Other Ancillary Services	X	X
5600	ANCILLARY STAFF - EMPLOYEE-RELATED EXPENSES	X	X
5610	Payroll Taxes (Ancillary)	X	X
5611	Payroll Taxes - FICA/Medicare (Ancillary)	X	X
5612	Payroll Taxes - Federal Unemployment Insurance (Ancillary)	X	X
5613	Payroll Taxes - State Unemployment Insurance (Ancillary)	X	X
5614	Payroll Taxes - Other (Ancillary)	X	X
5620	Insurance (Ancillary)	X	X
5621	Insurance - Health (Ancillary)	X	X

Chart of Accounts for Health Care Organizations

TABLE II

General - Detailed Format

Account Number	Description	Profit	Not-for-Profit
5622	Insurance - Dental (Ancillary)	X	X
5623	Insurance - Life (Ancillary)	X	X
5624	Insurance - Disability (Ancillary)	X	X
5625	Insurance - Workers' Compensation (Ancillary)	X	X
5626	Insurance - Other (Ancillary)	X	X
5630	Pension and Retirement Benefits (Ancillary)	X	X
5631	Pension (Ancillary)	X	X
5632	Deferred Compensation (Ancillary)	X	X
5633	Severance Plan (Ancillary)	X	X
5635	Professional Development (Ancillary)	X	X
5640	Books and Subscriptions (Ancillary)	X	X
5645	Dues and Memberships (Ancillary)	X	X
5650	Licenses (Ancillary)	X	X
5655	Meetings (Ancillary)	X	X
5660	Travel (Ancillary)	X	X
5665	Medical Reimbursement Plan (Ancillary)	X	X
5670	Vehicle (Ancillary)	X	X
5675	Parking (Ancillary)	X	X
5680	Telephones (Ancillary)	X	X
5685	Beepers (Ancillary)	X	X
5690	Meals and Entertainment (Ancillary)	X	X
5695	Other Benefits (Ancillary)	X	X
5700	EMPLOYEES - SALARIES	X	X
5710	Salaries - General Administrative	X	X
5715	Salaries - Business Office	X	X
5720	Salaries - Managed Care Administrative	X	X
5725	Salaries - Information Services	X	X

Chart of Accounts for Health Care Organizations

TABLE II

General - Detailed Format

Account Number	Description	Profit	Not-for-Profit
5730	Salaries - Housekeeping/ Maintenance / Security	X	X
5735	Salaries - Medical Receptionist	X	X
5740	Salaries - Medical Secretaries / Transcribers	X	X
5745	Salaries - Medical Records	X	X
5750	Salaries - Other Administrative Support	X	X
5755	Salaries - Registered Nurses	X	X
5760	Salaries - Licensed Practical Nurses	X	X
5765	Salaries - Medical Assistants / Nurses' Aids	X	X
5800	EMPLOYEES - EMPLOYEE-RELATED EXPENSES	X	X
5810	Payroll Taxes (Other)	X	X
5811	Payroll Taxes - FICA/Medicare (Other)	X	X
5812	Payroll Taxes - Federal Unemployment Insurance (Other)	X	X
5813	Payroll Taxes - State Unemployment Insurance (Other)	X	X
5814	Payroll Taxes - Other (Other)	X	X
5820	Insurance (Other)	X	X
5821	Insurance - Health (Other)	X	X
5822	Insurance - Dental (Other)	X	X
5823	Insurance - Life (Other)	X	X
5824	Insurance - Disability (Other)	X	X
5825	Insurance - Workers' Compensation (Other)	X	X
5826	Insurance - Other (Other)	X	X
5830	Pension and Retirement Benefits (Other)	X	X
5831	Pension (Other)	X	X
5832	Deferred Compensation (Other)	X	X
5833	Severance Plan (Other)	X	X
5835	Professional Development (Other)	X	X
5840	Books and Subscriptions (Other)	X	X

Chart of Accounts for Health Care Organizations

TABLE II

General - Detailed Format

Account Number	Description	Profit	Not-for-Profit
5845	Dues and Memberships (Other)	X	X
5850	Licenses (Other)	X	X
5855	Meetings (Other)	X	X
5860	Travel (Other)	X	X
5865	Medical Reimbursement Plan (Other)	X	X
5870	Vehicle (Other)	X	X
5875	Parking (Other)	X	X
5880	Telephones (Other)	X	X
5885	Beepers (Other)	X	X
5890	Meals and Entertainment (Other)	X	X
5895	Other Benefits (Other)	X	X
5900	Temporary Employee Salaries	X	X
5901	Physician Salaries	X	X
5902	Midlevel Provider Salaries	X	X
5903	Ancillary Staff Salaries	X	X
5904	Administrative and Other Staff	X	X
5910	Temporary Employee Benefits	X	X
5911	Physician Benefits	X	X
5912	Midlevel Provider Benefits	X	X
5913	Ancillary Staff Benefits	X	X
5914	Administrative and Other Staff	X	X
6000	**SERVICES AND GENERAL EXPENSE**	X	X
6100	Office and Administrative Expense	X	X
6110	Equipment Rentals (Admin)	X	X
6115	Equipment Maintenance (Admin)	X	X
6120	Telephone (Admin)	X	X
6130	Postage (Admin)	X	X

Chart of Accounts for Health Care Organizations

TABLE II

General - Detailed Format

Account Number	Description	Profit	Not-for-Profit
6140	Courier and Overnight Delivery (Admin)	X	X
6150	Security	X	X
6160	Library/Books and Subscriptions	X	X
6170	Advertising and Marketing	X	X
6180	General Business and Other Insurance	X	X
6181	Officers' and Directors' Liability	X	X
6182	Other Liability	X	X
6183	Reinsurance for Capitation Contracts	X	X
6184	Keyman and Overhead Insurance	X	X
6185	Malpractice Insurance	X	X
6186	Physicians	X	X
6187	Midlevel Providers	X	X
6188	Ancillary and Clinical Staff	X	X
6189	Global Coverage	X	X
6190	Printing (Admin)	X	X
6200	Copying (Admin)	X	X
6210	Medical Forms	X	X
6220	Answering Service	X	X
6230	Meals and Entertainment	X	X
6240	Cafeteria	X	X
6250	Employee Relations	X	X
6260	Physician Recruitment	X	X
6270	Nonphysician Recruitment	X	X
6300	Depreciation/Amortization	X	X
6301	Furniture and Fixtures	X	X
6302	Capital Leases	X	X
6303	Equipment	X	X
6304	Computers	X	X

Chart of Accounts for Health Care Organizations

TABLE II

General - Detailed Format

Account Number	Description	Profit	Not-for-Profit
6305	Vehicles	X	X
6306	Amortization	X	X
6307	Other Depreciation	X	X
6310	Accounting Services	X	X
6320	Legal Services	X	X
6330	Actuarial Services	X	X
6340	Pension Administration Expense	X	X
6350	Consulting Services	X	X
6360	Other Professional Services	X	X
6370	Medical Transcription	X	X
6380	Payroll Services	X	X
6390	Business Transportation	X	X
6400	General Supplies	X	X
6410	Taxes - Excise and Other Business Taxes	X	X
6420	Computer Supplies	X	X
6430	Computer Software	X	X
6440	Other Office and Administrative Expense	X	X
6500	Billing Expense	X	X
6510	Equipment Rentals (Billing)	X	X
6515	Equipment Maintenance (Billing)	X	X
6520	Electronic Data Processing	X	X
6530	Telephone (Billing)	X	X
6540	Postage (Billing)	X	X
6550	Courier and Overnight Delivery (Billing)	X	X
6560	Printing (Billing)	X	X
6570	Copying (Billing)	X	X
6580	Depreciation	X	X

Chart of Accounts for Health Care Organizations

TABLE II

General - Detailed Format

Account Number	Description	Profit	Not-for-Profit
6600	General Services	X	X
6650	Other Billing Expense	X	X
6700	Bad Debt Expense	X	X
6710	Accounts Receivable Write-Offs	X	X
6720	Collection Agency Write-Offs	X	X
6730	Collection Expenses	X	X
7000	**Clinical Expense**	X	X
7010	Drugs and Medications	X	X
7020	Medical Supplies	X	X
7021	Radiology	X	X
7022	Laboratory	X	X
7023	Other Ancillary Supplies	X	X
7030	Linen Supplies	X	X
7040	Uniforms and Laundry	X	X
7050	Patient Education	X	X
7060	Photography	X	X
7070	Biohazardous Waste Removal	X	X
7100	Equipment Rentals (Clinical)	X	X
7110	Equipment Maintenance (Clinical)	X	X
7120	Telephone (Clinical)	X	X
7130	Postage (Clinical)	X	X
7140	Medical Record Supplies	X	X
7150	Other Clinical Expense	X	X
7160	Depreciation (Clinical)	X	X
7161	General Clinical	X	X
7162	Radiology	X	X
7163	Laboratory	X	X

Chart of Accounts for Health Care Organizations

TABLE II

General - Detailed Format

Account Number	Description	Profit	Not-for-Profit
7500	Occupancy Expense	X	X
7510	Rent/Lease	X	X
7520	Condominium Assessments/Monthly Maintenance Fees	X	X
7530	General Maintenance	X	X
7540	Utilities	X	X
7541	Utilities - Water	X	X
7542	Utilities - Electricity	X	X
7543	Utilities - Waste Disposal	X	X
7544	Other Utilities	X	X
7550	Property Taxes	X	X
7560	Housekeeping/Maintenance Services	X	X
7570	Other Occupancy Expense	X	X
7580	Insurance (Occupancy)	X	X
7590	Depreciation (Occupancy)	X	X
7595	Amortization - Leasehold Improvements (Occupancy)	X	X
7600	Cost of Goods Sold - Medical Related	X	X
7700	PURCHASED SERVICES/MANAGEMENT FEES	X	X
7710	Medical Directorships	X	X
7720	General and Administrative Expense - Purchased Services	X	X
7730	Management Fees - MSO/PPMC	X	X
7731	Management Fees - Commercial	X	X
7732	Management Fees - Medicare	X	X
7733	Management Fees - Medicaid	X	X
7734	Management Fees - Other	X	X
7740	Management Company Incentive	X	X

Chart of Accounts for Health Care Organizations

TABLE II

General - Detailed Format

Account Number	Description	Profit	Not-for-Profit
7800	Purchased Services for HMO/PPO Patients - Professional and Medical	X	X
7810	FFS Purchased Services for HMO/PPO Patients	X	X
7811	FFS Purchased Services for HMO/PPO Patients - Physicians	X	X
7812	FFS Purchased Services for HMO/PPO Patients - Nonphysicians	X	X
7813	FFS Purchased Services for HMO/PPO Patients - Laboratory	X	X
7814	FFS Purchased Services for HMO/PPO Patients - Radiology	X	X
7815	FFS Purchased Services for HMO/PPO Patients - Hospital Inpatient	X	X
7816	FFS Purchased Services for HMO/PPO Patients - Hospital Emergency Room	X	X
7817	FFS Purchased Services for HMO/PPO Patients - Ambulance	X	X
7818	FFS Purchased Services for HMO/PPO Patients - Out-of-Area Emergency Care	X	X
7819	FFS Purchased Services for HMO/PPO Patients - Other Professional and Medic	X	X
7850	Sub-capitation Payments - Primary Care	X	X
7851	Sub-capitation Payments - Primary Care - Commercial	X	X
7852	Sub-capitation Payments - Primary Care - Medicare	X	X
7853	Sub-capitation Payments - Primary Care - Medicaid	X	X
7854	Sub-capitation Payments - Primary Care - Other	X	X
7860	Sub-capitation Payments - Specialty Care	X	X
7861	Sub-capitation Payments - Specialty Care - Commercial	X	X
7862	Sub-capitation Payments - Specialty Care - Medicare	X	X
7863	Sub-capitation Payments - Specialty Care - Medicaid	X	X
7864	Sub-capitation Payments - Specialty Care - Other	X	X
7870	Sub-capitation Payments - Hospitals	X	X
7880	Sub-capitation Payments - Other	X	X
8000	**PROVIDER-RELATED EXPENSES**		
8100	PHYSICIANS - SALARIES	X	X
8110	Salaries, Distributions and Incentives (Physician)	X	X
8120	Salaries - Owner/Stockholder (Physician)	X	X

Chart of Accounts for Health Care Organizations

General - Detailed Format

Account Number	Description	Profit	Not-for-Profit
8130	Distributions and Incentives (Physician)	X	X
8140	Global/Capitation Distributions (Physician)	X	X
8150	Employee Salaries (Physician)	X	X
8160	Employee Incentives (Physician)	X	X
8170	Administrative Salaries (Physician)	X	X
8180	Other Compensation (Physician)	X	X
8200	PHYSICIAN - EMPLOYEE-RELATED EXPENSES	X	X
8210	Payroll Taxes (Physician)	X	X
8211	Payroll Taxes - FICA/Medicare (Physician)	X	X
8212	Payroll Taxes - Federal Unemployment Insurance (Physician)	X	X
8213	Payroll Taxes - State Unemployment Insurance (Physician)	X	X
8214	Payroll Taxes - Other (Physician)	X	X
8220	Insurance (Physician)	X	X
8221	Insurance - Health (Physician)	X	X
8222	Insurance - Dental (Physician)	X	X
8223	Insurance - Life (Physician)	X	X
8224	Insurance - Disability (Physician)	X	X
8225	Insurance - Workers' Compensation (Physician)	X	X
8226	Insurance - Other (Physician)	X	X
8227	Insurance - Officers' Life (Physician)	X	X
8230	Pension and Retirement Benefits (Physician)	X	X
8231	Pension (Physician)	X	X
8232	Deferred Compensation (Physician)	X	X
8233	Severance Plan (Physician)	X	X
8235	Professional Development (Physician)	X	X
8240	Books and Subscriptions (Physician)	X	X
8245	Dues and Memberships (Physician)	X	X

Account Number	Description	Profit	Not-for-Profit
8250	Licenses (Physician)	X	X
8255	Meetings (Physician)	X	X
8260	Travel (Physician)	X	X
8265	Medical Reimbursement Plan (Physician)	X	X
8270	Vehicle (Physician)	X	X
8271	Leased Motor Vehicles (Physician)	X	X
8275	Parking (Physician)	X	X
8280	Telephone (Physician)	X	X
8285	Beepers (Physician)	X	X
8290	Meals and Entertainment (Physician)	X	X
8295	Other Benefits (Physician)	X	X
8300	MIDLEVEL PROVIDERS - SALARIES	X	X
8310	Salaries, Distributions and Incentives (Midlevel)	X	X
8320	Salaries - Owner/Stockholder (Midlevel)	X	X
8330	Distributions and Incentives (Midlevel)	X	X
8340	Global/Capitation Distributions (Midlevel)	X	X
8350	Employee Salaries (Midlevel)	X	X
8360	Employee Incentives (Midlevel)	X	X
8370	Administrative Salaries (Midlevel)	X	X
8380	Other Compensation (Midlevel)	X	X
8400	MIDLEVEL PROVIDERS - EMPLOYEE-RELATED EXPENSES	X	X
8410	Payroll Taxes (Midlevel)	X	X
8411	Payroll Taxes - FICA/Medicare (Midlevel)	X	X
8412	Payroll Taxes - Federal Unemployment Insurance (Midlevel)	X	X
8413	Payroll Taxes - State Unemployment Insurance (Midlevel)	X	X
8414	Payroll Taxes - Other (Midlevel)	X	X

Chart of Accounts for Health Care Organizations

TABLE II

General - Detailed Format

Account Number	Description	Profit	Not-for-Profit
8420	Insurance (Midlevel)	X	X
8421	Insurance - Health (Midlevel)	X	X
8422	Insurance - Dental (Midlevel)	X	X
8423	Insurance - Life (Midlevel)	X	X
8424	Insurance - Disability (Midlevel)	X	X
8425	Insurance - Workers' Compensation (Midlevel)	X	X
8426	Insurance - Other (Midlevel)	X	X
8430	Pension and Retirement Benefits (Midlevel)	X	X
8431	Pension (Midlevel)	X	X
8432	Deferred Compensation (Midlevel)	X	X
8433	Severance Plan (Midlevel)	X	X
8435	Professional Development (Midlevel)	X	X
8440	Books and Subscriptions (Midlevel)	X	X
8445	Dues and Memberships (Midlevel)	X	X
8450	Licenses (Midlevel)	X	X
8455	Meetings (Midlevel)	X	X
8460	Travel (Midlevel)	X	X
8465	Medical Reimbursement Plan (Midlevel)	X	X
8470	Vehicle (Midlevel)	X	X
8475	Parking (Midlevel)	X	X
8480	Telephones (Midlevel)	X	X
8485	Beepers (Midlevel)	X	X
8490	Meals and Entertainment (Midlevel)	X	X
8495	Other Benefits (Midlevel)	X	X
9000	**NONOP REVENUE & EXP; INCOME TAXES & OTHER EXP**	X	X
9100	Nonoperating Revenues	X	X
9110	Interest Income	X	X

Chart of Accounts for Health Care Organizations **TABLE II**

General - Detailed Format

Account Number	Description	Profit	Not-for-Profit
9120	Income from Long-Term Investments	X	X
9130	Property Rentals	X	X
9140	Unrealized Gains and Losses - Investments	X	X
9150	Realized Gains and Losses - Investments	X	X
9160	Donations Received (Nonoperating Revenue)	X	X
9170	Nonoperating Subsidy Income	X	X
9200	Nonoperating Expenses	X	X
9210	Interest Expense	X	X
9220	Contributions/Donations Expense	X	X
9230	Current Income Tax Expense (Recovery)	X	X
9231	Current Income Taxes - Federal	X	
9232	Current Income Taxes - State	X	
9233	Current Income Taxes - Other	X	
9240	Deferred Income Tax Expense (Recovery)	X	
9241	Deferred Income Taxes - Federal	X	
9242	Deferred Income Taxes - State	X	
9243	Deferred Income Taxes - Other	X	
9300	Other Income/Expense	X	X

Chart of Accounts for Health Care Organizations **TABLE III**

Crosswalk to the Medical Group Practice Chart of Accounts (1st edition, 1996)

NEW Account Number	NEW Description	PRIOR MGP COA Account Number
1000	**ASSETS**	
1110	Cash - Banks	1100 - 1140
1111	General Checking Accounts	1100
1112	Payroll Checking Accounts	1120
1113	Other Checking Accounts	1130 - 1140
1120	Cash - On hand	1150 - 1160
1121	Change Fund	1150
1122	Petty Cash	1160
1130	Cash - Restricted	1410
1200	Marketable Securities & Short-Term Investments	1170
1210	Valuation Allowance - Short-Term Investments	1180
1301	Accounts Receivable - Fee-for-Service Amounts	1200 - 1219
1302	Accounts Receivable - Prepaid Contracts	1220 - 1229
1320	Allowance for Estimated Uncollectible Receivables	1230
1321	Allowance for Bad Debts - Patient Accounts	1231
1322	Allowance for Contractual Adjustments	1240
1340	Notes Receivable - Short Term	1260
1350	Other Short-Term Receivables	1270 - 1290
1351	Interest Receivables	1271
1400	Supply Inventories	1310 - 1330
1420	Ancillary Department Supplies	1340 - 1370
1500	Prepaid Expenses	1380 - 1389
1550	Other Current Assets	1390
1600	INVESTMENTS - LONG-TERM RECEIVABLES	1400
1610	Long-Term Receivables	1420
1630	Long-Term Investments	1430
1635	Valuation Allowance - Long-Term Investments	1435
1640	Investments in Affiliates	1440
1650	Property Held for Future Use	1450
1710	REAL PROPERTY	1500
1711	Land	1510
1712	Land Improvements	1530
1713	Buildings	1540
1714	Capital Leases - Buildings	1560
1715	Leasehold Improvements	1570
1716	Construction in Progress	1580

Chart of Accounts for Health Care Organizations **TABLE III**

Crosswalk to the Medical Group Practice Chart of Accounts (1st edition, 1996)

NEW Account Number	NEW Description	PRIOR MGP COA Account Number
1717	Other Real Property	1590
1750	FURNITURE, FIXTURES & EQUIPMENT	1700
1751	Furniture and Fixtures	1710
1753	Equipment	1710
1755	Medical Equipment	1710
1790	Ancillary Service Equipment	1720 - 1740
1810	ACCUMULATED DEPRECIATION - REAL PROPERTY	1600
1812	Accum Depreciation - Land Improvements	1630
1813	Accum Depreciation - Buildings	1640
1814	Accum Depreciation - Capital Leases - Buildings	1660
1815	Accum Depreciation - Leasehold Improvements	1670
1817	Accum Depreciation - Other Real Property	1680 - 1690
1850	ACCUM DEPRECIATION - FURNITURE, FIXTURES & EQUIPMENT	1800
1851	Accum Depreciation - Furniture and Fixtures	1810
1853	Accum Depreciation - Equipment	1810
1855	Accum Depreciation - Medical Equipment	1810
1890	Other Accum Depreciation - Ancillary Service Equipment	1820-1840
1900	INTANGIBLE AND OTHER ASSETS	1900
1910	Organization Costs	1910
1920	Goodwill	1920
1930	Other Intangible Assets	1940
1950	Noncurrent Expenses Paid in Advance	1950
1960	Other Assets	1960 - 1990
2100	CURRENT LIABILITIES - PAYABLES	2100
2110	Accounts Payable	2110 - 2120
2120	Bank Overdrafts Payable	2180
2130	Other Current Liabilities Payable	2190
2160	Contract Claims Payable	2130
2200	CURRENT LIABILITIES - PAYROLL	2200
2210	Payroll Tax Withholdings Payable	2210 - 2240
2211	Federal Income Tax Withholdings Payable	2211
2212	State Income Tax Withholdings Payable	2212

Chart of Accounts for Health Care Organizations — TABLE III

Crosswalk to the Medical Group Practice Chart of Accounts (1st edition, 1996)

NEW Account Number	NEW Description	PRIOR MGP COA Account Number
2213	FICA/Medicare Tax Withholdings Payable	2213
2215	Other Tax Withholdings Payable	2214 - 2219
2220	Insurance Withholdings Payable	2220
2230	Other Payroll Withholdings Payable	2230 - 2240
2250	Accrued Payroll Liabilities	2250
2260	Other Payroll Liabilities	2260 - 2290
2300	CURRENT LIABILITIES - OTHER	2300
2310	Accrued Liabilities - Nonpayroll	2310 - 2320
2320	Notes and Loans Payable	2140
2330	Long-Term Debt - Current Portion	2150
2332	Capital Lease Obligation - Current Portion	2160
2333	Construction Contracts Payable	2170
2340	Advances from Settlements Due to Third-Party Agencies	2330 - 2339
2350	Patient Deposits	2340
2360	Claims Incurred But Not Reported	2350
2371	Deferred Revenue - Fee for Service	1250
2372	Deferred Revenue - Capitated or Prepaid Plan	2360
2375	Other Deferred Revenue	2370
2380	Deferred Income Taxes - Current Portion	2380
2390	Other Current Liabilities	2390
2400	LONG-TERM LIABILITIES	2400
2410	Long-Term Notes Payable	2410
2420	Construction Loans	2430
2430	Capital Lease Obligation - Long-Term Portion	2440
2440	Other Loans Payable - Long-Term Portion	2420
2450	Deferred Third-Party Revenue	2460
2460	Deferred Compensation	2470
2470	Deferred Income Taxes - Long-Term Portion	2480
2480	Other Long-Term Liabilities	2490
3000	**PARTNERS' EQUITY (PARTNERSHIP)**	2500
3010	Contributed Capital (Each Partner)	2510
3020	Undistributed Earnings	2520
3030	Partners' Drawing Accounts (Each Partner)	2530

Chart of Accounts for Health Care Organizations **TABLE III**

Crosswalk to the Medical Group Practice Chart of Accounts (1st edition, 1996)

NEW Account Number	NEW Description	PRIOR MGP COA Account Number
3000	**STOCKHOLDERS' EQUITY (CORPORATION)**	2600
3010	Preferred Stock	2610
3020	Common Stock	2620
3030	Capital Contributed in Excess of Par	2630
3040	Donated Capital	2640
3050	Allowance for Change in Net Unrealized Gains/Losses on Investments	2650
3060	Dividends and Distributions	2660
3070	Retained Earnings - Unappropriated	2670
3075	Retained Earnings - Appropriated	2680
3090	Treasury Stock	2690
3000	**NET ASSETS (NOT-FOR-PROFIT EQUITY)**	2700
3010	Unrestricted Net Assets	2710 - 2720
3030	Temporarily Restricted Net Assets	2730
3040	Permanently Restricted Net Assets	2740
4000	**REVENUES**	3000
4110	Gross Charges - Fee-for-Service (FFS)	3100
4120	Gross Charges - Discounted FFS Contracts	3200
4130	Gross Charges - FFS Equivalents for Capitation Plan Patients	3300
4150	Other Revenue	3400
4210	Fees Collected - FFS	3500
4220	Fees Collected - FFS for Managed Care	3600
4260	Capitated Premium Revenues - Other	3700
4292	Bad Debt Recovery	7750
4300	Patient Refunds	3900
4400	Fees Collected - Other Revenue	3800
4500	ADJUSTMENTS	4000
4510	Gross Charges - FFS Discount/Adjustment	4100
4520	Gross Charges - FFS for Managed Care Discount/Adjustment	4200
4530	Gross Charges - FFS Equivalents for Cap Plan Patients Adjustment	4300
4550	Other Revenue Discount/Adjustment	4400
4610	Courtesy Discount/Adjustment	4600
4620	Employee Discount/Adjustment	4700
4630	Charity Care Discount/Adjustment	4500
4700	Third-Party Settlements	4900
4800	Provision for Cash Basis Conversion	4800

Chart of Accounts for Health Care Organizations — TABLE III

Crosswalk to the Medical Group Practice Chart of Accounts (1st edition, 1996)

NEW Account Number	NEW Description	PRIOR MGP COA Account Number
5000	**OPERATING EXPENSES - Salary and Fringe Benefits**	5000
5500	ANCILLARY STAFF - SALARIES	5400 - 5490
5600	ANCILLARY STAFF - EMPLOYEE RELATED EXPENSES	5900 - 5990
5655	Meetings (Ancillary)	7420
5700	EMPLOYEES - SALARIES	5500 - 5800
5800	EMPLOYEES - EMPLOYEE RELATED EXPENSES	5900 - 5990
5855	Meetings (Other)	7420
6000	**SERVICES AND GENERAL EXPENSE**	6000
6110	Equipment Rentals (Admin)	6600 - 6690
6120	Telephone (Admin)	7610
6130	Postage (Admin)	7630
6140	Courier and Overnight Delivery (Admin)	7630
6160	Library/Books and Subscriptions	7670, 7650
6170	Advertising and Marketing	7620, 7710
6180	General Business and Other Insurance	7520
6181	Officers' and Directors' Liability	7500
6182	Other Liability	7500
6183	Reinsurance for Capitation Contracts	7530
6185	Malpractice Insurance	7510
6190	Printing (Admin)	7640
6210	Medical Forms	6150
6240	Cafeteria	7440
6250	Employee Relations	7430
6260	Physician Recruitment	7410
6270	Nonphysician Recruitment	7410
6300	Depreciation/Amortization	
6301	Furniture and Fixtures	6700 - 6790
6303	Equipment	6700 - 6790
6310	Accounting Services	7310 - 7320
6320	Legal Services	7330
6330	Actuarial Services	7380
6350	Consulting Services	7340
6360	Other Professional Services	7360, 7390

Chart of Accounts for Health Care Organizations

TABLE III

Crosswalk to the Medical Group Practice Chart of Accounts (1st edition, 1996)

NEW Account Number	NEW Description	PRIOR MGP COA Account Number
6390	Business Transportation	7690
6400	General Supplies	6100, 6140
6410	Taxes - Excise and Other Business Taxes	7680
6440	Other Office and Administrative Expense	7600 - 7700
6510	Equipment Rentals (Billing)	6600 - 6690
6520	Electronic Data Processing	7370
6530	Telephone (Billing)	7610
6540	Postage (Billing)	7630
6550	Courier and Overnight Delivery (Billing)	7630
6560	Printing (Billing)	7640
6700	Bad Debt Expense	7720
6710	Accounts Receivable Write-Offs	7730
6720	Collection Agency Write-Offs	7740
6730	Collection Expenses	7350
7010	Drugs and Medications	6110
7020	Medical Supplies	6120 - 6130
7023	Other Ancillary Supplies	6200 - 6290
7030	Linen Supplies	6170
7040	Uniforms and Laundry	7450
7050	Patient Education	7660
7100	Equipment Rentals (Clinical)	6600 - 6690
7120	Telephone (Clinical)	7610
7130	Postage (Clinical)	7630
7500	Occupancy Expense	6400 - 6490
7510	Rent/Lease	6400 - 6490
7560	Housekeeping/Maintenance Services	6160
7570	Other Occupancy Expense	6800 - 6900
7590	Depreciation (Occupancy)	6500 - 6590
7600	Cost of Goods Sold - Medical Related	6300 - 6390
7700	PURCHASED SERVICES/MANAGEMENT FEES	7000
7720	General and Administrative Expense - Purchased Services	7300
7800	Purchased Services for HMO/PPO Patients - Professional and Medical	7100 - 7290
8100	PHYSICIANS - SALARIES	5100 - 5160
8200	PHYSICIAN - EMPLOYEE RELATED EXPENSES	5200 - 5290
8210	Payroll Taxes (Physician)	5210
8220	Insurance (Physician)	5220

Chart of Accounts for Health Care Organizations — TABLE III

Crosswalk to the Medical Group Practice Chart of Accounts (1st edition, 1996)

NEW Account Number	NEW Description	PRIOR MGP COA Account Number
8230	Pension and Retirement Benefits (Physician)	5230
8235	Professional Development (Physician)	5240
8245	Dues and Memberships (Physician)	5250
8250	Licenses (Physician)	5250
8255	Meetings (Physician)	5260
8260	Travel (Physician)	5260
8265	Medical Reimbursement Plan (Physician)	5270
8270	Vehicles (Physician)	5280
8295	Other Benefits (Physician)	5290
8300	MIDLEVEL PROVIDERS - SALARIES	5300
8400	MIDLEVEL PROVIDERS - EMPLOYEE RELATED EXPENSES	5900 - 5990
8455	Meetings (Midlevel)	7420
9000	**NONOP REVENUE & EXP; INCOME TAXES & OTHER EXP**	8000
9100	Nonoperating Revenues	8100
9110	Interest Income	8110
9120	Income from Long-Term Investments	8120
9130	Property Rentals	8130
9140	Unrealized Gains and Losses - Investments	8140
9150	Realized Gains and Losses - Investments	8150
9200	Nonoperating Expenses	8200
9210	Interest Expense	8210
9230	Current Income Tax Expense (Recovery)	8300
9300	Other Income/Expense	8400, 8500

Chart of Accounts for Health Care Organizations

TABLE IV

General - Detailed Format

Your Account Number #	Description	Survey Account Number #	Your Account Amount $
	ASSETS	**1000**	
	Cash	1100	
	Cash - Banks	1110	
	General Checking Accounts	1111	
	Payroll Checking Accounts	1112	
	Other Checking Accounts	1113	
	Cash - On hand	1120	
	Change Fund	1121	
	Petty Cash	1122	
	Cash - Restricted	1130	
	Marketable Securities & Short-Term Investments	1200	
	Valuation Allowance - Short-Term Investments	1210	
	Accounts Receivable	1300	
	Accounts Receivable - Fee-for-Service Amounts	1301	
	Accounts Receivable - Prepaid Contracts	1302	
	Allowance for Estimated Uncollectible Receivables	1320	
	Allowance for Bad Debts - Patient Accounts	1321	
	Allowance for Contractual Adjustments	1322	
	Allowance for Bad Debts - Third-Party Payers	1323	
	Allowance for Charity Care	1324	
	Notes Receivable - Short Term	1340	
	Managed Care Contract - Bonus/Withhold	1345	
	Other Short-Term Receivables	1350	
	Interest Receivables	1351	
	Intercompany Receivables	1352	
	Due from Employees	1353	
	Due from Related Parties	1354	
	Supply Inventories	1400	
	Drugs and Medications	1401	
	Medical Supplies	1402	
	Administrative Supplies	1403	
	Forms	1404	
	Housekeeping and Maintenance Supplies	1405	
	Linen Supplies	1406	
	Other Supplies	1407	
	Ancillary Department Supplies	1420	
	Prepaid Expenses	1500	
	Prepaid Interest	1501	
	Prepaid Insurance	1502	
	Prepaid Rent	1503	

Chart of Accounts for Health Care Organizations

TABLE IV

General - Detailed Format

Your Account Number #	Description	Survey Account Number #	Your Account Amount $
	Prepaid Taxes	1504	
	Prepaid Dues	1505	
	Other Prepaid Expenses	1506	
	Other Current Assets	1550	
	INVESTMENTS - LONG-TERM RECEIVABLES	1600	
	Long-Term Receivables	1610	
	Long-Term Investments	1630	
	Valuation Allowance - Long-Term Investments	1635	
	Investments in Affiliates	1640	
	Property Held for Future Use	1650	
	PROPERTY, FURNITURE, FIXTURES & EQUIPMENT	1700	
	REAL PROPERTY	1710	
	Land	1711	
	Land Improvements	1712	
	Buildings	1713	
	Capital Leases - Buildings	1714	
	Leasehold Improvements	1715	
	Construction in Progress	1716	
	Other Real Property	1717	
	FURNITURE, FIXTURES & EQUIPMENT	1750	
	Furniture and Fixtures	1751	
	Capital Leases - Furniture and Fixtures	1752	
	Equipment	1753	
	Capital Leases - Equipment	1754	
	Medical Equipment	1755	
	Capital Leases - Medical Equipment	1756	
	Computer	1760	
	Computer - Hardware	1761	
	Computer - Software	1762	
	Computer - Other	1763	
	Capital Leases - Computer	1770	
	Capital Leases - Computer - Hardware	1771	
	Capital Leases - Computer - Software	1772	
	Capital Leases - Computer - Other	1773	
	Vehicles	1780	
	Vehicles	1781	
	Capital Leases - Vehicles	1782	
	Ancillary Service Equipment	1790	

Chart of Accounts for Health Care Organizations **TABLE IV**

General - Detailed Format

Your Account Number	Description	Survey Account Number	Your Account Amount
#		#	$
	Laboratory Equipment	1791	
	Radiology Equipment	1792	
	Physical Therapy Equipment	1793	
	Diagnostic Equipment	1794	
	Capital Leases - Ancillary Service Equipment	1795	
	Capital Leases - Laboratory Equipment	1796	
	Capital Leases - Radiology Equipment	1797	
	Capital Leases - Physical Therapy Equipment	1798	
	Capital Leases - Diagnostic Equipment	1799	
	ACCUMULATED DEPRECIATION - PROP, FURN, ETC.	1800	
	ACCUMULATED DEPRECIATION - REAL PROPERTY	1810	
	Accum Depreciation - Land Improvements	1812	
	Accum Depreciation - Buildings	1813	
	Accum Depreciation - Capital Leases - Buildings	1814	
	Accum Depreciation - Leasehold Improvements	1815	
	Accum Depreciation - Other Real Property	1817	
	ACCUM DEPRECIATION - FURNITURE, FIXTURES & EQUIPMENT	1850	
	Accum Depreciation - Furniture and Fixtures	1851	
	Accum Depreciation - Capital Leases - Furniture and Fixtures	1852	
	Accum Depreciation - Equipment	1853	
	Accum Depreciation - Capital Leases - Equipment	1854	
	Accum Depreciation - Medical Equipment	1855	
	Accum Depreciation - Capital Leases - Medical Equipment	1856	
	Accum Depreciation - Computer	1860	
	Accum Depreciation - Computer - Hardware	1861	
	Accum Depreciation - Computer - Software	1862	
	Accum Depreciation - Computer - Other	1863	
	Accum Depreciation - Capital Leases - Computer	1870	
	Accum Depreciation - Capital Leases - Computer Hardware	1871	
	Accum Depreciation - Capital Leases - Computer Software	1872	
	Accum Depreciation - Capital Leases - Computer - Other	1873	
	Accum Depreciation - Vehicles	1880	
	Accum Depreciation - Vehicles	1881	
	Accum Depreciation - Capital Leases - Vehicles	1882	
	Other Accum Depreciation - Ancillary Service Equipment	1890	
	Accum Depreciation - Laboratory Equipment	1891	
	Accum Depreciation - Radiology Equipment	1892	
	Accum Depreciation - Physical Therapy Equipment	1893	
	Accum Depreciation - Diagnostic Equipment	1894	

Chart of Accounts for Health Care Organizations

TABLE IV

General - Detailed Format

Your Account Number #	Description	Survey Account Number #	Your Account Amount $
	Accum Depreciation - Capital Leases - Ancillary Service Equipment	1895	
	Accum Depreciation - Capital Leases - Laboratory Equipment	1896	
	Accum Depreciation - Capital Leases - Radiology Equipment	1897	
	Accum Depreciation - Capital Leases - Physical Therapy Equipment	1898	
	Accum Depreciation - Capital Leases - Diagnostic Equipment	1899	
	INTANGIBLE AND OTHER ASSETS	1900	
	Organization Costs	1910	
	Accumulated Amortization - Organization Costs	1915	
	Goodwill	1920	
	Accumulated Amortization - Goodwill	1925	
	Other Intangible Assets	1930	
	Deposits	1940	
	Noncurrent Expenses Paid in Advance	1950	
	Noncurrent Interest Paid in Advance	1951	
	Noncurrent Insurance Paid in Advance	1952	
	Noncurrent Rent Paid in Advance	1953	
	Noncurrent Taxes Paid in Advance	1954	
	Noncurrent Dues Paid in Advance	1955	
	Other Noncurrent Expenses Paid in Advance	1956	
	Other Assets	1960	
	Cash Surrender Value of Life Insurance Policies	1961	
	LIABILITIES	**2000**	
	CURRENT LIABILITIES - PAYABLES	2100	
	Accounts Payable	2110	
	Bank Overdrafts Payable	2120	
	Other Current Liabilities Payable	2130	
	Intercompany Accounts Payable	2131	
	Accounts Payable - Employees	2132	
	Accounts Payable - Related Parties	2133	
	Accounts Payable - Other	2134	
	Contract Claims Payable	2160	
	CURRENT LIABILITIES - PAYROLL	2200	
	Payroll Tax Withholdings Payable	2210	
	Federal Income Tax Withholdings Payable	2211	
	State Income Tax Withholdings Payable	2212	
	FICA/Medicare Tax Withholdings Payable	2213	

Chart of Accounts for Health Care Organizations

TABLE IV

General - Detailed Format

Your Account Number #	Description	Survey Account Number #	Your Account Amount $
	Local Tax Withholdings Payable	2214	
	Other Tax Withholdings Payable	2215	
	Insurance Withholdings Payable	2220	
	Health Insurance Withholdings Payable	2221	
	Life Insurance Withholdings Payable	2222	
	State Disability Insurance Withholdings Payable	2223	
	Other Insurance Withholdings Payable	2224	
	Other Payroll Withholdings Payable	2230	
	401(k) Withholdings Payable	2231	
	Cafeteria Plan Withholdings Payable	2232	
	Court Mandated Child Support Withholdings Payable	2233	
	Other Payroll Withholdings Payable	2234	
	Accrued Payroll Liabilities	2250	
	Accrued Payroll	2251	
	Accrued Vacation, Holiday, & Sick Pay (Compensated Absences)	2252	
	Accrued FICA/Medicare Taxes Payable	2253	
	Accrued State Unemployment Taxes Payable	2254	
	Accrued Federal Unemployment Taxes Payable	2255	
	Accrued Retirement Plan Contribution	2256	
	Other Accrued Payroll Liabilities	2257	
	Other Payroll Liabilities	2260	
	CURRENT LIABILITIES - OTHER	2300	
	Accrued Liabilities - Nonpayroll	2310	
	Accrued Rent	2311	
	Accrued Interest	2312	
	Accrued Insurance	2313	
	Accrued Income Taxes (Federal/State)	2314	
	Accrued Property Taxes	2315	
	Accrued Franchise Taxes	2316	
	Other Accrued Liabilities	2317	
	Notes and Loans Payable	2320	
	Current Notes and Loans Payable - Vendors	2321	
	Current Notes and Loans Payable - Employees	2322	
	Current Notes and Loans Payable - Stockholders/Partners	2323	
	Current Other Notes and Loans Payable	2324	
	Bank Working Capital Line Outstanding	2325	
	Long-Term Debt - Current Portion	2330	
	Capital Lease Obligation - Current Portion	2331	
	Construction Contracts Payable	2332	

Chart of Accounts for Health Care Organizations

TABLE IV

General - Detailed Format

Your Account Number #	Description	Survey Account Number #	Your Account Amount $
	Other Loans Payable - Current Portion	2333	
	Advances from Settlements Due to Third-Party Agencies	2340	
	Patient Deposits	2350	
	Claims Payable Incurred But Not Reported	2360	
	Incurred But Not Reported Claims - Commercial	2361	
	Incurred But Not Reported Claims - Medicare	2362	
	Incurred But Not Reported Claims - Medicaid	2363	
	Other Claims Incurred But Not Reported	2365	
	Deferred Revenue	2370	
	Deferred Revenue - Fee for Service	2371	
	Deferred Revenue - Capitated or Prepaid Plan	2372	
	Other Deferred Revenue	2375	
	Deferred Income Taxes - Current Portion	2380	
	Other Current Liabilities	2390	
	LONG-TERM LIABILITIES	**2400**	
	Long-Term Notes Payable	2410	
	Construction Loans	2420	
	Capital Lease Obligation - Long-Term Portion	2430	
	Other Loans Payable - Long-Term Portion	2440	
	Deferred Third-Party Revenue	2450	
	Deferred Third-Party Revenue - Medicare	2451	
	Deferred Third-Party Revenue - Medicaid	2452	
	Deferred Third-Party Revenue - Other	2453	
	Deferred Compensation	2460	
	Severance Plan	2465	
	Deferred Income Taxes - Long-Term Portion	2470	
	Other Long-Term Liabilities	2480	
	Owners' Equity Accounts	**3000**	
	PARTNERS' EQUITY (PARTNERSHIP)	**3000**	
	Contributed Capital (Each Partner)	3010	
	Undistributed Earnings	3020	
	Partners' Drawing Accounts (Each Partner)	3030	
	Current Income/Loss	3040	
	STOCKHOLDERS' EQUITY (CORPORATION)	**3000**	
	Preferred Stock	3010	
	Common Stock	3020	

Chart of Accounts for Health Care Organizations

TABLE IV

General - Detailed Format

Your Account Number #	Description	Survey Account Number #	Your Account Amount $
	Capital Contributed in Excess of Par	3030	
	Donated Capital	3040	
	Allowance for Change in Net Unrealized Gains/Losses on Investments	3050	
	Dividends and Distributions	3060	
	Retained Earnings - Unappropriated	3070	
	Retained Earnings - Appropriated	3075	
	Current Income/Loss	3080	
	Treasury Stock	3090	
	NET ASSETS (NOT-FOR-PROFIT EQUITY)	**3000**	
	Unrestricted Net Assets	3010	
	Temporarily Restricted Net Assets	3030	
	Permanently Restricted Net Assets	3040	
	Current Surplus/Deficit	3050	
	LIMITED LIABILITY COMPANY/PARTNERSHIP	**3000**	
	Members' Capital/Limited Partners' Interest	3010	
	Members' Distributions/Limited Partners' Distributions	3020	
	Current Income/Loss	3030	
	INCOME STATEMENT ACCOUNTS		
	REVENUES	**4000**	
	GROSS CHARGES	4100	
	Gross Charges - Fee-for-Service (FFS)	4110	
	Gross Charges - Discounted FFS Contracts	4120	
	Gross Charges - FFS Equivalents for Capitation Plan Patients	4130	
	Other Gross Charges	4140	
	Other Revenue	4150	
	Fees Collected	4200	
	Fees Collected - FFS	4210	
	Fees Collected - FFS for Managed Care	4220	
	Capitated Premium Revenues - Commercial	4230	
	Capitated Premium Revenues - Medicare	4240	
	Capitated Premium Revenues - Medicaid	4250	
	Capitated Premium Revenues - Other	4260	
	Risk Sharing Revenue	4270	
	Hospital Risk Sharing - Commercial	4271	
	Hospital Risk Sharing - Medicare	4272	
	Hospital Risk Sharing - Medicaid	4273	

Chart of Accounts for Health Care Organizations

TABLE IV

General - Detailed Format

Your Account Number #	Description	Survey Account Number #	Your Account Amount $
	Hospital Risk Sharing - Pharmacy	4274	
	Hospital Risk Sharing - Other	4275	
	Other Managed Care Collected Revenues	4280	
	Copayments	4281	
	Coordination of Benefits	4282	
	Other Prepaid Professional Fees Collected	4283	
	Recoveries	4290	
	Reinsurance Recoveries	4291	
	Bad Debt Recovery	4292	
	Patient Refunds	4300	
	Fees Collected - Other Revenue	4400	
	Sales - Medical Related	4410	
	Patient Records Copying Reimbursement	4420	
	Fees Collected - Other	4430	
	Donations Received (Operating Revenue)	4450	
	Research/Clinical Studies Income	4460	
	Grant Revenue	4470	
	Miscellaneous Income	4480	
	Operating Subsidy Income	4490	
	ADJUSTMENTS	4500	
	Gross Charges - FFS Discount/Adjustment	4510	
	Gross Charges - Discounted FFS Contracts Adjustment	4520	
	Gross Charges - FFS Equivalents for Cap Plan Patients/Adjustment	4530	
	Other Gross Charges/Adjustments	4540	
	Other Revenue Discount/Adjustment	4550	
	Financial Hardship Care Discount/Adjustment	4600	
	Courtesy Discount/Adjustment	4610	
	Employee Discount/Adjustment	4620	
	Charity Care Discount/Adjustment	4630	
	Third-Party Settlements	4700	
	Provision for Cash Basis Conversion	4800	
	OPERATING EXPENSES - Salary and Fringe Benefits	**5000**	
	PHYSICIAN - SALARIES * * (See Accounts 8100 - 8400)	5100	
	PHYSICIAN - EMPLOYEE-RELATED EXPENSES *	5200	
	MIDLEVEL PROVIDERS - SALARIES *	5300	
	MIDLEVEL PROVIDERS - EMPLOYEE-RELATED EXPENSES *	5400	

Chart of Accounts for Health Care Organizations

TABLE IV

General - Detailed Format

Your Account Number #	Description	Survey Account Number #	Your Account Amount $
	ANCILLARY STAFF - SALARIES	5500	
	Salaries - Radiology	5510	
	Salaries - Laboratory	5520	
	Salaries - Optical	5530	
	Salaries - Physical Therapy	5540	
	Salaries - Other Ancillary Services	5550	
	ANCILLARY STAFF - EMPLOYEE-RELATED EXPENSES	5600	
	Payroll Taxes (Ancillary)	5610	
	Payroll Taxes - FICA/Medicare (Ancillary)	5611	
	Payroll Taxes - Federal Unemployment Insurance (Ancillary)	5612	
	Payroll Taxes - State Unemployment Insurance (Ancillary)	5613	
	Payroll Taxes - Other (Ancillary)	5614	
	Insurance (Ancillary)	5620	
	Insurance - Health (Ancillary)	5621	
	Insurance - Dental (Ancillary)	5622	
	Insurance - Life (Ancillary)	5623	
	Insurance - Disability (Ancillary)	5624	
	Insurance - Workers' Compensation (Ancillary)	5625	
	Insurance - Other (Ancillary)	5626	
	Pension and Retirement Benefits (Ancillary)	5630	
	Pension (Ancillary)	5631	
	Deferred Compensation (Ancillary)	5632	
	Severance Plan (Ancillary)	5633	
	Professional Development (Ancillary)	5635	
	Books and Subscriptions (Ancillary)	5640	
	Dues and Memberships (Ancillary)	5645	
	Licenses (Ancillary)	5650	
	Meetings (Ancillary)	5655	
	Travel (Ancillary)	5660	
	Medical Reimbursement Plan (Ancillary)	5665	
	Vehicle (Ancillary)	5670	
	Parking (Ancillary)	5675	
	Telephones (Ancillary)	5680	
	Beepers (Ancillary)	5685	
	Meals and Entertainment (Ancillary)	5690	
	Other Benefits (Ancillary)	5695	

Chart of Accounts for Health Care Organizations **TABLE IV**

General - Detailed Format

Your Account Number #	Description	Survey Account Number #	Your Account Amount $
	EMPLOYEES - SALARIES	**5700**	
	Salaries - General Administrative	5710	
	Salaries - Business Office	5715	
	Salaries - Managed Care Administrative	5720	
	Salaries - Information Services	5725	
	Salaries - Housekeeping/ Maintenance / Security	5730	
	Salaries - Medical Receptionist	5735	
	Salaries - Medical Secretaries / Transcribers	5740	
	Salaries - Medical Records	5745	
	Salaries - Other Administrative Support	5750	
	Salaries - Registered Nurses	5755	
	Salaries - Licensed Practical Nurses	5760	
	Salaries - Medical Assistants / Nurses' Aids	5765	
	EMPLOYEES - EMPLOYEE-RELATED EXPENSES	**5800**	
	Payroll Taxes (Other)	5810	
	Payroll Taxes - FICA/Medicare (Other)	5811	
	Payroll Taxes - Federal Unemployment Insurance (Other)	5812	
	Payroll Taxes - State Unemployment Insurance (Other)	5813	
	Payroll Taxes - Other (Other)	5814	
	Insurance (Other)	5820	
	Insurance - Health (Other)	5821	
	Insurance - Dental (Other)	5822	
	Insurance - Life (Other)	5823	
	Insurance - Disability (Other)	5824	
	Insurance - Workers' Compensation (Other)	5825	
	Insurance - Other (Other)	5826	
	Pension and Retirement Benefits (Other)	5830	
	Pension (Other)	5831	
	Deferred Compensation (Other)	5832	
	Severance Plan (Other)	5833	
	Professional Development (Other)	5835	
	Books and Subscriptions (Other)	5840	
	Dues and Memberships (Other)	5845	
	Licenses (Other)	5850	
	Meetings (Other)	5855	
	Travel (Other)	5860	
	Medical Reimbursement Plan (Other)	5865	
	Vehicle (Other)	5870	
	Parking (Other)	5875	

Chart of Accounts for Health Care Organizations

TABLE IV

General - Detailed Format

Your Account Number #	Description	Survey Account Number #	Your Account Amount $
	Telephones (Other)	5880	
	Beepers (Other)	5885	
	Meals and Entertainment (Other)	5890	
	Other Benefits (Other)	5895	
	Temporary Employee Salaries	5900	
	Physician Salaries	5901	
	Midlevel Provider Salaries	5902	
	Ancillary Staff Salaries	5903	
	Administrative and Other Staff	5904	
	Temporary Employee Benefits	5910	
	Physician Benefits	5911	
	Midlevel Provider Benefits	5912	
	Ancillary Staff Benefits	5913	
	Administrative and Other Staff	5914	
	SERVICES AND GENERAL EXPENSE	**6000**	
	Office and Administrative Expense	6100	
	Equipment Rentals (Admin)	6110	
	Equipment Maintenance (Admin)	6115	
	Telephone (Admin)	6120	
	Postage (Admin)	6130	
	Courier and Overnight Delivery (Admin)	6140	
	Security	6150	
	Library/Books and Subscriptions	6160	
	Advertising and Marketing	6170	
	General Business and Other Insurance	6180	
	Officers' and Directors' Liability	6181	
	Other Liability	6182	
	Reinsurance for Capitation Contracts	6183	
	Keyman and Overhead Insurance	6184	
	Malpractice Insurance	6185	
	Physicians	6186	
	Midlevel Providers	6187	
	Ancillary and Clinical Staff	6188	
	Global Coverage	6189	
	Printing (Admin)	6190	
	Copying (Admin)	6200	
	Medical Forms	6210	
	Answering Service	6220	
	Meals and Entertainment	6230	

Chart of Accounts for Health Care Organizations

TABLE IV

General - Detailed Format

Your Account Number #	Description	Survey Account Number #	Your Account Amount $
	Cafeteria	6240	
	Employee Relations	6250	
	Physician Recruitment	6260	
	Nonphysician Recruitment	6270	
	Depreciation/Amortization	6300	
	Furniture and Fixtures	6301	
	Capital Leases	6302	
	Equipment	6303	
	Computers	6304	
	Vehicles	6305	
	Amortization	6306	
	Other Depreciation	6307	
	Accounting Services	6310	
	Legal Services	6320	
	Actuarial Services	6330	
	Pension Administration Expense	6340	
	Consulting Services	6350	
	Other Professional Services	6360	
	Medical Transcription	6370	
	Payroll Services	6380	
	Business Transportation	6390	
	General Supplies	6400	
	Taxes - Excise and Other Business Taxes	6410	
	Computer Supplies	6420	
	Computer Software	6430	
	Other Office and Administrative Expense	6440	
	Billing Expense	6500	
	Equipment Rentals (Billing)	6510	
	Equipment Maintenance (Billing)	6515	
	Electronic Data Processing	6520	
	Telephone (Billing)	6530	
	Postage (Billing)	6540	
	Courier and Overnight Delivery (Billing)	6550	
	Printing (Billing)	6560	
	Copying (Billing)	6570	
	Depreciation	6580	
	General Services	6600	
	Other Billing Expense	6650	
	Bad Debt Expense	6700	

Chart of Accounts for Health Care Organizations

TABLE IV

General - Detailed Format

Your Account Number #	Description	Survey Account Number #	Your Account Amount $
	Accounts Receivable Write-Offs	6710	
	Collection Agency Write-Offs	6720	
	Collection Expenses	6730	
	Clinical Expense	**7000**	
	Drugs and Medications	7010	
	Medical Supplies	7020	
	Radiology	7021	
	Laboratory	7022	
	Other Ancillary Supplies	7023	
	Linen Supplies	7030	
	Uniforms and Laundry	7040	
	Patient Education	7050	
	Photography	7060	
	Biohazardous Waste Removal	7070	
	Equipment Rentals (Clinical)	7100	
	Equipment Maintenance (Clinical)	7110	
	Telephone (Clinical)	7120	
	Postage (Clinical)	7130	
	Medical Record Supplies	7140	
	Other Clinical Expense	7150	
	Depreciation (Clinical)	7160	
	General Clinical	7161	
	Radiology	7162	
	Laboratory	7163	
	Occupancy Expense	7500	
	Rent/Lease	7510	
	Condominium Assessments/Monthly Maintenance Fees	7520	
	General Maintenance	7530	
	Utilities	7540	
	Utilities - Water	7541	
	Utilities - Electricity	7542	
	Utilities - Waste Disposal	7543	
	Other Utilities	7544	
	Property Taxes	7550	
	Housekeeping/Maintenance Services	7560	
	Other Occupancy Expense	7570	
	Insurance (Occupancy)	7580	
	Depreciation (Occupancy)	7590	

Chart of Accounts for Health Care Organizations

TABLE IV

General - Detailed Format

Your Account Number #	Description	Survey Account Number #	Your Account Amount $
	Amortization - Leasehold Improvements (Occupancy)	7595	
	Cost of Goods Sold - Medical Related	7600	
	PURCHASED SERVICES/MANAGEMENT FEES	7700	
	Medical Directorships	7710	
	General and Administrative Expense - Purchased Services	7720	
	Management Fees - MSO/PPMC	7730	
	Management Fees - Commercial	7731	
	Management Fees - Medicare	7732	
	Management Fees - Medicaid	7733	
	Management Fees - Other	7734	
	Management Company Incentive	7740	
	Purchased Services for HMO/PPO Patients -	7800	
	Professional and Medical		
	FFS Purchased Services for HMO/PPO Patients	7810	
	FFS Purchased Services for HMO/PPO Patients - Physicians	7811	
	FFS Purchased Services for HMO/PPO Patients - Nonphysicians	7812	
	FFS Purchased Services for HMO/PPO Patients - Laboratory	7813	
	FFS Purchased Services for HMO/PPO Patients - Radiology	7814	
	FFS Purchased Services for HMO/PPO Patients - Hospital Inpatient	7815	
	FFS Purchased Services for HMO/PPO Patients - Hospital Emergency	7816	
	FFS Purchased Services for HMO/PPO Patients - Ambulance	7817	
	FFS Purchased Services for HMO/PPO Patients - Out-of-Area Emergen	7818	
	FFS Purchased Services for HMO/PPO Patients - Other Professional a	7819	
	Sub-capitation Payments - Primary Care	7850	
	Sub-capitation Payments - Primary Care - Commercial	7851	
	Sub-capitation Payments - Primary Care - Medicare	7852	
	Sub-capitation Payments - Primary Care - Medicaid	7853	
	Sub-capitation Payments - Primary Care - Other	7854	
	Sub-capitation Payments - Specialty Care	7860	
	Sub-capitation Payments - Specialty Care - Commercial	7861	
	Sub-capitation Payments - Specialty Care - Medicare	7862	
	Sub-capitation Payments - Specialty Care - Medicaid	7863	
	Sub-capitation Payments - Specialty Care - Other	7864	
	Sub-capitation Payments - Hospitals	7870	
	Sub-capitation Payments - Other	7880	

Chart of Accounts for Health Care Organizations

TABLE IV

General - Detailed Format

Your Account Number #	Description	Survey Account Number #	Your Account Amount $
	PROVIDER-RELATED EXPENSES	**8000**	
	PHYSICIANS - SALARIES	8100	
	Salaries, Distributions and Incentives (Physician)	8110	
	Salaries - Owner/Stockholder (Physician)	8120	
	Distributions and Incentives (Physician)	8130	
	Global/Capitation Distributions (Physician)	8140	
	Employee Salaries (Physician)	8150	
	Employee Incentives (Physician)	8160	
	Administrative Salaries (Physician)	8170	
	Other Compensation (Physician)	8180	
	PHYSICIAN - EMPLOYEE-RELATED EXPENSES	8200	
	Payroll Taxes (Physician)	8210	
	Payroll Taxes - FICA/Medicare (Physician)	8211	
	Payroll Taxes - Federal Unemployment Insurance (Physician)	8212	
	Payroll Taxes - State Unemployment Insurance (Physician)	8213	
	Payroll Taxes - Other (Physician)	8214	
	Insurance (Physician)	8220	
	Insurance - Health (Physician)	8221	
	Insurance - Dental (Physician)	8222	
	Insurance - Life (Physician)	8223	
	Insurance - Disability (Physician)	8224	
	Insurance - Workers' Compensation (Physician)	8225	
	Insurance - Other (Physician)	8226	
	Insurance - Officers' Life (Physician)	8227	
	Pension and Retirement Benefits (Physician)	8230	
	Pension (Physician)	8231	
	Deferred Compensation (Physician)	8232	
	Severance Plan (Physician)	8233	
	Professional Development (Physician)	8235	
	Books and Subscriptions (Physician)	8240	
	Dues and Memberships (Physician)	8245	
	Licenses (Physician)	8250	
	Meetings (Physician)	8255	
	Travel (Physician)	8260	
	Medical Reimbursement Plan (Physician)	8265	
	Vehicle (Physician)	8270	
	Leased Motor Vehicles (Physician)	8271	
	Parking (Physician)	8275	
	Telephone (Physician)	8280	

Chart of Accounts for Health Care Organizations

TABLE IV

General - Detailed Format

Your Account Number #	Description	Survey Account Number #	Your Account Amount $
	Beepers (Physician)	8285	
	Meals and Entertainment (Physician)	8290	
	Other Benefits (Physician)	8295	
	MIDLEVEL PROVIDERS - SALARIES	8300	
	Salaries, Distributions and Incentives (Midlevel)	8310	
	Salaries - Owner/Stockholder (Midlevel)	8320	
	Distributions and Incentives (Midlevel)	8330	
	Global/Capitation Distributions (Midlevel)	8340	
	Employee Salaries (Midlevel)	8350	
	Employee Incentives (Midlevel)	8360	
	Administrative Salaries (Midlevel)	8370	
	Other Compensation (Midlevel)	8380	
	MIDLEVEL PROVIDERS - EMPLOYEE-RELATED EXPENSES	8400	
	Payroll Taxes (Midlevel)	8410	
	Payroll Taxes - FICA/Medicare (Midlevel)	8411	
	Payroll Taxes - Federal Unemployment Insurance (Midlevel)	8412	
	Payroll Taxes - State Unemployment Insurance (Midlevel)	8413	
	Payroll Taxes - Other (Midlevel)	8414	
	Insurance (Midlevel)	8420	
	Insurance - Health (Midlevel)	8421	
	Insurance - Dental (Midlevel)	8422	
	Insurance - Life (Midlevel)	8423	
	Insurance - Disability (Midlevel)	8424	
	Insurance - Workers' Compensation (Midlevel)	8425	
	Insurance - Other (Midlevel)	8426	
	Pension and Retirement Benefits (Midlevel)	8430	
	Pension (Midlevel)	8431	
	Deferred Compensation (Midlevel)	8432	
	Severance Plan (Midlevel)	8433	
	Professional Development (Midlevel)	8435	
	Books and Subscriptions (Midlevel)	8440	
	Dues and Memberships (Midlevel)	8445	
	Licenses (Midlevel)	8450	
	Meetings (Midlevel)	8455	
	Travel (Midlevel)	8460	
	Medical Reimbursement Plan (Midlevel)	8465	
	Vehicle (Midlevel)	8470	
	Parking (Midlevel)	8475	

Chart of Accounts for Health Care Organizations

TABLE IV

General - Detailed Format

Your Account Number #	Description	Survey Account Number #	Your Account Amount $
	Telephones (Midlevel)	8480	
	Beepers (Midlevel)	8485	
	Meals and Entertainment (Midlevel)	8490	
	Other Benefits (Midlevel)	8495	
	NONOP REVENUE & EXP; INCOME TAXES & OTHER EXP	**9000**	
	Nonoperating Revenues	9100	
	Interest Income	9110	
	Income from Long-Term Investments	9120	
	Property Rentals	9130	
	Unrealized Gains and Losses - Investments	9140	
	Realized Gains and Losses - Investments	9150	
	Donations Received (Nonoperating Revenue)	9160	
	Nonoperating Subsidy Income	9170	
	Nonoperating Expenses	9200	
	Interest Expense	9210	
	Contributions/Donations Expense	9220	
	Current Income Tax Expense (Recovery)	9230	
	Current Income Taxes - Federal	9231	
	Current Income Taxes - State	9232	
	Current Income Taxes - Other	9233	
	Deferred Income Tax Expense (Recovery)	9240	
	Deferred Income Taxes - Federal	9241	
	Deferred Income Taxes - State	9242	
	Deferred Income Taxes - Other	9243	
	Other Income/Expense	9300	

Table V Look Up

Alphabetized Look Up Table for Balance Sheet Accounts	
ASSETS	**1000**
Accounts Receivable	**1300**
Accounts Receivable - Fee-for-Service Amounts	1301
Accounts Receivable - Prepaid Contracts	1302
Accum Depreciation - Buildings	1813
Accum Depreciation - Capital Leases - Furniture and Fixtures	1852
Accum Depreciation - Furniture and Fixtures	1851
Accum Depreciation - Capital Leases - Ancillary Service Equipment	1895
Accum Depreciation - Capital Leases - Buildings	1814
Accum Depreciation - Capital Leases - Computer	1870
Accum Depreciation - Capital Leases - Computer - Other	1873
Accum Depreciation - Capital Leases - Computer Hardware	1871
Accum Depreciation - Capital Leases - Computer Software	1872
Accum Depreciation - Capital Leases - Diagnostic Equipment	1899
Accum Depreciation - Capital Leases - Equipment	1854
Accum Depreciation - Capital Leases - Laboratory Equipment	1896
Accum Depreciation - Capital Leases - Medical Equipment	1856
Accum Depreciation - Capital Leases - Physical Therapy Equipment	1898
Accum Depreciation - Capital Leases - Radiology Equipment	1897
Accum Depreciation - Capital Leases - Vehicles	1882
Accum Depreciation - Computer	1860
Accum Depreciation - Computer - Hardware	1861
Accum Depreciation - Computer - Other	1863
Accum Depreciation - Computer - Software	1862
Accum Depreciation - Diagnostic Equipment	1894
Accum Depreciation - Equipment	1853
ACCUM DEPRECIATION - FURNITURE, FIXTURES & EQUIPMENT	1850
Accum Depreciation - Laboratory Equipment	1891
Accum Depreciation - Land Improvements	1812
Accum Depreciation - Leasehold Improvements	1815
Accum Depreciation - Medical Equipment	1855
Accum Depreciation - Other Real Property	1817
Accum Depreciation - Physical Therapy Equipment	1893
Accum Depreciation - Radiology Equipment	1892
Accum Depreciation - Vehicles	1881
Accum Depreciation - Vehicles (roll-up account)	1880
Accum Depreciation, Other - Ancillary Service Equipment	1890
Accumulated Amortization - Goodwill	1925
Accumulated Amortization - Organization Costs	1915
ACCUMULATED DEPRECIATION - PROP, FURN, ETC.	**1800**
ACCUMULATED DEPRECIATION - REAL PROPERTY	1810
Administrative Supplies	1403
Allowance for Bad Debts - Patient Accounts	1321
Allowance for Bad Debts - Third-Party Payers	1323
Allowance for Charity Care	1324
Allowance for Contractual Adjustments	1322

Table V Look Up

Alphabetized Look Up Table for Balance Sheet Accounts	
Allowance for Estimated Uncollectible Receivables	1320
Ancillary Department Supplies	1420
Ancillary Service Equipment	1790
Assets, Other	1960
Buildings	1713
Capital Leases - Ancillary Service Equipment	1795
Capital Leases - Buildings	1714
Capital Leases - Computer	1770
Capital Leases - Computer - Hardware	1771
Capital Leases - Computer - Other	1773
Capital Leases - Computer - Software	1772
Capital Leases - Diagnostic Equipment	1799
Capital Leases - Equipment	1754
Capital Leases - Furniture and Fixtures	1752
Capital Leases - Laboratory Equipment	1796
Capital Leases - Medical Equipment	1756
Capital Leases - Physical Therapy Equipment	1798
Capital Leases - Radiology Equipment	1797
Capital Leases - Vehicles	1782
Cash	1100
Cash - Banks	1110
Cash - On hand	1120
Cash - Restricted	1130
Cash Surrender Value of Life Insurance Policies	1961
Change Fund	1121
Checking Accounts, Other	1113
Computer	1760
Computer - Hardware	1761
Computer - Other	1763
Computer - Software	1762
Construction in Progress	1716
Current Assets, Other	1550
Deposits	1940
Diagnostic Equipment	1794
Drugs and Medications	1401
Due from Employees	1353
Due from Related Parties	1354
Equipment	1753
Forms	1404
Furniture and Fixtures	1751
FURNITURE, FIXTURES & EQUIPMENT	1750
General Checking Accounts	1111
Goodwill	1920
Housekeeping and Maintenance Supplies	1405
INTANGIBLE AND OTHER ASSETS	**1900**
Intangible Assets, Other	1930

Table V Look Up

Alphabetized Look Up Table for Balance Sheet Accounts	
Intercompany Receivables	1352
Interest Receivables	1351
INVESTMENTS - LONG-TERM RECEIVABLES	1600
Investments in Affiliates	1640
Laboratory Equipment	1791
Land	1711
Land Improvements	1712
Leasehold Improvements	1715
Linen Supplies	1406
Long-Term Investments	1630
Long-Term Receivables	1610
Maintenance and Housekeeping Supplies	1405
Managed Care Contract - Bonus/Withhold	1345
Marketable Securities & Short-Term Investments	1200
Medical Equipment	1755
Medical Supplies	1402
Noncurrent Dues Paid in Advance	1955
Noncurrent Expenses Paid in Advance	1950
Noncurrent Expenses Paid in Advance, Other	1956
Noncurrent Insurance Paid in Advance	1952
Noncurrent Interest Paid in Advance	1951
Noncurrent Rent Paid in Advance	1953
Noncurrent Taxes Paid in Advance	1954
Notes Receivable - Short Term	1340
Organization Costs	1910
Other Accum Depreciation - Ancillary Service Equipment	1890
Other Assets	1960
Other Checking Accounts	1113
Other Current Assets	1550
Other Intangible Assets	1930
Other Noncurrent Expenses Paid in Advance	1956
Other Prepaid Expenses	1506
Other Real Property	1717
Other Short-Term Receivables	1350
Other Supplies	1407
Payroll Checking Accounts	1112
Petty Cash	1122
Physical Therapy Equipment	1793
Prepaid Dues	1505
Prepaid Expenses	1500
Prepaid Expenses, Other	1506
Prepaid Insurance	1502
Prepaid Interest	1501
Prepaid Rent	1503
Prepaid Taxes	1504
Property Held for Future Use	1650

Table V Look Up

Alphabetized Look Up Table for Balance Sheet Accounts	
PROPERTY, FURNITURE, FIXTURES & EQUIPMENT	1700
Radiology Equipment	1792
REAL PROPERTY	1710
Real Property, Other	1717
Short-Term Investments & Marketable Securities	1200
Short-Term Receivables, Other	1350
Supplies, Other	1407
Supply Inventories	1400
Valuation Allowance - Long-Term Investments	1635
Valuation Allowance - Short-Term Investments	1210
Vehicles	1781
Vehicles (roll-up account)	1780
LIABILITIES	**2000**
401(k) Withholdings Payable	2231
Accounts Payable	2110
Accounts Payable - Employees	2132
Accounts Payable - Other	2134
Accounts Payable - Related Parties	2133
Accrued Federal Unemployment Taxes Payable	2255
Accrued FICA/Medicare Taxes Payable	2253
Accrued Franchise Taxes	2316
Accrued Income Taxes (Federal/State)	2314
Accrued Insurance	2313
Accrued Interest	2312
Accrued Liabilities - Nonpayroll	2310
Accrued Liabilitiesm, Other	2317
Accrued Payroll	2251
Accrued Payroll Liabilities	2250
Accrued Payroll Liabilities, Other	2257
Accrued Property Taxes	2315
Accrued Rent	2311
Accrued Retirement Plan Contribution	2256
Accrued State Unemployment Taxes Payable	2254
Accrued Vacation, Holiday, & Sick Pay (Compensated Absences)	2252
Advances from Settlements Due to Third-Party Agencies	2340
Bank Overdrafts Payable	2120
Bank Working Capital Line Outstanding	2325
Cafeteria Plan Withholdings Payable	2232
Capital Lease Obligation - Current Portion	2331
Capital Lease Obligation - Long-Term Portion	2430
Claims Incurred But Not Reported, Other	2365
Claims Payable Incurred But Not Reported	2360
Construction Contracts Payable	2332
Construction Loans	2420
Contract Claims Payable	2160

Table V Look Up

Alphabetized Look Up Table for Balance Sheet Accounts	
Court Mandated Child Support Withholdings Payable	2233
CURRENT LIABILITIES - OTHER	2300
CURRENT LIABILITIES - PAYABLES	2100
CURRENT LIABILITIES - PAYROLL	2200
Current Liabilities Payable, Other	2130
Current Liabilities, Other	2390
Current Notes and Loans Payable - Employees	2322
Current Notes and Loans Payable - Stockholders/Partners	2323
Current Notes and Loans Payable - Vendors	2321
Current Other Notes and Loans Payable	2324
Deferred Compensation	2460
Deferred Income Taxes - Current Portion	2380
Deferred Income Taxes - Long-Term Portion	2470
Deferred Revenue	2370
Deferred Revenue - Capitated or Prepaid Plan	2372
Deferred Revenue - Fee for Service	2371
Deferred Revenue, Other	2375
Deferred Third-Party Revenue	2450
Deferred Third-Party Revenue - Medicaid	2452
Deferred Third-Party Revenue - Medicare	2451
Deferred Third-Party Revenue - Other	2453
Federal Income Tax Withholdings Payable	2211
FICA/Medicare Tax Withholdings Payable	2213
Health Insurance Withholdings Payable	2221
Incurred But Not Reported Claims - Commercial	2361
Incurred But Not Reported Claims - Medicaid	2363
Incurred But Not Reported Claims - Medicare	2362
Insurance Withholdings Payable	2220
Insurance Withholdings Payable, Other	2224
Intercompany Accounts Payable	2131
Life Insurance Withholdings Payable	2222
Loans and Notes Payable	2320
Loans Payable, Other - Current Portion	2333
Loans Payable, Other - Long-Term Portion	2440
Local Tax Withholdings Payable	2214
Long-Term Debt - Current Portion	2330
LONG-TERM LIABILITIES	2400
Long-Term Liabilities, Other	2480
Long-Term Notes Payable	2410
Notes and Loans Payable	2320
Other Accrued Liabilities	2317
Other Accrued Payroll Liabilities	2257

Alphabetized Look Up Table for Balance Sheet Accounts	
Other Claims Incurred But Not Reported	2365
Other Current Liabilities	2390
Other Current Liabilities Payable	2130
Other Deferred Revenue	2375
Other Insurance Withholdings Payable	2224
Other Loans Payable - Current Portion	2333
Other Loans Payable - Long-Term Portion	2440
Other Long-Term Liabilities	2480
Other Payroll Liabilities	2260
Other Payroll Withholdings Payable	2234
Other Payroll Withholdings Payable	2230
Other Tax Withholdings Payable	2215
Patient Deposits	2350
Payroll Liabilities, Other	2260
Payroll Tax Withholdings Payable	2210
Payroll Withholdings Payable, Other	2234
Payroll Withholdings Payable, Other (roll-up account)	2230
Severance Plan	2465
State Disability Insurance Withholdings Payable	2223
State Income Tax Withholdings Payable	2212
Tax Withholdings Payable, Other	2215
Owners' Equity Accounts	
LIMITED LIABILITY COMPANY/PARTNERSHIP	**3000**
Current Income/Loss	3030
Members' Capital/Limited Partners' Interest	3010
Members' Distributions/Limited Partners' Distributions	3020
NET ASSETS (NOT-FOR-PROFIT EQUITY)	**3000**
Current Surplus/Deficit	3050
Permanently Restricted Net Assets	3040
Temporarily Restricted Net Assets	3030
Unrestricted Net Assets	3010
PARTNERS' EQUITY (PARTNERSHIP)	**3000**
Contributed Capital (Each Partner)	3010
Current Income/Loss	3040
Partners' Drawing Accounts (Each Partner)	3030
Undistributed Earnings	3020
STOCKHOLDERS' EQUITY (CORPORATION)	**3000**
Allowance for Change in Net Unrealized Gains/Losses on Investments	3050
Capital Contributed in Excess of Par	3030
Common Stock	3020
Current Income/Loss	3080
Dividends and Distributions	3060

Table V Look Up

Alphabetized Look Up Table for Balance Sheet Accounts	
Donated Capital	3040
Preferred Stock	3010
Retained Earnings - Appropriated	3075
Retained Earnings - Unappropriated	3070
Treasury Stock	3090

Table VI Look Up

Alphabetized Look Up Table for Income Statement Accounts		
REVENUES	**4000**	
Bad Debt Recovery	4292	
Capitated Premium Revenues - Commercial	4230	
Capitated Premium Revenues - Medicaid	4250	
Capitated Premium Revenues - Medicare	4240	
Capitated Premium Revenues - Other	4260	
Coordination of Benefits	4282	
Copayments	4281	
Donations Received (Operating Revenue)	4450	
Fees Collected	4200	
Fees Collected - FFS	4210	
Fees Collected - FFS for Managed Care	4220	
Fees Collected - Other	4430	
Fees Collected - Other Revenue	4400	
Grant Revenue	4470	
GROSS CHARGES	4100	
Gross Charges - Discounted FFS Contracts	4120	
Gross Charges - Fee-for-Service (FFS)	4110	
Gross Charges - FFS Equivalents for Capitation Plan Patients	4130	
Gross Charges, Other	4140	
Hospital Risk Sharing - Commercial	4271	
Hospital Risk Sharing - Medicaid	4273	
Hospital Risk Sharing - Medicare	4272	
Hospital Risk Sharing - Other	4275	
Hospital Risk Sharing - Pharmacy	4274	
Miscellaneous Income	4480	
Operating Subsidy Income	4490	
Other Gross Charges	4140	
Other Managed Care Collected Revenues	4280	
Other Prepaid Professional Fees Collected	4283	
Other Revenue	4150	
Patient Records Copying Reimbursement	4420	
Patient Refunds	4300	
Recoveries	4290	
Reinsurance Recoveries	4291	
Research/Clinical Studies Income	4460	
Revenue, Other	4150	
Risk Sharing Revenue	4270	
Sales - Medical Related	4410	
ADJUSTMENTS	4500	
Cash Basis Conversion, Provision for	4800	
Charity Care Discount/Adjustment	4630	

Table VI Look Up

Alphabetized Look Up Table for Income Statement Accounts		
Courtesy Discount/Adjustment	4610	
Employee Discount/Adjustment	4620	
Financial Hardship Care Discount/Adjustment	4600	
Gross Charges - Discounted FFS Contracts Adjustment	4520	
Gross Charges - FFS Discount/Adjustment	4510	
Gross Charges - FFS Equivalents for Cap Plan Patients/Adjustment	4530	
Gross Charges/Adjustments, Other	4540	
Other Gross Charges/Adjustments	4540	
Other Revenue Discount/Adjustment	4550	
Provision for Cash Basis Conversion	4800	
Revenue Discount/Adjustment, Other	4550	
Settlements, Third-Party	4700	
Third-Party Settlements	4700	
EXPENSES		
Accounting Services	6310	
Accounts Receivable Write-Offs	6710	
Actuarial Services	6330	
Administrative and General Expense - Purchased Services	7720	
Administrative and Office Expense	6100	
Administrative and Other Staff - Temporary Employee Benefits	5914	
Administrative and Other Staff - Temporary Employee Salaries	5904	
Administrative Salaries (Midlevel)	8370	
Administrative Salaries (Physician)	8170	
Advertising and Marketing	6170	
Amortization	6306	
Amortization - Leasehold Improvements (Occupancy)	7595	
Amortization/Depreciation	6300	
Ancillary and Clinical Staff - Malpractice Insurance	6188	
ANCILLARY STAFF - EMPLOYEE-RELATED EXPENSES	5600	
ANCILLARY STAFF - SALARIES	5500	
Ancillary Staff Benefits - Temporary Employee	5913	
Ancillary Staff Salaries - Temporary Employee	5903	
Answering Service (Admin)	6220	
Bad Debt Expense	6700	
Beepers (Ancillary)	5685	
Beepers (Midlevel)	8485	
Beepers (Other Employees)	5885	
Beepers (Physician)	8285	
Benefits, Other (Ancillary)	5695	
Benefits, Other (Midlevel)	8495	
Benefits, Other (Other Employees)	5895	

Table VI Look Up

Alphabetized Look Up Table for Income Statement Accounts		
Benefits, Other (Physician)	8295	
Billing (Department) Expense	6500	
Biohazardous Waste Removal	7070	
Books and Subscriptions (Ancillary)	5640	
Books and Subscriptions (Midlevel)	8440	
Books and Subscriptions (Other Employees)	5840	
Books and Subscriptions (Physician)	8240	
Business Transportation	6390	
Cafeteria (Admin)	6240	
Capital Leases - Depreciation/Amortization	6302	
Clinical Expense	**7000**	
Clinical Expense, Other	7150	
Collection Agency Write-Offs	6720	
Collection Expenses	6730	
Compensation, Other (Midlevel)	8380	
Compensation, Other (Physician)	8180	
Computer Software (Admin)	6430	
Computer Supplies (Admin)	6420	
Computers - Depreciation/Amortization	6304	
Condominium Assessments/Monthly Maintenance Fees	7520	
Consulting Services	6350	
Contributions/Donations Expense - Nonoperating	9220	
Copying (Admin)	6200	
Copying (Billing)	6570	
Cost of Goods Sold - Medical Related	7600	
Courier and Overnight Delivery (Admin)	6140	
Courier and Overnight Delivery (Billing)	6550	
Current Income Tax Expense (Recovery)	9230	
Current Income Taxes - Federal	9231	
Current Income Taxes - Other	9233	
Current Income Taxes - State	9232	
Deferred Compensation (Ancillary)	5632	
Deferred Compensation (Midlevel)	8432	
Deferred Compensation (Other Employees)	5832	
Deferred Compensation (Physician)	8232	
Deferred Income Tax Expense (Recovery)	9240	
Deferred Income Taxes - Federal	9241	
Deferred Income Taxes - Other	9243	
Deferred Income Taxes - State	9242	
Depreciation - Laboratory (Clinical)	7163	
Depreciation - Radiology (Clinical)	7164	
Depreciation (Billing)	6580	
Depreciation (Clinical)	7160	

Table VI Look Up

Alphabetized Look Up Table for Income Statement Accounts		
Depreciation (Occupancy)	7590	
Depreciation, Other	6307	
Depreciation/Amortization	6300	
Directors' and Officers' Liability Insurance	6181	
Distributions and Incentives (Midlevel)	8330	
Distributions and Incentives (Physician)	8130	
Donations Received (Nonoperating Revenue)	9160	
Drugs and Medications	7010	
Dues and Memberships (Ancillary)	5645	
Dues and Memberships (Midlevel)	8445	
Dues and Memberships (Other Employees)	5845	
Dues and Memberships (Physician)	8245	
Electricity, Utilities	7542	
Electronic Data Processing	6520	
Employee Incentives (Midlevel)	8360	
Employee Incentives (Physician)	8160	
Employee Relations (Admin)	6250	
Employee Salaries (Midlevel)	8350	
Employee Salaries (Physician)	8150	
EMPLOYEES - EMPLOYEE-RELATED EXPENSES	5800	
EMPLOYEES - SALARIES	5700	
Entertainment and Meals (Ancillary)	5690	
Entertainment and Meals (Midlevel)	8490	
Entertainment and Meals (Other Employees)	5890	
Entertainment and Meals (Physician)	8290	
Equipment - Depreciation/Amortization	6303	
Equipment Maintenance (Admin)	6115	
Equipment Maintenance (Billing)	6515	
Equipment Maintenance (Clinical)	7110	
Equipment Rentals (Admin)	6110	
Equipment Rentals (Billing)	6510	
Equipment Rentals (Clinical)	7100	
FFS Purchased Services - Commercial	7811	
FFS Purchased Services - Medicaid	7813	
FFS Purchased Services - Medicare	7812	
FFS Purchased Services - Other	7814	
FFS Purchased Services for HMO/PPO Patients	7810	
Furniture and Fixtures - Depreciation/Amortization	6301	
General and Administrative Expense - Purchased Services	7720	
General Business and Other Insurance	6180	
General Clinical - Depreciation	7161	
General Maintenance	7530	
General Services (Billing)	6600	

Table VI Look Up

Alphabetized Look Up Table for Income Statement Accounts		
General Supplies (Admin)	6400	
Global Coverage - Malpractice Insurance	6189	
Global/Capitation Distributions (Midlevel)	8340	
Global/Capitation Distributions (Physician)	8140	
Housekeeping/Maintenance Services	7560	
Incentives and Distributions (Midlevel)	8330	
Incentives and Distributions (Physician)	8130	
Income from Long-Term Investments	9120	
Insurance (Midlevel)	8420	
Insurance - Dental (Ancillary)	5622	
Insurance - Dental (Midlevel)	8422	
Insurance - Dental (Other Employees)	5822	
Insurance - Dental (Physician)	8222	
Insurance - Disability (Ancillary)	5624	
Insurance - Disability (Midlevel)	8424	
Insurance - Disability (Other Employees)	5824	
Insurance - Disability (Physician)	8224	
Insurance - Health (Ancillary)	5621	
Insurance - Health (Midlevel)	8421	
Insurance - Health (Other Employees)	5821	
Insurance - Health (Physician)	8221	
Insurance - Life (Ancillary)	5623	
Insurance - Life (Midlevel)	8423	
Insurance - Life (Other Employees)	5823	
Insurance - Life (Physician)	8223	
Insurance - Officers' Life (Physician)	8227	
Insurance - Other (Ancillary)	5626	
Insurance - Other (Midlevel)	8426	
Insurance - Other (Other Employees)	5826	
Insurance - Other (Physician)	8226	
Insurance - Workers' Compensation (Ancillary)	5625	
Insurance - Workers' Compensation (Midlevel)	8425	
Insurance - Workers' Compensation (Other Employees)	5825	
Insurance - Workers' Compensation (Physician)	8225	
Insurance (Ancillary)	5620	
Insurance (Occupancy)	7580	
Insurance (Other Employees)	5820	
Insurance (Physician)	8220	
Interest Expense - Nonoperating	9210	
Interest Income - Nonoperating Revenues	9110	
Keyman and Overhead Insurance	6184	
Laboratory - Depreciation (Clinical)	7163	
Laboratory - Medical Supplies (Clinical)	7022	
Laundry and Uniforms (Clinical)	7040	

Table VI Look Up

Alphabetized Look Up Table for Income Statement Accounts		
Lease/Rent	7510	
Leased Motor Vehicles (Physician)	8271	
Legal Services	6320	
Liability Insurance, Other	6182	
Library/Books and Subscriptions	6160	
Licenses (Ancillary)	5650	
Licenses (Midlevel)	8450	
Licenses (Other Employees)	5850	
Licenses (Physician)	8250	
Linen Supplies (Clinical)	7030	
Maintenance/Housekeeping Services	7560	
Malpractice Insurance	6185	
Management Company Incentive	7740	
Management Fees - Commercial	7731	
Management Fees - Medicaid	7733	
Management Fees - Medicare	7732	
Management Fees - MSO/PPMC	7730	
Management Fees - Other	7734	
Marketing and Advertising	6170	
Meals and Entertainment (Admin)	6230	
Meals and Entertainment (Ancillary)	5690	
Meals and Entertainment (Midlevel)	8490	
Meals and Entertainment (Other Employees)	5890	
Meals and Entertainment (Physician)	8290	
Medical Directorships	7710	
Medical Forms (Admin)	6210	
Medical Record Supplies	7140	
Medical Reimbursement Plan (Ancillary)	5665	
Medical Reimbursement Plan (Midlevel)	8465	
Medical Reimbursement Plan (Other Employees)	5865	
Medical Reimbursement Plan (Physician)	8265	
Medical Supplies (Clinical)	7020	
Medical Transcription	6370	
Meetings (Ancillary)	5655	
Meetings (Midlevel)	8455	
Meetings (Other Employees)	5855	
Meetings (Physician)	8255	
Memberships and Dues (Ancillary)	5645	
Memberships and Dues (Midlevel)	8445	
Memberships and Dues (Other Employees)	5845	
Memberships and Dues (Physician)	8245	
Midlevel Provider Benefits - Temporary Employee	5912	
Midlevel Provider Salaries - Temporary Employee	5902	
MIDLEVEL PROVIDERS - EMPLOYEE-RELATED EXPENSES	8400	

Table VI Look Up

Alphabetized Look Up Table for Income Statement Accounts		
MIDLEVEL PROVIDERS - EMPLOYEE-RELATED EXPENSES	5400	
Midlevel Providers - Malpractice Insurance	6187	
MIDLEVEL PROVIDERS - SALARIES	8300	
MIDLEVEL PROVIDERS - SALARIES *	5300	
Motor Vehicles, Leased (Physician)	8271	
NONOP REVENUE & EXP; INCOME TAXES & OTHER EXP	**9000**	
Nonoperating Expenses	9200	
Nonoperating Revenues	9100	
Nonoperating Subsidy Income	9170	
Nonphysician Recruitment	6270	
Occupancy Expense	7500	
Occupancy Expense, Other	7570	
Office and Administrative Expense	6100	
Officers' and Directors' Liability Insurance	6181	
OPERATING EXPENSES - Salary and Fringe Benefits	**5000**	
Other Ancillary Supplies (Clinical)	7023	
Other and General Business Insurance	6180	
Other Benefits (Ancillary)	5695	
Other Benefits (Midlevel)	8495	
Other Benefits (Other Employees)	5895	
Other Benefits (Physician)	8295	
Other Billing Expense	6650	
Other Clinical Expense	7150	
Other Compensation (Midlevel)	8380	
Other Compensation (Physician)	8180	
Other Depreciation	6307	
Other Liability Insurance	6182	
Other Occupancy Expense	7570	
Other Office and Administrative Expense	6440	
Other Professional Services	6360	
Other Utilities	7544	
Overnight and Courier Delivery (Admin)	6140	
Overnight and Courier Delivery (Billing)	6550	
Parking (Ancillary)	5675	
Parking (Midlevel)	8475	
Parking (Other Employees)	5875	
Parking (Physician)	8275	
Patient Education (Clinical)	7050	
Payroll Services	6380	
Payroll Taxes - Federal Unemployment Insurance (Ancillary)	5612	
Payroll Taxes - Federal Unemployment Insurance (Midlevel)	8412	
Payroll Taxes - Federal Unemployment Insurance (Other Employees)	5812	

Table VI Look Up

Alphabetized Look Up Table for Income Statement Accounts		
Payroll Taxes - Federal Unemployment Insurance (Physician)	8212	
Payroll Taxes - FICA/Medicare (Ancillary)	5611	
Payroll Taxes - FICA/Medicare (Midlevel)	8411	
Payroll Taxes - FICA/Medicare (Other Employees)	5811	
Payroll Taxes - FICA/Medicare (Physician)	8211	
Payroll Taxes - Other (Ancillary)	5614	
Payroll Taxes - Other (Midlevel)	8414	
Payroll Taxes - Other (Other Employees)	5814	
Payroll Taxes - Other (Physician)	8214	
Payroll Taxes - State Unemployment Insurance (Ancillary)	5613	
Payroll Taxes - State Unemployment Insurance (Midlevel)	8413	
Payroll Taxes - State Unemployment Insurance (Other Employees)	5813	
Payroll Taxes - State Unemployment Insurance (Physician)	8213	
Payroll Taxes (Ancillary)	5610	
Payroll Taxes (Midlevel)	8410	
Payroll Taxes (Other Employees)	5810	
Payroll Taxes (Physician)	8210	
Pension (Ancillary)	5631	
Pension (Midlevel)	8431	
Pension (Other Employees)	5831	
Pension (Physician)	8231	
Pension Administration Expense	6340	
Pension and Retirement Benefits (Ancillary)	5630	
Pension and Retirement Benefits (Midlevel)	8430	
Pension and Retirement Benefits (Other Employees)	5830	
Pension and Retirement Benefits (Physician)	8230	
Photography (Clinical)	7060	
PHYSICIAN - EMPLOYEE-RELATED EXPENSES	8200	
PHYSICIAN - EMPLOYEE-RELATED EXPENSES *	5200	
PHYSICIAN - SALARIES *	5100	
Physician Benefits - Temporary Employee	5911	
Physician Recruitment	6260	
Physician Salaries - Temporary Employee	5901	
Physicians - Malpractice Insurance	6186	
PHYSICIANS - SALARIES	8100	
Postage (Admin)	6130	
Postage (Billing)	6540	
Postage (Clinical)	7130	
Printing (Admin)	6190	
Printing (Billing)	6560	
Professional Development (Ancillary)	5635	
Professional Development (Midlevel)	8435	
Professional Development (Other Employees)	5835	

Table VI Look Up

Alphabetized Look Up Table for Income Statement Accounts		
Professional Development (Physician)	8235	
Professional Services, Other	6360	
Property Rentals - Nonoperating Revenues	9130	
Property Taxes	7550	
PROVIDER-RELATED EXPENSES	**8000**	
Purchased Services for HMO/PPO Patients - Professional and	7800	
PURCHASED SERVICES/MANAGEMENT FEES	7700	
Radiology - Depreciation	7162	
Radiology - Medical Supplies (Clinical)	7021	
Realized Gains and Losses - Investments	9150	
Recruitment, Nonphysician	6270	
Recruitment, Physician	6260	
Reinsurance for Capitation Contracts	6183	
Rent/Lease	7510	
Retirement and Pension Benefits (Ancillary)	5630	
Retirement and Pension Benefits (Midlevel)	8430	
Retirement and Pension Benefits (Other Employees)	5830	
Retirement and Pension Benefits (Physician)	8230	
Salaries - Business Office	5715	
Salaries - General Administrative	5710	
Salaries - Housekeeping/ Maintenance / Security	5730	
Salaries - Information Services	5725	
Salaries - Laboratory	5520	
Salaries - Licensed Practical Nurses	5760	
Salaries - Managed Care Administrative	5720	
Salaries - Medical Assistants / Nurses' Aids	5765	
Salaries - Medical Receptionist	5735	
Salaries - Medical Records	5745	
Salaries - Medical Secretaries / Transcribers	5740	
Salaries - Optical	5530	
Salaries - Other Administrative Support	5750	
Salaries - Other Ancillary Services	5550	
Salaries - Owner/Stockholder (Midlevel)	8320	
Salaries - Owner/Stockholder (Physician)	8120	
Salaries - Physical Therapy	5540	
Salaries - Radiology	5510	
Salaries - Registered Nurses	5755	
Salaries, Distributions and Incentives (Midlevel)	8310	
Salaries, Distributions and Incentives (Physician)	8110	
Security	6150	

Table VI Look Up

Alphabetized Look Up Table for Income Statement Accounts		
SERVICES AND GENERAL EXPENSE	**6000**	
Severance Plan (Ancillary)	5633	
Severance Plan (Midlevel)	8433	
Severance Plan (Other Employees)	5833	
Severance Plan (Physician)	8233	
Sub-capitation Payments - Hospitals	7870	
Sub-capitation Payments - Other	7880	
Sub-capitation Payments - Primary Care	7850	
Sub-capitation Payments - Primary Care - Commercial	7851	
Sub-capitation Payments - Primary Care - Medicaid	7853	
Sub-capitation Payments - Primary Care - Medicare	7852	
Sub-capitation Payments - Primary Care - Other	7854	
Sub-capitation Payments - Specialty Care	7860	
Sub-capitation Payments - Specialty Care - Commercial	7861	
Sub-capitation Payments - Specialty Care - Medicaid	7863	
Sub-capitation Payments - Specialty Care - Medicare	7862	
Sub-capitation Payments - Specialty Care - Other	7864	
Subscriptions and Books (Ancillary)	5640	
Subscriptions and Books (Midlevel)	8440	
Subscriptions and Books (Other Employees)	5840	
Subscriptions and Books (Physician)	8240	
Taxes - Excise and Other Business Taxes	6410	
Telephone (Admin)	6120	
Telephone (Ancillary)	5680	
Telephone (Billing)	6530	
Telephone (Clinical)	7120	
Telephone (Midlevel)	8480	
Telephone (Other Employees)	5880	
Telephone (Physician)	8280	
Temporary Employee Benefits	5910	
Temporary Employee Salaries	5900	
Travel (Ancillary)	5660	
Travel (Midlevel)	8460	
Travel (Other Employees)	5860	
Travel (Physician)	8260	
Uniforms and Laundry (Clinical)	7040	
Unrealized Gains and Losses - Investments	9140	

Table VI Look Up

Alphabetized Look Up Table for Income Statement Accounts		
Utilities	7540	
Utilities - Electricity	7542	
Utilities - Waste Disposal	7543	
Utilities - Water	7541	
Utilities, Other	7544	
Vehicles - Depreciation/Amortization	6305	
Vehicles (Ancillary)	5670	
Vehicles (Midlevel)	8470	
Vehicles (Other Employees)	5870	
Vehicles (Physician)	8270	
Waste Disposal, Utilities	7543	
Water, Utilities	7541	

INDEX

A

ABC accounting system 109
Academic medical centers
  future of 187
Accounting for contributions 154
Accounting methods 3, 130
Accounts receivable 36
  Detail 153
Accrual 3
Accumulated depreciation 42
Activity-Based Costing (ABC) 107
  accounting 109
  converting plan into design 113
  financial costing format 111
  implementing design 126
  planning process 110
Activity-Based Costing Exhibits:
  Allocating Indirect Costs (5.4) 118
  Assigning Direct Costs (5.3) 116
  Category Map (5.1) 112
  Component Expense Worksheet (5.8) 125
  Cost Per CPT Code (5.7) 123
  Defining Points of Service (5.2) 114
  Provider Expense Allocation (5.5) 119
  Total Production Units (5.6) 122
Adapting COAs to PSPA
  Cost category structure 241
  Operating Expenses (13.5) 234
  Salaries (13.4) 232
Adjustments 70
Allocating indirect costs 118
Allocation of indirect expenses 118
Allowance 36
Ancillary department supplies 38
Ancillary staff — employee related expenses 75
Ancillary staff — salaries 74
Application to MGMA Surveys 146
Asset detail (selected accounts) 192
Assets
  Description 34
  in an accrual-based system 134
Assigning direct costs 116

B

Bad debt expense 88
Balance sheet 38
Balance Sheet Account Descriptions Exhibits:
  Assets (3.1) 47-49
  Liabilities (3.2) 55-56
  Limited Liability Company/Partnership (3.6) 62
  Net Assets (Not-for-Profit) Equity (3.5) 61
  Stockholders' Equity (Corporation) (3.4) 58
Basic field 2, 13
Benchmarking 219
Billing Expense 88
Bureau of Primary Health Care (BPHC) 161

C

Capital contributed in excess of par 58
Capital lease 40
Capitalization
  criteria for 41
Capitated premium revenue 208
Case studies for academic medical practices 179
Cash basis accounting 5
Cash in banks 34
Cash on hand 35
Cash restricted 35
Change fund 35
Charity care
  guidelines 150
Chart format 14
Clinical expense 89
Coding structure 2
Coding Structure Exhibits:
  Chart of Accounts — General, Detailed Format (2.1) 16-27
  Summary Format (2.2) 28-33
Common stock 58
Community Health Centers
  account numbers 162
  cost report requirements 161
  departments 169
  financial statement audit 160
  funding agency requirements 160
  managed care requirements 162
  reporting requirements 160
  salary expense 164
  Sites 168
  tax requirements 160
  tracking grants, contracts, donations & organizational units 165
Community Health Centers Exhibits:
  Departments (8.11) 170
  Federal Grant Programs (8.8) 168
  Funds (8.7) 167
  Grants and Contracts Receivable (8.4) 166
  Other Grants and Contracts (8.9) 168
  Refundable Advances (8.5) 166
  Salaries (8.3) 165
  Sites (8.10) 169
Comparability 9
Components of provider compensation expense 226
Conceptual framework for financial reporting 2
Conservatism 9
Consistency 9
Corporate background 178
Cost of goods sold — medical related 92
Cost report requirements 161
Criteria for capital leases 40
Current assets 34
Current liabilities — payroll 50
Current liabilities (selected accounts) 197

D

Defining points of service and centers of activity 114
Defining the ownership types 148
Departmental segments
  application to tracking 169
Descriptive terms 111
Developing cost analysis 119
Development of Accounting Standards
  evolution of accepted of practice 2
Dividends and distribution 59

E

Employees — employee related expenses 79
Employees — salaries 78
Entity 7
Equity 155
Equity relationships 198
Expenses 200

F

Faculty Practice Plans
- activities survey 218
- business decisions 172
- chart of accounts and management continuum 180
- industry summary 178
- physician compensation structures 173

Faculty Practice Plans Exhibits:
- Physician Compensation Structure (9.1) 175
- Physician Revenues Expense (9.2) 177
- Spread Sheet of Performance (9.3) 182-184

FASB 2
Federal grant programs 167
- sample 168

Fees collected 65
Fees collected — other revenue 68
Financial Accounting Standards Board (FASB) 148
Financial hardship care discount/ adjustment 72
Financial statement audit requirements 160
Financial statements 7
Financing institutions 1
Flexibility of structure 1
Focusing on costs 107
Full disclosure 9
Fully integrated delivery systems 213
Funding agency requirements 160
Funds
- tracking for restrictions 167
- sample 167

Furniture, fixtures & equipment 41
Future of academic medical centers 187

G

General checking accounts 35
General ledger crosswalks 200
Generally Accepted Accounting Principles (GAAP) 2, 3, 5, 190
Going-concern 8
Grants and contracts receivable 166
Group practices 210

H

Historical cost basis 3
HMOs 1
Hospital Based Physician Practice
- Assets 191
- determining salaries 200
- equity relationships 198
- general ledger crosswalks 200
- liabilities 196
- overall account structure 190
- Revenues 199

Hospital Based Physician Practice Exhibits:
- Assets, Detail(10.2) 192-194
- Current Liabilities (10.4) 197-198
- Practice Codes (10.1) 191
- Revenues (103) 195-196

How to adapt the COA for CHCs 162

I

Impact on compensation systems 210
Incentive compensation plan 174
Income Statement Accounts 14
- revenue 137

Income Statement of Accounts Exhibits:
- Adjustments (4.2) 93
- Billing Expenses (4.6) 89
- Clinical Expenses (4.7) 91
- Income Statement Accounts (4.1) 70
- Nonop Revenue Expenses (4.11) 106
- Occupancy Expenses (4.8) 93
- Operating Expenses (4.3) 77
- Provider Related Expenses (4.10) 103-104

Purchased Services/Management Fees (4.0) 95
Salaries (4.4) 82
Services and General Expense (4.5) 87
Income tax method of accounting 6, 215
Independent practice associations (IPA) 203, 205
Industry summary 178
In-kind goods and services 167
Intangible and other assets
deposits 45
goodwill 45
noncurrent expenses paid in advance 46
organization costs 45
Integrated Delivery Systems
assets 207
adapting the COA 202
definition 203
expenses 209
group practices 210
income tax accounting 215
independent practice association 205
liabilities 208
multilocations groups 211
multispecialty groups 211
revenues 208
Integrated Delivery Systems Exhibit:
Balance Sheet (11.1) 206-207
Internal revenue service 1
Investments
in affiliates 39
In securities 153

K

Key areas for not-for-profit HCOs
charity care 150

L

Liabilities 49, 135, 196
Current — payroll 50
integrated delivery systems 208
Limited Liability company/partnership 61
Long-lived assets 4
Long-term assets 34
Long-term investments 39
Long-term liabilities 53
Long-term receivables 38

M

Malpractice expenses 230, 234
Malpractice insurance 84
Managed care requirements 162
Managed care contract
Bonus/withhold 37
Management of reporting for multiple sites 168
Management service organizations 212
Marketable securities & short-term investments 35
Medical foundations 216
MGMA Surveys 217
Assessments 220
data comparison/standardization 219
internal and external benchmarks 220
MGMA Surveys Exhibit:
Data Requirements for Cost Survey (12.1) 221-223
Midlevel providers — employee related expenses 100
Midlevel providers — salaries 99
Modified cash basis of accounting 6, 130
Monetary units 8
Multilocation groups
expense allocations 212
legal implications 212
management service organizations 212
Multispecialty groups 211
expense allocations 211
legal implications 212

N

Net assets (not-for-profit equity) 60, 156
- current surplus/deficit 61
- permanently restricted 61

Nonfederal grant and contract services 168
Nonop revenue & expenses 104
Nonoperating revenue 155
- detail 104
- revenues and expenses 146

Notes receivable — short-term 37
Not-for-Profit CHOs 150
- accounting for contributions 154
- chart of accounts 156
- differentiating bad debts from charity service 150
- equity 155
- investment in securities 153
- reporting requirements for the IRS 156

Not-for-Profit CHOs Exhibits:
- Account Receivable for Charity Services (7.1) 153
- Balance Sheets (7.2) 154
- Net Assets (Not-for-Profit) Equity (7.4) 156
- Nonoperating Revenue — Detail (7.3) 155
- Operating Expenses — Salaries (7.5) 157-158

O

Objectives of financial reporting 149
Objectivity 8
Occupancy expense 91
Office and administrative expense 83
Operating expenses 74, 141
Other Comprehensive Basis of Accounting (OCBOA) 4
Other income/expense 106
Overhead expenses 233
Owners' equity 136
Owners' equity accounts 56

P

Partially integrated systems
- first-tier integration 203
- second-tier integration 204

Partners' equity 57
Patient refunds 68
Payroll checking accounts 35
Petty cash 35
Physician — employee related expense 97
Physician compensation structures 173
Physician services practice analysis (PSPA) 224
Physician vs. provider 225
Physician-hospital organization (PHO) 204
Physicians — salaries 96
Preferred stock 58
Prepaid expenses 38
Preparing for the unexpected 108
Professional courtesy discounts 139
Property held for future use 39
Property, furniture, fixtures & equipment 39
Provider compensation expenses 226
Provider expense allocation 119
Provider expenses 144
Provider-related expenses 95
Provision for cash-basis conversion 73
PSPA
- cost category structure 225
- cost input screen 235
- overhead expenses 233
- physician vs. provider 225

PSPA Exhibits:
- Direct Provider Expense (13.1) 228-229
- Expenses (13.2) 230
- Malpractice Expense (13.3) 243 (13.6) 235
- Operating Expense (13.5) 234
- Salaries (13.4) 232

Purchased services for HMO/PPO patient 94
Purchased services/management fees 93

R

Real property 39
Recoveries 68
Refundable advances — grants and contracts 166
Reimbursement scenarios 108
Reporting requirements
  tax requirements 160
Resource-based relative value scale 107
Retained Earnings
  unappropriated/ appropriated 59
Revenue from the sale of goods 3
Revenue recognition 214
Revenues 63, 199
  donations received 69
  fees collected 65
  fees collected for medical-related activities 68
  Grants 69
  gross charges 63
  operating subsidy income 69
  Recoveries 68
  research/clinical studies income 69
  risk sharing 67
  selected accounts 195
RVU components 225

S

Salary and fringe benefits 74
School of Thought #1 227
School of Thought #2 231
Services and general expense 83, 143
Short-term receivables
  due from related parties 37
Sites (Sample)169
Small Group Practices
  account structure 132
  accounting methods 130
  assets 133
  definition 129
  income statement accounts 137
  nonoperating revenue and expenses 146
  operating expenses 141
  owner equity 136
  Revenue 137
  services and general expenses 143
  use of accounting data 131
Small Group Practices Exhibits:
  Accounting Structure (Utilities) (8.1) 132
  Accumulated Depreciation (6.3) 135
  Adjustments (6.8) 139
  Assets (Accrual-Based System) (6.2) 134-135
  Liabilities (6.4) 136
  Nonoperating Revenue Expenses (6.12) 146
  Operating Expenses (6.9) 142
  Partners' Equity (Partnership) (6.5) 137
  Provider-Related Expenses (6.11) 145
  Services and General Expenses (6.10) 143
  Stockholders' Equity (Corporation) (6.6) 137
Standard COA for academic practices 171
State and federal regulatory authorities 1
Statement of Financial Accounting Concepts (SFAC) 149
Statement of Financial Position 34
  Accounts 13
Stockholders' equity 58
Summary categories 2
Summary format 28
Supply inventories 37
Surveys 218

T

Temporary employee benefits 81
Temporary employee salaries 81
Third-party payers 1
Third-party settlements 72
Timeliness 10

Total production units 122
Total utilization cost 126

U

U.S. Government Printing Office (GPO)
disk from 121
Use of accounting data for small groups 131

V

Valuation allowance
long-term investment 39
short-term investment 36